# SPIRITUAL RESOURCES
# IN FAMILY THERAPY

# SPIRITUAL RESOURCES
# IN FAMILY THERAPY

## SECOND EDITION

*edited by*
# FROMA WALSH

THE GUILFORD PRESS
New York    London

© 2009 The Guilford Press
A Division of Guilford Publications, Inc.
370 Seventh Avenue, Suite 1200, New York, NY 10001
www.guilford.com

Printed in the United States of America

This book is printed on acid-free paper.

Last digit is print number:   9   8   7

**Library of Congress Cataloging-in-Publication Data**

Spiritual resources in family therapy / edited by Froma Walsh.—2nd ed.
    p. cm.
  Includes bibliographical references and index.
  ISBN 978-1-60623-022-0 (hardcover: alk. paper)
  ISBN 978-1-60623-908-7 (paperback: alk. paper)
    1. Family psychotherapy—Religious aspects.   2. Spirituality.   3. Psychology
and religion.   I. Walsh, Froma.
  RC488.5.S69 2009
  616.89′156—dc22

                                    2008042097

*To my loving parents, whose spirits shine down to light my path:*

In the rising sun and its going down,
 we remember them;
In the blowing of the wind and in the chill of winter,
 we remember them;
In the opening of buds and in the rebirth of spring,
 we remember them;
In the rustling of leaves and in the beauty of autumn,
 we remember them;
In the beginning of the year and when it ends,
 we remember them;
When we are weary and in need of strength,
 we remember them;
When we are lost and sick at heart,
 we remember them;
When we have joys we wish to share,
 we remember them;
So long as we live, they too shall live,
For they are now a part of us,
 as we remember them.

—Memorial Prayers, *Rabbi's Manual,*
Central Conference of American Rabbis

# About the Editor

**Froma Walsh, MSW, PhD,** is the Mose and Sylvia Firestone Professor Emerita in the School of Social Service Administration and the Department of Psychiatry, Pritzker School of Medicine at the University of Chicago. She is also Co-Director of the University-affiliated Chicago Center for Family Health, a past president of the American Family Therapy Academy, and past editor of the *Journal of Marital and Family Therapy*. Dr. Walsh has received many honors for her distinguished contributions and leadership in the field of family therapy, including awards from the Division of Family Psychology of the American Psychological Association, the American Family Therapy Academy, the American Association for Marriage and Family Therapy, the American Orthopsychiatric Association, and the Society for Pastoral Care Research. Her books include *Strengthening Family Resilience, Second Edition*; *Normal Family Processes: Growing Diversity and Complexity, Third Edition*; *Living Beyond Loss: Death in the Family, Second Edition*; *Women in Families: Framework for Family Therapy*; and the first edition of *Spiritual Resources in Family Therapy*. She is a frequent speaker and international consultant on resilience-oriented professional training, practice, and research.

# Contributors

**Herbert Anderson, PhD,** Pacific Lutheran Theological Seminary, Berkeley, California

**Harry J. Aponte, LCSW, LMFT,** private practice and Programs in Couple and Family Therapy, Drexel University, Philadelphia, Pennsylvania

**Mary Jo Barrett, MSW,** Center for Contextual Change and School of Social Service Administration, University of Chicago, Chicago, Illinois

**Nancy Boyd-Franklin, PhD,** Graduate School of Applied and Professional Psychology, Rutgers—The State University of New Jersey, Piscataway, New Jersey

**Yvette Castillo, PhD,** Department of Education, West Texas A & M University, Canyon, Texas

**William J. Doherty, PhD,** Department of Family Social Science, University of Minnesota, St. Paul, Minnesota

**Melissa Elliott, MSN, LMFT,** University of Virginia Health System, Charlottesville, Virginia

**Celia Jaes Falicov, PhD,** Department of Psychiatry, University of California—San Diego, San Diego, California

**Mona DeKoven Fishbane, PhD,** Chicago Center for Family Health, Chicago, Illinois

**Janet Froeschle, PhD,** Department of Education, West Texas A & M University, Canyon, Texas

**Jerry Gale, PhD,** Department of Child and Family Development, University of Georgia, Athens, Georgia

**Terry D. Hargrave, PhD,** Department of Marriage and Family Therapy, Fuller Theological Seminary, Pasadena, California

**Evan Imber-Black, PhD,** Ackerman Institute for the Family and Department of Psychiatry, Albert Einstein College of Medicine, New York, New York

**Hugo Kamya, MDiv, MSW, PhD,** Simmons College School of Social Work, Boston, Massachusetts

**Tonya Walker Lockwood, PsyD,** private practice, Washington, DC

**Wayne Muller, DDiv,** Bread for the Journey, Mill Valley, California

**Alice de V. Perry, MDiv, DMin,** Yale Divinity School, New Haven, Connecticut; Andover Newton Theological School, Newton, Massachusetts; and Milford Pastoral Counseling Center, Milford, Connecticut

**Shanthi Ranganathan, PhD,** T T Raganathan Clinical Research Foundation, TTK Hospital, Chennai, India

**Janine Roberts, EdD,** Emerita, School of Education, University of Massachusetts, Amherst, Massachusetts

**John S. Rolland, MD,** Department of Psychiatry, Pritzker School of Medicine, University of Chicago, and Chicago Center for Family Health, Chicago, Illinois

**Dyaa Saymah, MA,** Mental Health National Program, World Health Organization, Gaza, Palestinian Territories, Israel

**Fred Taylor, DDiv,** formerly of For Love of Children, Washington, DC

**Froma Walsh, MSW, PhD,** Emerita, School of Social Service Administration, University of Chicago, and Chicago Center for Family Health, Chicago, Illinois

**Kaethe Weingarten, PhD,** Department of Psychology, Harvard Medical School, and Program in Family, Trauma, and Resilience, The Family Institute of Cambridge, Cambridge, Massachusetts

**Steven J. Wolin, MD,** George Washington University and Project Resilience, Washington, DC

**Sybil Wolin, PhD,** Project Resilience, Washington, DC

**Lorraine M. Wright, RN, PhD,** Emerita, Faculty of Nursing, University of Calgary, Calgary, Alberta, Canada

**Hasan Zeyada, MA,** Gaza Community Mental Health Programme, Gaza, Palestinian Territories, Israel

# Preface

Spirituality is a powerful dimension of human experience involving transcendent beliefs and practices that foster meaning, well-being, and connectedness. A spiritual worldview orients individuals and their families over the life course and across the generations. It provides larger values and purpose, guides daily actions and relationships, and strengthens resilience in overcoming adversity. A growing body of research documents the powerful influence of personal faith, prayer and meditation, and a faith community on physical, emotional, and relational well-being and on recovery from illness and trauma. Spiritual distress or a spiritual void in one's life and relationships can contribute to suffering and block positive growth. Yet, until recently, spirituality was regarded as "off limits" in clinical training and practice, leaving most therapists and counselors uncertain how to approach it, if at all.

The first edition of this volume filled a crucial need in the literature: opening family therapy to the spiritual dimension and bringing a broad, multifaith perspective. This second edition deepens and extends that base for all practitioners working with couples and families—mental health, health care, human service, and pastoral care professionals. It describes more fully how faith beliefs and practices influence suffering and coping and how spiritual resources can be tapped to foster personal and relational healing and resilience. The contributing authors, all leading family systems scholars, educators, and practitioners, bring valuable knowledge and expertise in working with a wide range of clinical situations. Expanded and updated throughout, the new edition features five new chapters on death and loss, refugee trauma, meditation practices, use of rituals, and forgiveness. Attention is given to the many diverse spiritual orientations in today's society, from Jewish, Christian, Islamic, Buddhist, and Hindu faiths to indigenous spiritual beliefs and practices, particularly those of Native American, Latin American, Asian, and African traditions.

The focus of the volume is on the lived experience of spirituality in couple and family relationships. This is especially important in light of the growing diversity of faith beliefs and practices in families through conversion, interfaith marriage, and the blending of approaches. Recent survey data reveal a dramatically changing religious landscape in North America. Nearly 40% of Americans have left the faith tradition of their upbringing. Religious affiliation has been shifting and congregational membership, attendance at worship services, and adherence to doctrine have been declining. Yet spirituality—transcendent values and practices that are both broader and more personal—is more important than ever. In our turbulent world, there is a deep yearning for spiritual faith, practices, and communities that offer shelter, meaning, nourishment, and connection. Increasingly, individuals, couples, and families are creatively forging their own spiritual paths, often combining elements within and across faith orientations to fit their lives and relationships.

In this book, we consider the many varied ways spiritual resources can be tapped both within and outside organized religion: through strong religious and humanistic values; in personal faith and a relationship with God or a Higher Power; in practices of prayer, meditation, and rituals; by involvement in a faith community; in communion with nature; through music and the creative arts; and in service and social action to benefit others and our environment.

Spirituality can be expressed most profoundly in loving human relationships. At the heart of this volume, chapters address the many ways spiritual meaning and connection can be fostered between intimate partners and "kindred spirits"; in parent–child bonds; in caring for elders and those with special needs; in supportive kin and community networks; and through compassionate engagement with others in our larger world. All faith traditions teach the values and practice of love, kindness, honor, mutual respect, harmony, genuineness, compassion, and forgiveness. These are essential elements for healthy couple and family relationships and are consonant with core principles in therapeutic work to strengthen couples and families in distress.

Spiritual belief systems, intertwined with culture and life circumstances, influence how family members define problems, view causes and solutions, and make meaning of adversity and suffering. They also influence how family members approach coping, acceptance, and change, and where members turn for help. As helping professionals, we need to understand how trauma or persistent hardship affect the spirit and how constraining beliefs, negative religious experiences, or a spiritual void may contribute to distress and block healing. We need to address denigrating or abusive practices and injustices that wound the mind, body, and spirit. Therapists can also foster greater understanding, acceptance, and relational healing in couples and families where religious differences fuel misunderstanding, conflict, or estrangement.

This volume is designed to be a valuable sourcebook to inform and inspire the integration of spirituality in all therapeutic work with couples and families:

- To explore the meaning and significance of spiritual beliefs and practices in their lives.
- To understand spiritual sources of suffering and constraints to positive growth.
- To identify and draw on spiritual resources for healing and resilience that fit clients' values and preferences.

The authors approach spirituality not as a special topic but as it is interwoven in all aspects of people's lives and in the therapeutic process—from family heritage to personal beliefs, practices, and relationships—influencing the experience of problems, coping, and help seeking. Distinct from texts that prescribe a particular spiritual approach rooted in the therapist's religious convictions, the authors in this volume bring varied spiritual vantage points to inform clinical assessment and intervention. All are grounded in a strengths-based family systems orientation and a collaborative approach to practice.

This volume also encourages all helping professionals to examine their own spiritual positions, since the therapeutic process and goals involve the interaction of core beliefs of therapists and clients. Faulty assumptions or inattention to spiritual influences may undermine therapeutic efforts or lead to inappropriate aims. Just as we have recognized that therapists inescapably carry their personal, professional, and larger cultural values and cannot be neutral, so must we be aware of our values and biases and take care not to impose our own spiritual position. It is also important to build linkages between pastoral care and clinical services for mutual referral, consultation, and collaboration in areas of expertise. If we are to understand the clients we serve and assist in their healing and growth, it is crucial to understand their spiritual beliefs, attend to their concerns, and respond to their spiritual needs.

Part I in this volume provides an overview. Chapter 1 surveys the dramatically changing landscape of religion and spirituality in North America and examines the growing diversity and significance of spiritual beliefs and practices for individuals, couples, and families over the life course. Chapter 2 surveys the increasing research evidence on the significance of spiritual beliefs, practices, and faith community for health and recovery from medical crises, trauma, substance abuse, and major life challenges. Guidelines and cautions are offered for the inclusion of the spiritual dimension in clinical practice to address spiritual sources of distress and to draw on spiritual resources for healing and resilience.

In Part II, chapters illuminate the importance of spiritual resources for families in overcoming life challenges and in strengthening their relationships. Lorraine M. Wright reveals how illness and suffering invite us into the spiritual domain and presents her integrative approach to healing. Froma Walsh examines the ways in which spiritual beliefs and practices of varied faith traditions come to the fore with death, dying, and concerns about afterlife. Steven J. Wolin and colleagues present Buddhist, Christian, Jewish, Hindu, and Islamic perspectives on resilience in facing adversity. Harry J. Aponte urges therapists to attend to the need for spiritual sustenance of families in poor, underserved, minority communities. Nancy Boyd-Franklin and Tonya Walker Lockwood discuss the significance of faith and congregational involvement for the resilience of African American families. Celia Jaes Falicov examines the intertwining of formal religion and traditional spiritual beliefs and practices for immigrant families in their approach to health and mental health problems. Mona DeKoven Fishbane considers the value in Jewish tradition—honor thy father and mother—and its relevance for therapy to repair grievances in intergenerational relations. Herbert Anderson offers his vision for spirituality in contemporary family life, grounded in core values such as justice in couple relationships.

In Part III, the authors present a rich abundance of ways to integrate spirituality in clinical practice. William J. Doherty focuses on the interweaving of moral, spiritual, and clinical issues. Evan Imber-Black describes the therapeutic use of rituals. Jerry Gale offers meditation approaches for relational connectedness in couples and families. Mary Jo Barrett finds spiritual resources invaluable in client healing from relational trauma and in preventing therapist compassion fatigue. Hugo Kamya invites indigenous spiritual traditions into his therapeutic work with refugee youth from Sudan and links them with faith communities and faith-based services. Terry D.

Hargrave, Janet Froeschle, and Yvette Castillo survey the value of forgiveness in Christian, Jewish, and Islamic teachings and describe leading clinical approaches to forgiveness in wounded relationships. Melissa Elliott describes ways to open therapeutic conversations to a personal relationship with God in her work with deeply religious Christians. Kaethe Weingarten offers insightful observations on the essence of the therapeutic bond and the process of healing as a profoundly spiritual experience. Janine Roberts presents useful exercises for therapists, trainees, and clients to examine their values and explore their spiritual life journey. Finally, Alice de V. Perry and John S. Rolland expand the therapeutic frame to encourage social justice initiatives for client and community empowerment, healing, and hope.

Broad in scope, this volume presents valuable knowledge and practice guidelines for practitioners to develop a spiritual pluralism, with understanding and respect for the varied faith beliefs and practices of clients in our increasingly diverse society. In each chapter, the authors bring their expertise, wisdom, and creativity to inform and inspire a therapeutic process that fosters deeper meaning, wholeness, and connection for healing, well-being, and resilience.

# Acknowledgments

I would like to express my deep appreciation to all of the authors who have contributed such stimulating chapters in the new edition of this volume. We are all indebted to our families, our colleagues, and the clients who have inspired our work, and we have all found that the spirit is nourished and grows through such meaningful connections.

I want to express my gratitude for the highly dedicated and responsive staff of The Guilford Press, in particular, Senior Editor Jim Nageotte and his assistant, Jane Keislar. I thank John Rolland, MD, and Janet Goeking, MA, for their valuable feedback on drafts and Rob Gellman, PhD, for his assistance in reviewing the growing research literature on spirituality and sexual orientation. I especially value my ongoing conversations with my daughter, Claire Whitney, LMSW, MIA, for her profound questions and insights on the diversity and complexity of religion and spirituality.

Most of all, I am grateful to my parents, Mary Jo Bourassa and George Weisberg, who wove together multihued strands of disparate faith traditions, embodying a richly textured spirituality in all aspects of their lives and relationships. Through their example, I gained appreciation for many varied spiritual paths. In facing tremendous adversity, their deep and abiding spirituality was a wellspring for their love, their compassion for others, and their resilience.

> May we walk with grace
> And may the light of the universe
> Shine upon our path
> —ANONYMOUS

# Contents

## III. SPIRITUALITY IN THERAPEUTIC PRACTICE

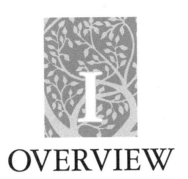

# OVERVIEW

# Religion, Spirituality, and the Family
## Multifaith Perspectives

### FROMA WALSH

> Love is the most powerful
> and still the most unknown energy of the world.
> —TEILHARD DE CHARDIN

Over the millennia and across cultures, people have lit candles, prayed together, meditated, and quietly turned to faith for solace, strength, and connectedness in their lives. Spiritual beliefs and practices anchor and nourish families and their communities. At times of crisis and with prolonged adversity, they foster recovery and resilience. Today, the vast majority of individuals and their families adopt some form of expression for their spirituality, whether within or outside formal religion. Many who seek help for physical, emotional, or interpersonal problems are also in spiritual distress. Therefore, as therapists and human service professionals, we need to attend to the spiritual dimension of human experience if we are to understand the needs and suffering of our clients and assist in their healing and growth.

Spirituality is not simply a special topic. Rather, like culture and ethnicity, it involves streams of experience that flow through all aspects of our lives, from family heritage to personal belief systems, rituals and practices, and shared faith communities. Spiritual beliefs influence ways of coping with adversity, the experience of suffering, and the meaning of symptoms.

They also influence how people communicate about their problems and pain; their beliefs about the causes and future course; their attitudes toward professional helpers—in pastoral care, mental health, health care, and human services—as well as faith healers; the treatments they seek; and their preferred pathways in problem solving or recovery. Moreover, psychotherapy itself, long considered a healing art, can be a profoundly spiritual experience for both clients and therapists, yet this has been a hidden aspect of our work. The very essence of the therapeutic relationship and meaningful change is ultimately spiritual in nature, fostering transformation, wholeness, and relational connection.

Therapists and trainees across professional disciplines have begun to show keen interest in exploring and developing the spiritual dimension of our practice. This overview chapter examines the growing diversity and significance of religion and spirituality for individuals, couples, and families today. Chapter 2 then suggests ways to include spirituality in clinical practice to understand spiritual sources of distress and to tap spiritual resources for healing, recovery, and resilience.

## SPIRITUALITY IN A CHANGING WORLD

There has been a growing interest in spirituality throughout North America as people have sought greater meaning, harmony, and connection in their lives (Bibby, 2002; Miller & Thoresen, 2003). Over recent decades, tumultuous social and economic dislocations have generated widespread insecurity. Our harried, fragmented, and materialistic culture leaves many disconnected and unfulfilled, contributing to a spiritual malaise (Lerner, 2007). Marriage and family life have become more challenging. With increasing diversity, changing gender roles, and varied family structures over an extended life course, family members seek transcendent values and practices for greater coherence in their lives (Walsh, 2003b, 2006).

Moreover, major disasters, war, and widespread terrorist attacks shatter illusions of invulnerability and heighten awareness of the precariousness of life. In times of crisis and tragedy, people turn to their loved ones and to spiritual resources for meaning, solace, and strength in facing an uncertain future. Life was never more secure in earlier times; yet in our era, some are alarmed by a seeming collapse of universal moral values and seek spiritual moorings. The rise in religious fundamentalism in many parts of the world expresses, in part, a desire to restore traditions that provide clear structure and absolute certainties in the midst of rapid social change. Buffeted by global forces seemingly beyond control or comprehension, we yearn for inner peace, for a sense of coherence in our fragmented lives, and for more mean-ingful connection with others. It is no wonder that so many Americans have been turning to spiritual resources for resilience, blending varied religious traditions, and seeking new spiritual pathways to fit their lives.

## DEFINING RELIGION AND SPIRITUALITY

It is important to clarify our understanding of the terms *religion* and *spiri-tuality*, which are often used interchangeably. *Religion* can be defined as an organized, institutionalized belief system, set of practices, and faith commu-nity. *Spirituality*, an overarching construct, refers to a dimension of human experience involving personal transcendent beliefs and practices, within or outside formal religion, through family and cultural heritage, and in con-nection with nature and humanity.

Most research and discourse until recently have focused on religious beliefs, practices, and congregational affiliation (e.g., Gallup and Pew sur-veys). More attention is needed to the broader and more personal expressions of spirituality, as people are increasingly seeking and shaping their own varied spiritual pathways.

### Religion: Organized Belief System

*Religion* is an organized belief system that includes shared, institutionalized, moral values, practices, involvement in a faith community, and, for most, belief in God or a Higher Power. Through sacred scriptures and teachings, religions provide standards and prescriptions for individual virtue, relational conduct, and family life grounded in core beliefs. Congregational affiliation provides the guidance of clergy and a community of shared faith, as well as support in times of crisis. Rituals and ceremonies carry profound signifi-cance, connecting individuals and families with their larger community, its history, and its survival over adversity. Religious belief systems provide faith explanations of past history and present experiences. For many, they predict the future and offer pathways toward understanding the ultimate meanings of life and existence (Campbell & Moyers, 1988).

### Spirituality: Transcendent Beliefs and Practices

*Spirituality* is a dimension of human experience involving transcendent beliefs and practices. It is the heart and soul of religion (Pargament, 2007). Spirituality can also be experienced outside formal religious structures, and is both broader and more personal (Elkins, 1990). Spiritual resources might include practices of prayer, meditation, or traditional faith healing rituals and participation in a faith community. Many people who do not consider themselves "religious" lead deeply spiritual lives and find spiritual nourishment in varied ways. Some find renewal and connection through nature and the creative arts; others find meaning and purpose through secular humanism, service to others, and social activism.

One simple yet profound definition of *spirituality* is "that which connects one to all there is" (Griffith & Elliott Griffith, 2002). It involves an active investment in an internal set of values. It fosters a sense of meaning, wholeness, harmony, and connection with others—a unity with all life, nature, and the universe (Wright, Watson, & Bell, 1996). One's spirituality may involve belief in a supreme being, a divine spirit within all living things, or an ultimate human condition toward which we strive.

Spirituality invites an expansion of consciousness, along with personal responsibility for and beyond oneself, from local to global concerns. A child's moral awareness evolves out of spiritual belief systems (Coles, 1997). Morality involves the activity of informed conscience—judging right and wrong based on principles of justice, decency, and compassion (Doherty, 1995; see Chapter 11, this volume). Moral or ethical values spur us to go beyond virtuous conduct to respond to the suffering of others; to dedicate efforts to right injustice; and to repair and improve conditions in our world (see Perry & Rolland, Chapter 20, this volume). At their best, they promote humanity.

## Spirit

Universally, the spirit is seen as our vital essence, the source of life and power. In many languages the word for *spirit* and *breath* is the same: in Greek, *pneuma*; in Hebrew, *reach* ("ray-akh"); in Latin, *spiritus*; and in Sanskrit, *prana* (Weil, 1994). We are *inspired* by great teachers, scriptures and hymns, works of art, and the magnificence of nature. We *aspire* to become our best selves. We *expire* with our last breath at death, when, for religious believers, our spirit is released to an afterlife.

## Soul

Similarly, the soul has been seen over the ages as the source of human genuineness, depth, joy, sorrow, and mystery. In many religions, the soul is also a metaphor expressing the relationship between human beings and God: To tend to the soul is to restore and strengthen that connection.

Herbert Anderson, a theological authority on marriage and the family (see Chapter 10, this volume), describes the soul as our visualizing center, guiding how we live with others and ourselves. Yet we can't quite locate it: We sense something as true or profound in our "gut." Anderson notes that the literal translation of Proverbs 23:16 is "my kidneys will rejoice when your lips speak what is right" (1994, p. 209). He adds that because the human being is a unity, soul or kidney may also refer to the individual as a whole.

Taking a double view, Anderson (1994) describes the soul as being everywhere but nowhere—in every cell of the body and also capable of self-transcendence. In this view, we are both soul-filled bodies and embodied souls, linked to earth and sky. Similarly, Thomas Moore (1992) observes that if we are to care for the soul, then "we will have to know the sky and earth as well as human behavior" (p. 20).

Such perspectives are strikingly akin to Native American and First Nation spirituality. Black Elk, a Holy Man of the Lakota tribe, recounting the tragic decades of the Custer battle and the Wounded Knee Massacre, revealed the spiritual source of resilience that sustained Native American tribes: their system of beliefs based in a vision of the unity of all creation. "All living things . . . are children of one mother, Mother Earth, and their father is one Spirit. We are related to all things: the stars in the universe and the grasses of the earth" (Neihardt, 1932/1979, p. 5).

Many scholars and therapists regard the wounding or neglect of the soul as a primary source of the maladies of our times, afflicting individuals and society with symptoms such as obsessions, addictions, violence, sexual abuse, and loss of meaning and hope (see Aponte [Chapter 6], Barrett [Chapter 14], Kamya [Chapter 15], and Weingarten [Chapter 18], this volume). Moore (1992) asserts that the mental health field tries to isolate and eradicate these symptoms, but much suffering that is given pathological labels may also be understood as maladies of the soul, of overwhelming loss and disconnection. We refer to someone in despair as a "lost soul," without hope or community, struggling to survive. Much of the suffering that therapists treat involves deep yearnings for meaning and connection. When we lose ourselves in a multitude of activities and petty concerns, we endanger the soul. Tending to the soul involves purposeful activity and restful replenishing.

We can only glimpse the soul and cannot penetrate its essence. More process and substance, the language of soul is not technical or scientific but rather embodied in poetry, art, and music. Imagination is the expression of soul; it involves the making of meaningful memory, linking the past, present, and future; the individual with the community and all that is beyond.

The soul also involves vulnerability and uncertainty. As humans we are all susceptible to being wounded; we grapple with the meaning of our lives and with our own mortality. We nourish the soul by living without pretense or armor, approaching all experience with openness, courage, and compassion.

## INCREASING RELIGIOUS AND SPIRITUAL PLURALISM

Americans are among the most religious people in the world. In 2007 surveys, 83% of all adults said that religion is important in their lives, 56% regarded it as very important, and nearly 33% considered it the most important part of their lives (Gallup, Inc., 2008[1]). Over recent decades, religion has been in transformation (Smith, 2005), with growing diversity and personal choice of faith beliefs and practices.

The United States was founded by religious dissidents on the principle of respect and tolerance for diversity of faith (Gaustad & Schmidt, 2002). Christianity has remained dominant, as it has in Canada (Lindner, 2008); however, the religious landscape in North America has been changing dramatically over recent decades both through immigration and the increasing desire to seek varied spiritual pathways.

### Religious Identification

Over 80% of Americans identify as Christian (Gallup, Inc., 2008). Nearly 50% are Protestant, with membership shifting in recent years from mainline denominations to evangelical churches, many nondenominational. Twenty-three percent are Roman Catholic. Additionally, 2% identify as Mormon (Church of Jesus Christ of the Latter-Day Saints) and 0.8% are Eastern Orthodox (e.g., Greek or Russian).

Over 40% of Christians describe themselves as evangelical, "born again," or fundamentalist, which are overlapping groups (Gallup, Inc., 2008). The influence of the Christian right, a coalition combining fundamentalist visions of religion with a politically and socially conservative agenda, has been waning. Evangelical Christians are politically diverse and increasingly broad in focus on human rights, poverty, and environmental concerns (Greeley & Hout, 2006).

The non-Christian proportion of the United States has been rising, from 3.6% in 1900, to nearly 15% by 2000 (Gallup, 2002). Over 2% of Americans consider themselves to be Jewish, ranging widely in beliefs and practices from Orthodox, Conservative, Reform, and Reconstructionist branches to secular humanism, identification with parentage or upbringing, and connection to the history and heritage of the Jewish people (Mayer, Kosmin, & Keysar, 2002). Those who identify as Buddhists, Muslims, and Hindus are near 1% each and increasing. Others follow ancient traditions such as Native American, Sikh, Shinto, and Tao. Some are drawn to religions that present a universality of faiths, such as Unitarian/Universalist and Baha'i, which avows "many lamps; one light."

### Faith Communities

Formal denominational affiliation and congregational membership have been declining in recent years in North America, especially in Canada (Pew Forum on Religion and Public Life, 2008; Lindner, 2008). In the United States, 62% say they are members of "a church or synagogue," although attendance at worship services is less regular than in the past, particularly by men. Yet there are over 2,000 denominations plus countless independent congregations (Lindner, 2008), with nearly 500,000 churches, temples, mosques, and other places of worship—from small storefronts to megachurches drawing tens of thousands of congregants.

Beyond places of worship, congregations that flourish are vibrant communities of faith, offering a wide range of programs, with flexible schedules and childcare, to fit the needs of overburdened families. In addition to prayer and scripture reading groups, choir singing, potluck suppers, and social gatherings, they encourage involvement in community service, from volunteer support in faith-affiliated hospitals and social service agencies, to local and global activism for causes such as disaster recovery, HIV-AIDS prevention, social justice, human rights, peace efforts, and the environment. Many offer "cradle to grave" services including marriage and parenting skills, childcare and eldercare, teen clubs, computer and job skills training, preventive health care, mental health counseling, and senior activities. Clergy and pastoral counselors provide spiritual guidance through times of adversity. In religious support groups, members gain strength and a sense of interdependence. Internet services provide information, promote connection, and rally prayers and support for those in need.

## INTERTWINING OF RELIGIOUS
## AND CULTURAL INFLUENCES

Religion and culture are interwoven in all aspects of spiritual experience (McGoldrick, Giordano, & Garcia-Preto, 2005). Frank McCourt (1998) experienced his Irish Catholic upbringing as a faith that seemed "mean, scrimped, and life-denying" (p. 64). He formed the image of an angry, vengeful God "who'd let you have it upside your head if you strayed, transgressed, coveted. . . . He had His priests preaching hellfire and damnation from the pulpit and scaring us to death" (p. 64). In traveling to Italy, McCourt was struck by the differences: "Statues and pictures of the Virgin Mary in the Irish churches seemed disembodied and she seemed to be saying, 'Who is this kid?' In contrast, Italian art portrayed a voluptuous, maternal Mary with a happy infant Jesus at her bosom" (p. 64). McCourt wondered: "Was it the weather? Did God change His aspect as He moved from the chilly north to the vineyards of Italy?" (p. 64). He thought that, all in all, he'd prefer the Italian expression of Catholicism to the Irish one.

Spiritual beliefs and practices vary greatly across and within cultures. African Americans are far more likely than all other groups to consider religion important, from personal faith and connection with God to active congregational participation (Gallup & Lindsay, 1999). Many are involved in historically Black churches (e.g., AME, African Methodist Episcopal) that have been vital resources during and since the time of slavery. African Americans practice their faith fervently and look to it for strength in dealing with adversity (see Boyd-Franklin & Lockwood, Chapter 7, this volume).

Hispanics are transforming the religious landscape in the United States, especially the Catholic Church, through their growing numbers and their practice of a distinctive form of Christianity (Pew Hispanic Project and the Pew Forum on Religion and Public Life, 2007). Two-thirds of Latinos identify as Roman Catholic—now one-third of all Catholics in the U.S. Over half of Catholic Latinos find religious expressions associated with the Pentecostal and charismatic movements. Also, growing numbers are converting from Catholic to evangelical churches, primarily for a more direct, personal experience of God.

For the great majority of Latinos, regardless of religious preference, God is an active force in everyday life. Most identify with spirit-filled religion or renewalist movements emphasizing God's ongoing intervention in daily human affairs through the Holy Spirit. Many say they have experienced such occurrences as divine healing, miracles, transpersonal encounters (with angels, demons, and other spiritual visitations), and direct revelations from God. Most Latinos pray every day, have religious objects in their home, and attend religious services at least monthly. Latino-oriented churches are flourishing; two-thirds of Hispanics attend churches with Latino clergy and services in Spanish. This trend is prevalent among not only recent immigrants but also native-born and English-speaking Latinos, suggesting that it involves a broad and lasting form of cultural and spiritual identification (see Falicov, Chapter 8, this volume).

Immigrants from Latin America, Southeast Asia, and Africa commonly follow traditional spiritual beliefs and practices alongside Christianity, comingling African and indigenous influences, as do many Latinos in *santería* and *espiritismo* (Comas-Díaz, 1981; see Falicov [Chapter 8] and Kamya [Chapter 15], this volume). Most turn to the church for weddings, christenings, and funerals, yet tend to personalize their connection with God through special relationships with saints or spiritual guides, and show faith and gratitude through offerings, prayers, and rituals. Many believe in an invisible world inhabited by good and evil spirits who influence human behavior and can either protect or harm, prevent or cause illness, and be influenced by good or evil deeds. Incense, candles, and powders, alleged to have mystical properties, are used to cure illness and ward off the "evil eye."

Differences are found between families from rural, traditional backgrounds and those from urban, educated, and middle-class settings. Religious expression is further influenced by race, recent immigration, and acceptance or marginalization by the dominant culture. Religious prejudice or discrimination can lead family members to suppress identification.

It is crucial not to link religion and ethnicity reflexively, and to guard against stereotypes. Contrary to popular belief, only one-third of Arab Americans are Muslim; many are Christian. U.S. Muslims include African Americans, as well as immigrants from the Middle East, North and sub-Saharan Africa, South Asia, and Indonesia. Although they face strong discrimination, Muslim Americans are largely assimilated, happy with their lives, and moderate with respect to many issues that have divided Muslims and Westerners around the world (Pew Forum on Religion and Public Life, 2007).

Immigrants from Southeast Asia may be Christian or bring Eastern religious and ancient animist traditions. Refugees from the former Yugoslavia who are Croatian, Bosnian, or Kosovar, are also Orthodox Christian, Catholic, or Muslim—differences that carry heavy historical meaning (i.e., the 13th-century imposition of Islam by invading Turks) that fueled hatred and bloodshed across the generations. In our work with Bosnian and Kosovar refugee families who fled "ethnic cleansing," it was important to be mindful of the religious aspect of their trauma and their resilience (Walsh, 2006).

In a predominantly Christian nation of European origins, we must be cautious not to superimpose the template of Western European values on other belief systems and practices that may not be understood in Christian terms. It is crucial not to judge diverse faith orientations, particularly those of non-Christian, non-European, and indigenous cultures, such as African healing traditions, as inferior or primitive (Somé, 1998). Early European American conquerors viewed Native American tribes as savage heathens and regarded their spiritual beliefs and practices as pagan witchcraft. Such attitudes led to government and religious missionary programs to educate and acculturate Indians in Christianity and Western ways, eradicating their tribal language, religion, and customs. Children were forcibly taken from their families and tribes and sent to boarding schools, where they were stripped of their cultural identity and religious heritage. Today, Native American youth are returning in large numbers to the spiritual roots of their ancestors, seeking identity and worth in their spiritual communities (Bucko, 2007; Deloria, 1994).

Religious intolerance and extremism have spawned hatred and violence. Although Muslim terrorists proclaim religious adherence, Islamic Law forbids suicide and the killing of innocent people (Nasr, 2002). In the United States, violent acts have also been committed by members of White supremacist, extremist Christian groups that espouse racism and religious intolerance. Imposition of the dogmatic belief that there is only one "true religion" has led to catastrophic consequences throughout human times, such as holy wars, including the Crusades and the Spanish Inquisition, to convert, subjugate, or annihilate nonbelievers (Marty, 2005).

## COMMON RELIGIOUS BELIEFS AND PRACTICES

Belief in God is strong among Americans. In 2007 surveys, 86% said they believe in God, a Higher Power, or a Universal spirit. Only 6% are atheists, nonbelievers in the existence of God, and 8% are agnostic, or uncertain (Gallup, 2008). Conceptions of God vary widely; some think of God as a "force" that maintains a balance in nature. Most believe in a personal God, who watches over and judges people, guiding them in making decisions. Most believe that God performs miracles today. Many say they have felt the presence of God at various times and believe that God has a plan for their lives. The closer people feel to God, the better they feel about themselves and others.

Most Americans believe that they will be called before God on Judgment Day to answer for their sins. The vast majority believes in an afterlife: 81% believe in heaven, and 75% believe in angels, whereas nearly 70%

believe in hell and the devil (Gallup, 2008; see Walsh, Chapter 4, this volume). Most people say their religious beliefs help them to solve problems, to respect themselves and others, to help those in need, and keep them from doing things they know they shouldn't do. However, there is often a gap between people's faith and knowledge of their religion and its core tenets. Although over 90% of homes contain a Bible, 58% of Americans couldn't name five of the Ten Commandments; furthermore, 10% thought Joan of Arc was Noah's wife. Nearly half of all teens thought Moses was one of the twelve Apostles (Prothero, 2007)!

Public attitudes across a set of social issues such as gay marriage, gay adoption of children, abortion, and stem cell research have become more moderate (Pew Forum on Religion and Public Life, 2006). The most conservative on these issues are White evangelical Protestants, men, Blacks, those over 65, and those less educated.

Such issues can be contentious in couple and family relationships. Yet we must be cautious not to assume that particular individuals or families adhere to doctrines of their religion. On reproductive rights, most Americans (73%) view abortion as morally wrong in at least some circumstances. Yet across the ideological spectrum, two-thirds support finding common ground: making abortion available but rare. Among Catholics, over 60% believe that those who have abortions can still be good Catholics. Over 75% of Catholics disagree with the Church refusal to sanction divorce and remarriage (Gallup & Lindsay, 1999). There is a growing gap between personal faith and adherence to institutionalized religious systems. Most people regard decisions such as birth control, abortion, divorce, and assisted dying as matters between themselves, their loved ones, and God. In all, most Americans are highly independent in their spiritual lives (Pew Forum on Religion & Public Life, 2006).

## Prayer, Meditation, and Rituals

Prayer has strong meaning for Americans: 90% pray in some fashion at least weekly; 75% pray daily (Gallup & Lindsay, 1999; Gallup, Inc., 2008). For most, prayer originates in the family, is centered in the home, and grows in importance over the life course. Prayer at bedtime and saying grace or giving thanks to God before meals are common practices. Most people report that they pray whenever they feel the need. As one African American woman said, "My own father died when I was 18 months old and so I had to talk to my father in heaven and rely on him to guide me throughout my life." She added, "You need that higher power to help you when you have deaths in the family or your children get into trouble. If I didn't always have Him to talk to, I never would have made it through."

Prayers serve many functions. Daily prayers express praise and gratitude. Almost all people pray for their family's health and happiness; very few pray for bad tidings for others. People commonly pray for strength, wisdom, or courage in facing life challenges. Many pray to seek forgiveness for sins, wrongdoing, or harm to others. Some request intercession or miracles in dire situations, such as when a loved one's life is at risk. Others pray that God's will be done.

Prayer generates feelings of hope and peace. Most who pray believe it makes them better persons. Nearly all report that their prayers have been heard and answered. One in four reports a voice or vision as a result of prayer. Most say they received what they hoped for, as well as divine inspiration or a feeling of being led by God. Yet one in five persons has been angered or disappointed when prayers have not been answered, most often when a requested miracle did not occur. Some (30%) have had long periods of time when they stopped praying, mostly because they got out of the habit. A few (10%) stopped because they lost their faith, were angry with God or their church, or felt their prayers had not been answered (Gallup & Lindsay, 1999).

Every religion values some form of prayer or meditation. Many people who are not religious also practice meditation for physical, psychological, and spiritual well-being. It may involve silent contemplation, mindfulness practices, chanting, reading sacred or inspirational texts, reciting a rosary or a mantra, or rituals, such as lighting candles or incense. Catholics commonly offer prayers to patron Saints for guidance or intercession with God. Hindu meditation and offerings to various gods take place most often in the home, where small statues and shrines are placed. One of the five pillars of Islam is observance of ritual prayer, facing Mecca, five times daily. For Muslims, one reason to pray is to express praise and gratitude for life itself. Another reason is to keep life in perspective, which is considered the most difficult lesson people must learn (Nasr, 2002). Across faiths, shared meditative experiences foster genuine and empathic bonds, reduce defensive reactivity, and deepen couple and family bonds (see Gale, Chapter 13, this volume).

Rituals and ceremonies serve invaluable functions in connecting individuals with their families and communities, as well as guiding them through life passage and times of adversity (Imber-Black, Roberts, & Whiting, 2003; see Imber-Black, Chapter 12, this volume). Rituals celebrate or commemorate important events in family life and faith traditions. They also connect a particular celebration or tragedy with all human experience, a birth or death with all others.

## *Patriarchy and Changing Gender Role Relations*

Patriarchy, an ancient and enduring cultural pattern embedded in most religious traditions, has been a dominant force. At its worst, it has sanctioned the subordination and abuse of women and children (Bottoms, Shaver, Goodman, & Qin, 1995; Bowman, 1983; Bridges & Spilka, 1992). In Genesis 3:16, Eve was admonished, "In pain you shall bring forth children; yet your desire shall be for your husband, and he shall rule over you." In the New Testament, St. Paul told women, "Wives, be submissive to your husbands" (Colossians 3:18). Confucius (551–479 B.C.) boldly proclaimed, "one hundred women are not worth a single testicle." The Hindu Code of Manu (c. 100 A.D.) declared, "In childhood a woman must be subject to her father; in youth to her husband; and when her husband is dead, to her sons. A woman must never be free of subjugation." A legacy of this devaluation in some parts of the world, such as China and India, has been the practice of infanticide, abandonment and, with modern technology, abortion of unwanted daughters. With the preference for sons, the one-child mandate in China since the 1980s has produced a gross imbalance in the numbers of young men to women.

Over recent decades, traditional gender role relations have been in transformation in couples and families. In the United States, evangelical and mainline Protestant churches have markedly different ideological positions on these changes, with evangelicals holding to patriarchal expectations for the husband/father to be the "spiritual head" of the family. Yet, as Wilcox (2004) finds, the actual family behavior of Christian men who are married with children does not differ greatly. Mainline Protestant men, whom Wilcox terms "new men," take a more egalitarian position on the sharing of household responsibilities than do their conservative peers; and they take a more involved approach with their children than do men with no religious affiliation. Wilcox finds that Evangelical men tend to be "soft patriarchs": authoritative yet not as authoritarian as past generations. Their parenting style involves both strict discipline and warm, expressive interactions, and they tend to be more affectionate and dedicated to their wives and children than mainline Christian and secular men (Wilcox, 2004; see also Anderson, Chapter 10, this volume; on Latter-Day Saint marriage and family life, see Dollahite, 2007).

Within conservative sects, most women support traditional family role relations, adhering to their deep faith convictions when they are treated with respect and valued for their centrality in family life as mothers, caregivers, and keepers of the hearth. However, tensions rise when relationships are highly skewed in power, privilege, and control. Men who are more conservative than their wives are more likely to act violently toward them when conflict arises as women assert their needs or challenge authority (Sullivan, 2001).

Harmful patterns of denigration and abuse lead women increasingly to separate and divorce; they also alienate many from their religious roots. Some have found new meaning and esteem through more progressive churches and faiths, such as Baha'i, that promote the equality of men and women in family life and society. Some turn to holistic or Earth-based spiritualities. Feminist scholars have challenged androcentric interpretation of scriptures, such as the Bible and the Koran (Bakhtiar, 2007). The theologian Frymer-Kensky (cited in Murphy, 1998) asserts that the complex, multifaceted nature of God, combining all the attributes that went into the making of humankind, set a standard of unity, without sex or class division, that should be an inspiration to all.

### Gender Identity and Sexual Orientation

The condemnation of homosexuality in religious doctrine has been a source of deep anguish for lesbian, gay, bisexual, and transgendered (LGBT) persons. Some denominations have adopted a loving acceptance of gay persons as human beings created by God, yet abhor same-sex practices as unnatural and sinful. Such a dualistic position perpetuates stigma and shame, producing a deep schism in an individual's gender identity that wounds the soul. Even those who avow to "hate the sin, but love the sinner" engender a sense of conflict between their sexual orientation and full participation in religious life.

Many LGBT persons abandon their childhood faith, feeling that to accept themselves, they must reject their religion (Yip, 2002). They may still confront heterosexist religiosity in their family, kin, and social network; in their community; or in dealings with health care, workplace, or other, larger systems. Longstanding public opposition to same-sex marriage and adoption by gays and lesbians is declining. Those who have a friend or family member who is gay are twice as likely to be supportive (Pew Forum on Religion and Public Life, 2006, 2008).

Increasingly, many religious groups have been challenging traditional orthodoxy for the full acceptance of persons and relationships of diverse sexual orientation as human rights issues for equality and social justice. Many offer broadly inclusive ministries to meet spiritual needs, such as Unitarian and Metropolitan Community Churches. Many local congregations of varying denominations welcome LGBT members despite the official positions of their larger institution.

The diversity among LGBT individuals, couples, and families requires an especially broad definition of religion, faith, and spirituality. The challenges presented by religious dogma have not undermined the importance of spirituality. Some LGBT Christians and their families reconcile their spiritual and sexual identities through a personal relationship with a God that loves them unconditionally (Lease & Shulman, 2003). The HIV-AIDS crisis, the proliferation of families headed by same-sex partners, and the heated debates on same-sex marriage and gay clergy have intensified spiritual explorations (Davidson, 2000; Smith & Horne, 2007; Tan, 2005). Many show resilience in forging their own spiritual pathways by seeking out gay-inclusive faith communities and focusing on self-exploration and spiritual growth (Roseborough, 2006). Others turn to alternative faiths that emphasize personal, versus institutional, authority over spiritual matters, including Eastern and Earth-spirited faiths (Yip, 2002).

## *Spiritual Resources through Nature, the Arts, and Activism*

Spiritual resources are all around us. Many find spiritual connection and nourishment through communion with nature—in a walk at sunrise or the rhythm of waves on the shore; in tending a garden or a bond with a companion animal (Walsh, 2009). Such everyday experiences take us into the moment and beyond ourselves, making us feel at one with other life and the universe. Many are drawn to visit places with high spiritual energy— sacred mountains, shrines, cathedrals, mosques, and temples; sites of past civilizations; places of natural beauty and wonder. Living in harmony with nature and the environment is at the heart of the spirituality of indigenous communities.

Across cultures, people are inspired by art, poetry, and drama that communicate our common humanity. Music, both sacred and secular, can offer a powerful transcendent experience. Native Americans say, "to watch us dance is to hear our hearts speak." African American gospel "spirituals," blues, jazz, and "soul music" are creative expressions forged out of the cauldron of slavery, racism, and impoverished conditions, transcending those scarring experiences through the resilience of the human spirit.

Many who don't consider themselves religious do find spiritual meaning through nature, the arts, or activism. The author Alice Walker (1997) combined all three in her spiritual journey. Her beloved mother, devoted to her rural church, was active in bringing children in need into her home and looking out for the welfare of others in their struggling African American community. Walker dropped out of the church at age 13, feeling that the structure and teachings were oppressive. Finding that nature nourished her soul, she became what she calls a "born-again pagan" experiencing spirituality through the land. Her activist spirit found powerful expression in her writing and work in movements for social justice, following her mother's footsteps, yet on her own path.

## Broad Spectrum of Faith Beliefs and Practices

The wide spectrum of faiths today has been called a "supermarket" of religions, attesting to their strength and vitality. A broader spirituality is expected to continue in significance over the coming decades, shaped less by institutions and more by the people who are seeking meaning and connection. They commonly pick and choose among spiritual beliefs and practices from their faith tradition and from other sources to fit their lives. Canadian sociologist Reginald Bibby (2002) calls this trend "religion à la carte." Many immigrants blend traditional or indigenous beliefs and practices with Christianity. Others combine Buddhist teachings with their Jewish or Christian heritage. As spiritual diversity within families increases, most are taking a broader, multifaith, holistic perspective. Most Americans believe that all religions are essentially good and that nonreligious people can lead ethical lives. Although affiliation and adherence to formal religion has been declining, what matters for most is deep personal spirituality, guided by transcendent values that are lived out in daily life, relationships, and concern for others (Wendel, 2003).

## From Spiritual Diversity to Pluralism

The terms *pluralism* and *diversity* are sometimes used synonymously. However, as Eck (2006) clarifies, diversity refers simply to many differences— splendid, colorful, perhaps threatening. For instance, she observes that located on the same street in one neighborhood, there are diverse faith communities: a Vietnamese Catholic church, a Cambodian Buddhist temple, a Ukranian Orthodox church, a Muslim Community Center, a Disciples of Christ church, and a Hindu temple. Pluralism involves the engagement and relationship with one another that creates a common society from multifaith diversity.

America's growing spiritual diversity is generating a new period of bridge building as varied faith communities forge linkages with one another (see Harvard's Pluralism Project at *www.pluralism.org*). Interfaith dialogues tackle issues such as teen pregnancy; coalitions work to fight hunger and homelessness. More than the tolerance of differences, pluralism requires some knowledge of our differences and our commonalities. Rather than relinquishing the distinctiveness of one's own tradition of faith to reach the "lowest common denominator," it involves a broad inclusiveness of people of every faith, and of none, nurturing constructive dialogue, mutual understanding, and connectedness.

## THE IMPORTANCE OF SPIRITUALITY IN FAMILY LIFE

Spirituality is deeply interwoven in all aspects of family life. A growing body of research has been examining the influences of spiritual beliefs, practices, and congregational involvement on family functioning, parenting styles, family dynamics, and intergenerational bonds (Bailey, 2002; Mahoney, Pargament, Tarakeshwar, & Swank, 2001; Marks, 2006; Snarey & Dollahite, 2001; Snider, Clements, & Vazsonyi, 2004). Scholars are exploring the adaptation of a wide range of faith traditions for contemporary families (Browning & Clairmont, 2007). Studies of highly religious families are examining the role of religion in couple conflict (Lambert & Dollahite, 2006; Marsh & Dallos, 2001) and parent–child interactions (Marks, 2004).

Those who regard religion as the most important influence in their lives and receive a great deal of comfort from their faith are far more likely to feel close to their families, to find their jobs fulfilling, and to be hopeful about the future. In public surveys, over 80% say that religion was important in their family of origin when they were growing up, and nearly 75% report that their family relationships have been strengthened by religion in their home (Gallup & Lindsay, 1999). From a family systems perspective, there is a mutual influence between spirituality and the family: Meaningful spiritual beliefs and practices can strengthen families and their members; in turn, their shared spiritual experiences strengthen members' faith. Likewise, harsh or oppressive spiritual beliefs and practices can wound family members, their spirits, and their relationships; in turn, those who have been injured often turn away from their faith.

### *Transcendent Values*

Family process research has found that transcendent spiritual beliefs and practices foster healthy family functioning (Beavers & Hampson, 2003; Stinnett & DeFrain, 1985). A system of values and shared beliefs that transcends the limits of family members' experience and knowledge enables better acceptance of the inevitable risks and losses in living and loving fully.

Family values became a hotly debated topic in political discourse over recent decades as many religious conservatives contended that the changing family forms and gender roles led to the demise of the family. Today, there is less polarization and wide recognition that faith traditions need to adapt to the growing complexity and diversity of family life (Browning, Miller-McLemore, Couture, Lyon, & Franklin, 2001; Browning & Clairmont, 2007; Edgell, 2005; Houseknecht & Pankhurst, 2000). It is crucial to move beyond the faulty assumption that one family model is the "paragon of virtue" and that all others are inherently damaging (Stacey, 1996). Abundant research confirms that the vast majority of children fare well when raised in a variety of kinship arrangements, and by gay as well as straight parents. What matters most are stable, caring, committed bonds and family processes that support optimal functioning and positive growth (Walsh, 2003b). By becoming more broadly inclusive toward contemporary couples and families, faith institutions and communities can be more responsive to their diverse relational and spiritual needs.

The vast majority of families raise their children with strong values. Some contemporary values break with tradition, such as regarding men and women as equal partners in family life (see Anderson, Chapter 10, this volume). Still, most couples and families uphold traditional values of commitment, responsibility, and investment in raising healthy children. Most value a spiritual dimension in their lives that fosters personal and relational well-being, positive growth, and concern for others. Most are giving and forgiving in their personal relationships. Of interest, survey respondents (Gallup & Lindsay, 1999) have ranked family ties, loyalty, and traditions as the main factors thought to strengthen the family; next were moral and spiritual values, which far outranked family counseling and parent training classes.

## Spirituality across the Family Life Cycle

Religion and spirituality profoundly influence individual and family development. They involve dynamic processes that ebb and flow, shifting in meaning over the life course and across the generations (Hood, Spilka, Hunsberger, & Gorsuch, 2003; Worthington, 1989).

In all religions, the family is central in rites that mark the birth of a new member, entry into the adult community, marriage vows, and the death of a loved one. For instance, the practice of Judaism is centered on the family observance of rituals, from weekly *Shabbat* (Sabbath) to the holidays in the Jewish calendar year and rites of passage across the life cycle. Each ritual carries significant meaning that connects family members with their larger community and with the history and survival of the Jewish people and their covenant with God.

*Couple Relationships*

In the family life cycle, marriage often brings religious considerations to the fore. Conflict may arise over whether to have a religious ceremony. Even partners of the same faith may differ in their particular denomination, degree of observance, or preferences for clergy and vows. Families of origin may exert pressures for wedding plans in line with their own convictions, or they may not attend, if offended. This can fuel intergenerational conflicts and in-law triangles that reverberate for years.

When spouses are similar with respect to religious affiliation, beliefs, and practices, they report greater personal well-being, more relationship satisfaction, less abuse, and lower likelihood of divorce (Myers, 2006). Couple relationships are enhanced by the sharing of meaningful spiritual practices, such as holiday rituals (Fiese & Tomcho, 2001).

Until recent decades, many religions prohibited interfaith marriage. Families strongly discouraged their children from marrying someone of even another denomination. As society has become more open, interfaith marriage has become widespread (Waite & Lewin, 2008). Acceptance has increased with the support of interfaith movements and the blurring of racial and ethnic barriers. However, the high rate of intermarriage by Jews (over half) is of deep concern to their community, and families may react with a sense of disappointment and loss, if not outright disapproval.

For interfaith couples, religious beliefs can complicate relationship issues and generate conflict. Under stress, tolerance for differences can erode, particularly if one way is upheld as right, true, or morally superior. In some cases, the choice of a spouse from a different religious background may express rebellion against parental values and authority (Friedman, 1985). The acceptance or disapproval by families of origin can strongly influence the success or failure of the marriage and intergenerational relations.

Divorce and remarriage can be fraught with religious complications. For Orthodox Jews, a woman wishing to remarry must obtain a "get," or written permission, from her ex-spouse, although a man is not required to do so. The Catholic Church regards marriage as a sacrament that is indissoluble. The church does not recognize divorce. An annulment (granted with proof that the marriage was invalid or unconsummated) is required for remarriage in the church. These strict rulings have led many Catholics to leave the church. Some couples decide to live together without legal remarriage or religious rites. When annulments are granted, even over objections of a former spouse and children, they may be deeply wounded at the invalidation of their prior family life and legitimacy. It is crucial to explore such conflict-laden religious issues.

## Parent–Child Relationships

A growing number of studies find that parent–child relationships benefit from spiritual resources. Consonant with the "lived experience" of religion and spirituality, when parents are congruent in transmitting and following their spiritual values in family life and interactions with their children—practicing and parenting what they preach—and when they engage in meaningful spiritual practices together, children are more likely to internalize similar beliefs and practices, to find them to be a resource, and to feel more positive about their relationships (Marks, 2004). Involvement in religious communities is a strong protective factor for at-risk adolescent single mothers and their children, with lower depression and child abuse, and higher socioemotional adjustment and educational and job attainment (Carothers, Borkowski, Lefevre, & Whitman, 2005). Data from the National Longitudinal Study of Adolescent Health (Pearce & Haynie, 2004) show that when both mothers and their adolescent children consider religion important and attend religious services, the child is less often delinquent. Religion tends to be protective when shared among family members.

The vast majority of parents want their children to have some religious upbringing (Gallup & Lindsay, 1999). With the birth of the first child, some couples who viewed religion as unimportant in their lives find that one or both partners care deeply about it for their children. Often the children bring their parents back to their religious roots. One secular Jewish couple was surprised when their 12-year-old son requested a bar mitzvah. In interfaith marriages, or with intrafaith differences in degree of observance, conflicts may arise over decisions about rituals such as circumcision, christening, baptism, or confirmation. Here again, the older generation, now as grandparents, may make their religious preferences strongly known. Previous acceptance of their children's choice of a nontraditional wedding or an interfaith marriage may shift when they consider the moral development and religious identification of their grandchildren. This is an especially salient concern in the Jewish community. Studies suggest that if the non-Jewish partner converts to Judaism, children are more likely to grow up with a Jewish identity and practice their faith.

Most teenagers say it is important for parents and young children to attend religious services together (Gallup & Lindsay, 1999). Like their parents, the vast majority of teenagers believe in God and that God loves them.

Three out of four teens say they pray when alone. Youths of diverse faiths express interest in discussing life's meaning and how to make moral decisions (Coles, 1990, 1997). Most parents and children show increasing religious tolerance and favor courses in public schools to provide nondevotional instruction about various world religions.

## Adulthood and Later Life

Young adults, particularly those in college, often distance from their religious upbringing. Some simply become less involved and lose faith, while others more actively question or cut off from their family religious traditions. Many explore other spiritual paths in search of meaning, faith, and commitment. Some who choose to convert or "marry out" may seek to rebalance the family's ethnic or religious orientation, moving away from some values and toward others. In some cases, this may express an attempt to separate and differentiate from their family of origin (Friedman, 1985). Parents may interpret such a choice as a rejection of them and their heritage. Some may wish to cut off from religious or parental upbringing that they experienced as oppressive, but more often this choice is a natural outgrowth of broader social contacts in our multicultural society.

Middle to later life is a time of growing saliency of spirituality, as family members grapple with questions about the meaning of life and face the death of loved ones and their own mortality (Erikson, Erikson, & Kivnick, 1986; Lyons, 2005; Walsh, 1999; see Walsh, Chapter 4, this volume). With parental chronic illness, despite physical decline and caregiving burdens, a deeper intimacy and spiritual bond may develop between parents and the adult children involved in their care. Spiritual resources are particularly important for caregivers of elders with dementia (Smith & Harkness, 2002). In the lesbian, gay, bisexual, and transgender (LGBT) community, the impact of the HIV-AIDS epidemic and the aging of leaders in the Gay Rights movement have increased the importance of spirituality (Maher, 2006). As gay persons age, they often engage in a process of existential questioning, complicated by legal and religious battles for equal rights, that leads to deeper explorations of faith, spirit, and soul.

With aging and retirement, most people shift priorities to make more time for their spiritual life. Active participation in a faith community, prayer and meditation, time spent in nature, and service to others tend to become increasingly important. As individuals reflect on their lives, they focus more on their connections with those who came before them and with future generations. Surely the wisdom of elders is deepened by their growing spirituality.

## Spirituality, Connectedness, and Resilience: Many Pathways

Faith is inherently relational from our earliest years, when the most fundamental convictions about life are shaped within caregiving relationships. Intimate bonds with authentic communication ("I and Thou") are expressions of spirituality and offer pathways for spiritual growth (Buber, 1921/1970; Fishbane, 1998), as in the Quaker adage "I lift thee and thou lifts me." We experience deep connections with "kindred spirits" and "soul mates." Caring bonds with partners, family members, and close friends can nourish spiritual well-being; in turn spirituality deepens and expands our connections with others. It can be spiritually enriching to share intimacy, to care for an infant or a frail elder, to befriend others or to receive the loving kindness of strangers. The intimate bond with a loving God strengthens many people in their darkest hours (see Elliott, Chapter 17, this volume).

Faith, intimacy, and resilience are interwoven (Higgins, 1994). Love sustains people's lives, infuses them with meaning, and supports faith in overcoming adversity. Viktor Frankl (1946/1984), in recounting his experiences in Nazi prison camps, was sustained by his deep connection with his wife, by visualizing her image: "I didn't even know if she were still alive. I knew only one thing—which I have learned well by now: Love goes very far beyond the physical person of the beloved. It finds its deepest meaning in his spiritual being, his inner self" (pp. 59–60).

The transcendent connectedness of family and community is forged through shared values, commitment, and mutual support through adversity. In contrast to the highly individualized concept of human autonomy centered on the "self" in Western societies, most cultures worldwide view the person as embedded within the family and larger community. African theologian John Mbiti (1970) describes this sociocentric view of human experience: "I am because we are." We need to keep this broad outlook toward spirituality as it is experienced within faith traditions and through many aspects of people's lives. Banding together in community service or social activism can be a transformative expression of spirituality (see Perry & Rolland, Chapter 20, this volume).

Faith, in its many communal expressions, fuels the resilient spirit in families. As Anderson affirms (see Chapter 10, this volume), human systems, like families, are meaning making communities with directionality and a life of their own. For that reason, each family has its own spirituality. Despite the diversity of perspectives, the broad aim of spirituality remains constant: to be open to the transcendent dimension of life and all relationships, both in ordinary, everyday activity and in the midst of adversity.

In our rapidly changing world, religion is less often a given that people are born into and accept unquestioningly. Increasingly, individuals, couples, and families are seeking their own spiritual pathways for meaning and connection, and they choose among beliefs and practices to fit their lives. This combining of varied elements has been likened to a platter of "religious linguini" (Deloria, 1994). As spiritual pluralism increases within families, many are creating their own recipes for spiritual nourishment.

## NOTE

1. It is difficult to obtain accurate statistics on the lived experience of spirituality and religion. In interpreting the percentages of individuals who report specific beliefs and practices, it must be kept in mind that nearly 80% of Americans are Christian; thus, high (or low) percentages reflected predominantly Christian views. Over more than 60 years, Gallup Polls have provided reliable and widely cited surveys of individual religious identity, beliefs, and practices (see Gallup & Lindsay, 1999). Recent Gallup survey data can be found on the website *www. gallup.com.*

The Pew Forum on Religion and Public Life (*www.religions.pewforum.org*) provides a wide range of information and survey data. Their 2008 *U.S. Religious Landscape Survey* focused on "affiliation" (belonging to a particular denomination and attending worship services regularly); they note that 16% of Americans were "unaffiliated," but that does not mean religion and spirituality were unimportant in people's lives (Lindner, 2008). Their data are not directly comparable with Gallup Poll findings on religious identification. Also of note, both surveys have used only the term *religious* and have not used the term *spiritual,* which might not capture the more varied ways in which Americans tap spiritual resources.

The Pluralism Project at Harvard University (*www.pluralism.org/resources*) offers a treasure trove of information on the wide spectrum of religious orientations in America today, multifaith perspectives, and interfaith initiatives (see also Eck, 2006).

A resource website for journalists, *religionsource* (*www.religionsource.org/contents/resourcesstatistics.aspx*), offers links to a number of online providers of religious statistics.

beliefnet (*www.beliefnet.org*) is the largest spiritual website offering the general public a wide variety of multifaith and spiritual resources to help meet spiritual needs, including articles, devotionals, sacred text searches, message boards, prayer circles, and photo galleries.

## REFERENCES

Anderson, H. (1994). The recovery of the soul. In B. Childs & D. Waanders (Eds.), *The treasure in earthen vessels: Explorations in theological anthropology* (pp. 208–223). Louisville, KY: Westminster Press/John Knox Press.

Bailey, C. E. (2002). The effects of spiritual beliefs and practices on family functioning: A qualitative study. *Journal of Family Psychotherapy, 13*(1–2), 127–144.

Bakhtiar, L. (2007). *Sublime Koran*. Chicago: Kazi Publications.

Beavers, W. R., & Hampson, R. B. (2003). Measuring family competence: The Beavers systems model. In F. Walsh (Ed.), *Normal family processes* (3rd ed., pp. 549–580). New York: Guilford Press.

Bibby, R. W. (2002). *Restless gods: The renaissance of religion in Canada*. Toronto: Stoddart.

Bottoms, B. L., Shaver, P. R., Goodman, G. S., & Qin, J. (1995). In the name of God: A profile of religion-related child abuse. *Journal of Social Issues, 51*, 85–111.

Bowman, M. (1983, November/December). Why we burn: Sexism exorcised. *The Humanist*, 28–29.

Bridges, R. A., & Spilka, B. (1992). Religion and the mental health of women. In J. F. Schumaker (Ed.), *Religion and mental health* (pp. 43–53). New York: Oxford University Press.

Browning, D., & Clairmont, D. A. (Eds.). (2007). *American religions and the family: How faith traditions cope with modernization and democracy*. New York: Columbia University Press.

Browning, D., Miller-McLemore, B., Couture, P., Lyon, K., & Franklin, R. (2001). *From culture wars to common ground: Religion and the American family* (2nd ed.). Louisville, KY: Westminster Press/John Knox Press.

Buber, M. (1970). *I and thou* (Kaufmann translation). New York: Charles Scribner's Sons. Original work published 1921

Bucko, R. (2007). Native American families and religion. In D. S. Browning & D. A. Clairmont (Eds.), *American religions and the family* (pp. 70–86). New York: Columbia University Press.

Campbell, J., & Moyers, B. (1988). *The power of myth*. New York: Doubleday.

Carothers, S. S., Borkowski, J. G., Lefever, J. B., & Whitman, T. L. (2005). Religiosity and the socio-emotional adjustment of adolescent mothers and their children. *Journal of Family Psychology, 19*(2), 263–275.

Coles, R. (1990). *The spiritual life of children*. Boston: Houghton Mifflin.

Coles, R. (1997). *The moral intelligence of children*. New York: Random House.

Comas-Díaz, L. (1981). Puerto Rican *espiritismo* and psychotherapy. *American Journal of Orthopsychiatry, 51*, 636–645.

Davidson, M. (2000). Religion and spirituality. In K. J. Bieschke, R. M. Perez, & K. A. DeBord (Eds.), *Handbook for counseling and psychotherapy with lesbian, gay, bisexual, and transgender clients* (pp. 409–433). Washington DC: American Psychological Association.

Deloria, V., Jr. (1994). *God is red: A native view of religion* (2nd ed.). Golden, CO: Fulcrum.

Doherty, W. J. (1995). *Soul searching: Why psychotherapy must promote moral responsibility*. New York: Basic Books.

Dollahite, D. C. (2007). Latter-Day Saint marriage and family life. In D. S. Browning & D. A. Clairmont (Eds.), *American religions and the family: How faith traditions cope with modernization and democracy* (pp. 124–150). New York: Columbia University Press.

Eck, D. (2006). *On common ground: World religions in America.* New York: Columbia University Press.

Edgell, P. (2005). *Religion and family in a changing society.* Princeton, NJ: Princeton University Press.

Elkins, D. (1990, June). On being spiritual without necessarily being religious. *Association for Humanistic Psychology Perspective,* pp. 4–6.

Erikson, E. H., Erikson, J. M., & Kivnick, H. (1986). *Vital involvement in old age.* New York: Norton.

Fiese, B. H., & Tomcho, T. J. (2001). Finding meaning in religious practices: The relation between holiday rituals and marital satisfaction. *Journal of Family Psychology, 15*(4), 597–609.

Fishbane, M. D. (1998). I, thou, and we: A dialogue approach to couples therapy. *Journal of Marital and Family Therapy, 24,* 41–58.

Frankl, V. (1984). *Man's search for meaning.* New York: Simon & Schuster. (Original work published 1946)

Friedman, E. H. (1985). *Generation to generation: Family process in church and synagogue.* New York: Guilford Press.

Gallup, G. H., Jr. (2002). *The Gallup Poll: Public Opinion 2001.* Washington, DC: Scholarly Resources.

Gallup, G. H., Jr., & Lindsay, D. M. (1999). *Surveying the religious landscape: Trends in U.S. beliefs.* Harrisburg, PA: Morehouse.

Gallup, Inc. (2008). *Religion* (survey data summaries). Retrieved 3/14/08 from *www.gallup.com/poll/1690/religion.* Princeton, NJ: Author.

Gaustad, E. S., & Schmidt, L. E. (2002). *The religious history of America* (Rev. ed.). New York: HarperCollins.

Greeley, A., & Hout, M. (2006). *The facts about conservative Christians.* Chicago: University of Chicago Press.

Griffith, J. L., & Elliott Griffith, M. (2002). *Encountering the sacred in psychotherapy.* New York: Guilford Press.

Higgins, G. O. (1994). *Resilient adults: Overcoming a cruel past.* San Francisco: Jossey-Bass.

Hood, R. W., Spilka, B., Hunsberger, B., & Gorsuch, R. (2003). *The psychology of religion: An empirical approach* (3rd ed.). New York: Guilford Press.

Houseknecht, S. K., & Pankhurst, J. G. (Eds.). (2000). *Family, religion, and social change in diverse societies.* New York: Oxford University Press.

Imber-Black, E., Roberts, J., & Whiting, R. (Eds.). (2003). *Rituals in families and family therapy* (2nd ed.). New York: Norton.

Lambert, N., & Dollahite, D. (2006). How religiosity helps couples prevent, resolve, and overcome marital conflict. *Family Relations, 55*(4), 439–449.

Lease, S. H., & Shulman, J. L. (2003). A preliminary investigation of the role of religion for family members of lesbian, gay male, or bisexual individuals. *Counseling and Values, 47*, 195–209.

Lerner, M. (2007). *The left hand of God: Healing America's political and spiritual crisis.* New York: HarperCollins.

Lindner, E. W. (2008). *Yearbook of American and Canadian churches: 2008* (73rd ed.). New York: National Council of Churches in the USA.

Lyons, L. (May 31, 2005). *Faith accompanies most Americans through life.* Retrieved March 12, 2008, from *www.gallup.com/poll/16522/faith-accompanies-most-americans-through-life.aspx*.

Maher, M. J. (2006). A voice in the wilderness: Gay and lesbian religious groups in the western United States. *Journal of Homosexuality, 51*(4), 91–117.

Mahoney, A., Pargament, K., Tarakeshwar, N., & Swank, A. (2001). Religion in the home in the 1980s and 1990s: A meta-analytic review and conceptual analysis of links between religion, marriage, and parenting. *Journal of Family Psychology, 15*(4), 559–596.

Marks, L. (2004). Sacred practices in highly religious families: Christian, Jewish, Mormon, and Muslim perspectives. *Family Process, 43*(2), 217–231.

Marks, L. (2006). Religion and family relational health: Overview and conceptual model. *Journal of Religion and Health, 45*(4), 603–618.

Marsh, R., & Dallos, R. (2001). Roman Catholic couples: Wrath and religion. *Family Process, 40*(3), 343–360.

Marty, M. E. (2005). *When faiths collide.* Malden, MA: Blackwell.

Mayer, E., Kosmin, B. A., & Keysar, A. (2002). *American Jewish Identity Survey 2001.* New York: Center for Jewish Studies, City University of New York.

Mbiti, J. S. (1970). *African religions and philosophy.* Garden City, NY: Anchor Books.

McCourt, F. (1998, December). God in America: When you think of God—What do you see? *Life, 21*(13), 60–74.

McGoldrick, M., Giordano, J., & Garcia-Preto, N. (Eds.). (2005). *Ethnicity and family therapy* (3rd ed.). New York: Guilford Press.

Miller, W. R., & Thoresen, C. E. (2003). Spirituality, religion, and health. *American Psychologist, 58*(1), 24–35.

Moore, T. (1992). *Care of the soul: A guide for cultivating depth and sacredness in everyday life.* New York: HarperCollins.

Murphy, C. (1998). *The word according to Eve: Women and the Bible in ancient times.* Boston: Houghton Mifflin.

Myers, S. (2006). Religious homogamy and marital quality: Historical and generational patterns. *Journal of Marriage and the Family, 68*(2), 292–304.

Nasr, S. H. (2002). *The heart of Islam: Enduring values for humanity.* New York: HarperCollins.

Neihardt, J. (1979). *Black Elk speaks: Being the life story of a Holy Man of the Oglala Sioux.* Lincoln: University of Nebraska Press. (Original work published 1932)

Pargament, K. I. (2007). *Spiritually integrated psychotherapy: Understanding and addressing the sacred.* New York: Guilford Press.

Pearce, L. D., & Haynie, D. L. (2004). Intergenerational religious dynamics and adolescent delinquency. *Social Forces, 82*(4), 1533–1572.

Pew Forum on Religion and Public Life. (2006, August 3). *Public divided on social issues, but no "culture war."* Retrieved from *religions.pewforum.org.*

Pew Forum on Religion and Public Life. (2007, May 22). *Muslim Americans: Middle class and mostly mainstream.* Retrieved March 14, 2008, from *religions.pewforum. org.*

Pew Forum on Religion and Public Life. (2008). U.S. Religious Landscape Survey. Retrieved February 26, 2008, from *religions.pewforum.org.*

Pew Hispanic Project and the Pew Forum on Religion and Public Life (April 25, 2007). *Changing faiths: Latinos and the transformation of American religion.* Retrieved February 26, 2008, from *religions.pewforum.org.*

Prothero, S. (2007). *Religious literacy: What every American needs to know—and doesn't.* New York: HarperCollins.

Roseborough, D. (2006). Coming out stories framed as faith narratives or stories about spiritual growth. *Pastoral Psychology, 55,* 47–59.

Smith, A. L., & Harkness, J. (2002). Spirituality and meaning: A qualitative inquiry with caregivers of Alzheimer's disease. *Journal of Family Psychotherapy, 13,* 1–2, 87–108.

Smith, B., & Horne, S. (2007). Gay, lesbian, bi-sexual, and transgendered (GLBT) experiences with earth-spirited faith. *Journal of Homosexuality, 52*(3/4), 235–249.

Smith, T. W. (2005). *Spiritual and religious transformation in America: The National Spiritual Transformation Study* (GSS Topical Report No. 37). Chicago: National Opinion Research Center.

Snarey, J. R., & Dollahite, D. C. (2001). Varieties of religion—family linkages. *Journal of Family Psychology, 15*(4), 646–651.

Snider, J. B., Clements, A., & Vazsonyi, A. T. (2004). Late adolescent perceptions of parent religiosity and parenting processes. *Family Process, 43*(4), 489–502.

Somé, M. P. (1998). *The healing wisdom of Africa.* New York: Tarcher/Putnam.

Stacey, J. (1996). *In the name of the family: Rethinking family values in the postmodern age.* Boston: Beacon Press.

Stinnett, N., & DeFrain, J. (1985). *Secrets of strong families.* Boston: Little, Brown.

Sullivan, K. T. (2001). Understanding the relationship between religiosity and marriage: An investigation of the immediate and longitudinal effects of religiosity on newlywed couples. *Journal of Family Psychology, 15*(4), 610–626.

Tan, P. P. (2005). The importance of spirituality among gay and lesbian individuals. *Journal of Homosexuality, 49*(2), 135–144.

Waite, L. J., & Lewin, A. C. (in press). Religious intermarriage and conversion in the United States: Patterns and changes over time. In C. Ellison & R. Hummer (Eds.), *Religion, families, and health in the United States: New directions in population-based research.* New Brunswick, NJ: Rutgers University Press.

Walker, A. (1997). *Anything we love can be saved: A writer's activism*. New York: Random House.

Walsh, F. (1999). Families in later life: Challenges and opportunities. In B. Carter & M. McGoldrick (Eds.), *The expanded family life cycle* (3rd ed., pp. 307–326). Needham Heights, MA: Allyn & Bacon.

Walsh, F. (2003a). Family resilience: Framework for clinical practice. *Family Process, 42*(1), 1–18.

Walsh, F. (2003b). *Normal family processes: Growing diversity and complexity* (3rd ed.). New York: Guilford Press.

Walsh, F. (2006). *Strengthening family resilience* (2nd ed.). New York: Guilford Press.

Walsh, F. (2009). The relational significance of companion animals. *Family Process, 48*(4), 462–480.

Weil, A. (1994). *Spontaneous healing*. New York: Knopf.

Wendel, R. (2003). Lived religion and family therapy: What does spirituality have to do with it? *Family Process, 42*(1), 165–179.

Wilcox, W. B. (2004). *Soft patriarchs, new men: How Christianity shapes fathers and husbands*. Chicago: University of Chicago Press.

Worthington, E. L., Jr. (1989). Religious faith across the lifespan: Implications for counseling and research. *Counseling Psychologist, 17*, 555–612.

Wright, L., Watson, W. L., & Bell, J. M. (1996). *Beliefs: The heart of healing in families and illness*. New York: Basic Books.

Yip, A. K. T. (2002). The persistence of faith among non-heterosexual Christians: Evidence for the neo-secularization thesis of religious transformation. *Journal for the Scientific Study of Religion, 41*(2), 199–212.

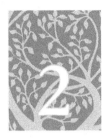

# Integrating Spirituality in Family Therapy

## Wellsprings for Health, Healing, and Resilience

### FROMA WALSH

> May we see not only with our two eyes but with
> the one eye which is our heart.
>
> —BLACK ELK

Most families and couples who come for therapy or counseling are seeking more than symptom reduction, problem solving, or communication skills; they are seeking deeper meaning and connections in their lives. For many, spiritual distress contributes to their physical, emotional, and relational problems. For some, the interplay of religion and culture has been oppressive and harmful. Surveys find that the vast majority of Americans want their physicians, therapists, and counselors to address their spiritual concerns. Yet clinicians are only beginning to include this vital dimension in their practice.

There is growing interest in spirituality by mental health professionals, including family therapists. Still, most feel ill equipped in their training, constrained from broaching the subject with clients, and uncomfortable when it does arise. Clients, sensing that spirituality doesn't belong in the clinical context, may censor themselves from bringing this aspect of their lives into the therapeutic conversation. This chapter addresses ways to move beyond constraints to include spirituality in clinical practice in order to understand spiritual sources of distress and to tap spiritual resources for healing, recovery, and resilience.


## OVERCOMING CONSTRAINTS

Throughout the mental health field, until only recently, religion was regarded as a taboo subject to be checked at the office door by both client and therapist. It was even more taboo than broaching such topics as sex, money, or death. Spirituality and religion were purposefully omitted in clinical training, practice, and research. Several influences contributed to this inattention, including the deliberate separation of secular and sacred domains; concerns about therapists' influence; and the schism between science and faith (Prest & Keller, 1993).


### Secular and Sacred Domains: Building Connection and Collaboration

One assumption has been that spirituality is not the proper domain of mental health professionals. As the field of mental health developed over the 20th century, rigid boundaries were upheld to keep spiritual issues "off limits" from psychotherapy. Therapists were trained not to intrude into clients' "private" spiritual matters or personal relationship with their God. Spiritual distress was seen to exist in a separate realm from physical and psychosocial distress, and was restricted to the domain of pastoral care. Likewise, spiritual healing approaches were deemed to be outside the province of mental health and health care. It was expected that faith-based healers and secular professionals should each tend to their own matters. Although many marriage and family therapists came from pastoral counseling traditions, most mental health professionals were trained to adhere to their professional role and boundaries.

There has been growing recognition that these are complementary domains, which overlap and need to be bridged in work with couples and families (Stander, Piercy, MacKinnon, & Helmeke, 1994). For instance, military chaplains and family life chaplains play a crucial role in individual and relational counseling, particularly for service personnel in combat zones and those undergoing the stressful readjustment to family and civilian life. Because of the stigma of mental illness in the military, most who are suffering emotional or relational distress turn to their chaplains rather than seeking mental health services when both may be needed.

It is crucial to build connections between mental health professionals and those with expertise in pastoral care for mutual referral, consultation, and ongoing collaboration (Doehring, 2007; Weaver, Koenig, & Larson, 1997). In one partnership, Stanley, Markman, and colleagues (2001) have linked effectively with clergy and lay leaders to provide their evidence-based premarital program (education and communication skills training) to couples in the community. Clinicians also need to become acquainted with local multifaith congregational resources and faith-based health care and human services that fit clients' needs and spiritual preferences (Koenig, 2005; see Kamya, Chapter 15, this volume). In one initiative, a Catholic community of Sisters in Saskatoon, Canada, collaborated with Catholic Family Services to sponsor a successful Family-to-Family Mentorship Program in which parish families volunteer to invest in a yearlong involvement with a local family that is struggling (McRae & Walker, 2007).

### Power and Influence: Fostering Collaboration and Empowerment

A related barrier to integration involves the potential in the therapeutic relationship for vulnerable clients, in distress, to be swayed to adopt their therapists' spiritual orientations. Concerns about therapists' influence (or actual proselytizing) stem from recognition of the power of therapists and the dependent position of clients. Therefore, professionals were trained to remain objective and unbiased. To protect clients, they were advised to be cautious not to reveal their own spiritual values or practices. However, it is impossible to be neutral or value-free (Walsh, 2003). Inescapably, all therapeutic work involves the interaction of therapists' and clients' value systems. Just as other aspects of culture (e.g., ethnicity, social class, and gender) influence client and therapist constructions of norms, problems, and solutions, so too does the spiritual dimension of experience. What we ask and pursue— or do not—influences the therapeutic relationship, process, and outcome. Therefore, therapists need to gain awareness of their own religious and spiritual beliefs and biases. It is also crucial to be cautious and open about any dual relationships they have, such as active involvement or a leadership role in a religious community (Hill, Mamalakis, Butler, & Gardner, 2001).

We best respect our clients not by avoiding discussion of spirituality altogether but by demonstrating active interest in exploring and understanding *their* values, practices, and concerns. Surveys find that patients are less interested in their therapists' spirituality and more interested in addressing their own spiritual issues. As they do so, it is important to understand their constraining beliefs and to affirm and encourage those that foster well-being. At times, therapists have an ethical responsibility *not* to take a neutral stance, but to challenge specific beliefs or practices that are harmful to clients or their loved ones. It is important for therapists to be aware of their own influence and work collaboratively, reflecting power back in ways that foster resilience and empowerment within clients, their family relationships, and their communities (Walsh, 2006).

## Science and Faith: A Biopsychosocial–Spiritual Orientation

Historically, the physical, psychological, and the spiritual were viewed as interconnected. In fact, *psyche* was the Greek word for spirit. Mental disorders are still seen and treated as possession by spirits in many traditional cultures (see Falicov, Chapter 8, this volume). Over the centuries, faith healers and shamans have held highly influential roles in their communities, taking a holistic approach to human distress for physical, emotional, and spiritual healing (Eliade, Trask, & Doniger, 2004). Likewise, priests, ministers, rabbis, and other religious advisers have tended to physical and emotional suffering, as well as relational problems, of their congregants. Eastern religions and medicine have throughout time integrated the body, mind, and spirit in health and healing.

However, in 20th-century Western cultures, the fields of medicine and mental health severed the connections. Freud's (1927/1961) scorn for religion as offering no more than comforting illusions strongly influenced the exclusion of spirituality from psychotherapy theory and practice. (See Simpkinson & Simpkinson [1999] for an annotated bibliography of leading voices in psychology, from William James to Carl Jung, Viktor Frankl, and Jerome Frank, who maintained strong spiritual perspectives in their work.)

The scientific paradigm and medical model emerged as the dominant epistemology in the field of mental health, along with skepticism toward the inclusion of spiritual influences in research and practice. Mental health professions sought greater scientific credibility and status through evidence-based practice, distancing from aspects of client experience, therapeutic process, and outcome that presumably could not be observed and measured.

Now, over a decade of quantitative studies have found abundant evidence of spiritual influences in mental health and physical well-being (Hill & Pargament, 2003; Koenig, 2005; Koenig, McCullough, & Larson, 2001). Increasingly, possibilities are being pursued for the integration of science and spirituality in addressing couple and family relationships (Baucom, 2001). Qualitative studies are yielding greater understanding of the role of faith beliefs and practices in overcoming adversity and in problem construction and solutions. The inclusion of spiritual issues in the revised *Diagnostic and Statistical Manual of Mental Disorders* (DSM-IV) is indicative of a growing recognition of their importance in mental health assessment and treatment. In DSM-IV, the Religion or Spiritual Problems category (V Code 62.89) can be used "when the focus of clinical attention is a religious or spiritual problem. Examples include distressing experiences that involve loss or questioning of faith, or questioning of spiritual values that may not necessarily be related to an organized church or religious institution" (American Psychiatric Association, 1994, p. 685).

Debates persist concerning the integration of science and religion. Yet Albert Einstein, considered the greatest scientist of the 20th century, wrote in his memoirs: "Science without religion is lame—religion without science is blind" (1931, p. 355). He envisioned a broad spirituality providing complementarity rather than contradiction between the domains of science and religion: "The religion of the future will be a cosmic religion. It should transcend a personal God and avoid dogma and theology . . . based on a religious sense arising from the experience of all things natural and spiritual as a meaningful unity" (p. 355).

## HEALING AND TREATMENT

Although psychotherapists, like health care professionals, are considered specialists in the healing arts, many are uncomfortable with the notion of healing. In part, it carries spiritual connotations of the therapist as healer, with special power to cure others, much like faith healers or the laying on of hands. While the scientific paradigm has become dominant in health care and mental health fields, healing remains at the heart of all medical and therapeutic practice.

Family therapists have approached healing in terms of a therapeutic relationship that encourages clients' own inherent healing potential. This collaborative approach is at the core of strength-based and resilience-oriented practice (Walsh, 2006). Distinct from curing or problem resolution, healing is seen as a natural process in response to injury or trauma. Sometimes people heal physically but don't heal emotionally, mentally, or spiritually; badly strained relationships may remain unhealed. Some may recover from an illness or loss but may not regain a spirit to live and love fully. Yet we are able to heal psychosocially and spiritually even when we do not heal physically, or when a traumatic event cannot be reversed. The literal meaning of *healing* is becoming whole. For the psychiatrist Carl Jung (1933, 1958), wholeness includes the sacred dimension, which is at the heart of healing.

Healing and treatment are quite different concepts. *Healing* involves a gathering of resources within the person, the family, and the community, and is fostered through a collaborative therapeutic relationship. *Treatment* is externally administered by experts to reduce or eradicate individual disorders or family dysfunction. Medical and psychiatric treatment paradigms focus on therapist knowledge, skills, and strategies to alter individual and family pathology. Western scientific medicine has been focused on identifying external agents of disease and developing technological weapons to defeat them. Metaphors of war are prominent: fighting germs; combating illness; aggressive treatments to destroy disease. An unbalanced focus on pathology rather than health contributes to despair (Weil, 1994).

In contrast, medicine in Eastern religious and philosophical traditions is grounded in a set of beliefs about healing processes and the importance of harmonious balance in mind–body–spirit interactions. The healing system is a functional system, not an assemblage of structures. Chinese medicine, for instance, explores ways of increasing our energy (*chi*) for internal resilience and resistance to disease. This belief in strengthening protective processes assumes that the body has a natural ability to heal and grow stronger. Holistic approaches to medicine and psychotherapy are drawing on these convictions to decrease pain and foster greater well-being (e.g., Kabat-Zinn, 2003).

Similarly, family resilience-oriented practice approaches tap psychosocial–spiritual resources so that when exposed to harmful influences or trauma, members are less vulnerable, can readily heal, and can experience positive growth (Walsh, 2006). Resources for diagnosis, self-repair, and regeneration exist in all of us; they can be activated as need arises. Emphasis has shifted from earlier focus on therapist techniques to tap into the family's own healing resources. In strengthening resilience, we inspire people to believe in their own possibilities for the relief of suffering and renewal of life passage. Our faith in clients' desires to be healthy and their potential for healing and growth can encourage their best efforts.

## INTEGRATING SPIRITUALITY
## IN CLINICAL PRACTICE

The general public has expressed a need for mental health and health care professionals to attend to the spiritual dimension of their lives. Over 80% of survey respondents preferred to have their own spiritual practices and beliefs integrated into any counseling process; 75% wanted physicians and therapists to address spiritual issues as part of their care. Half of older adults say they want their doctors to pray with them as they face death (Gallup & Lindsay, 1999). When therapists neglect the potential relevance of clients' spiritual beliefs and practices, and when clients hold back spiritual concerns, therapy can leave them feeling fragmented (Griffith & Elliott Griffith, 2002). It is time to integrate spirituality in clinical practice (Koenig, 2007).

Wright, Watson, and Bell (1996) have urged systems-oriented professionals to conceptualize persons as biopsychosocial–spiritual beings. As we integrate spirituality and other aspects of our experience, we can advance a truly holistic view of families, their suffering, and their healing potential. Gregory Bateson, our most visionary systems theorist, taught us to look for the "patterns that connect" and to see mind and nature as a necessary unity (Bateson, 1979).

Among early pioneers in family therapy, Virigina Satir stood out in embracing a broad spirituality in her view of healthy family functioning and in her practice approach (Satir, 1972/1988). Ivan Boszormenyi-Nagy's (1987) contextual family therapy emphasizes the ethical dimension and issues of justice in intergenerational relationships. In *Soul Searching*, William Doherty (1995) criticized psychotherapy's overemphasis on self-interest and called for clinicians' greater sensitivity to the moral responsibilities in loving relationships and communities (see Doherty, Chapter 11, this volume). His message resonates with Viktor Frankl's (1955) view that both therapist and client ethical convictions are powerful resources to draw upon in the therapeutic process.

Over the past decade, a number of family therapists have begun to bring spiritual perspectives into practice (e.g., Anderson & Worthen, 1997; Becvar, 1996; Carlson & Erickson, 2002; Fishbane, 1998; Prest & Keller, 1993; Walsh, 1999, 2006). Helmeke and Sori (2006) offer an array of practical suggestions and activities. Some therapists offer ways to work with very religious couples and families of varied faiths (Butler & Harper, 1994; Daneshpour, 1998; Griffith & Elliott Griffith, 2002; Joanides, 1996). Lambert and Dollahite (2006) suggest ways that the beliefs and practices of highly religious Christian, Jewish, and Muslim couples can help them to prevent problems, resolve conflicts, and achieve reconciliation.

### Exploring the Spiritual Dimension in Clinical Assessment

Just as family therapists have recognized the importance of inquiring about ethnicity and other cultural influences, clinical assessment should routinely explore the spiritual dimension of clients' lives. It is helpful to open discussion by clarifying our use of the terms *religion* and *spirituality*, which are distinct yet overlapping concepts (see Walsh, Chapter 1, this volume). *Religion* refers to formal, organized faith traditions and their shared beliefs, practices, and faith communities. *Spirituality* refers more broadly to a dimension of human experience, involving transcendent values, beliefs, and practices for meaning, harmony, and connection, which may be expressed within or outside religion. It is important to convey respect for people of all faith perspectives, as well as for those who are not religious.

As I discussed in Chapter 1, most Americans express a religious identification or preference, although, increasingly, they may not follow all tenets of their faith tradition or attend worship services regularly. Many have left the religion of their upbringing and converted to other denominations. Many others are not affiliated with a particular denomination or congregation but maintain strong personal faith and practices such as prayer, meditation, and service to others. Still others may not consider themselves at all "religious," they may identify as secular humanist, existentialist, agnostic, or atheist, yet live by strong transcendent values. Both religious and nonreligious people find spiritual nourishment in a variety of ways, most often through nature, the creative arts, and community/social activism. Increasingly, individuals and their families combine beliefs and practices within or among spiritual orientations to fit their lives. Therefore, therapists need to understand the lived experience of religion and spirituality for each client (Wendel, 2003) and take a broad view of potential spiritual resources.

The religious or spiritual orientation of clients and their families of origin should be noted on the family genogram (McGoldrick, Gerson, & Petry, 2007). Significant changes can be tracked on a family timeline. Several schemas for detailed spiritual histories, genograms, and ecograms have been proposed for more comprehensive assessment (for comparison and guidelines, see Hodge, 2005a, 2005b). These tools are especially useful for therapists' own exploration.

Table 2.1 suggests some fruitful lines of inquiry in exploring the spiritual dimension of individual, couple, and family experience. Particular attention should be focused on exploring two major areas:

- Ways that religious/spiritual beliefs or experiences might contribute to current distress.
- Ways that past, current, or potential spiritual resources might be drawn upon to ease distress, resolve problems, and strengthen resilience in dealing with adversity.

It is important to explore the personal, family, and cultural meaning and significance of faith beliefs, practices, congregational involvement, and nonreligious expressions of spirituality. Therapists should clarify, for

TABLE 2.1. Exploring the Spiritual Dimension: Sources of Distress and Resources for Well-being, Healing, and Resilience

---

Start by grounding in individual, couple, and family experience of religion/spirituality:

1. *Religious identification, affiliation*—Organized, institutionalized faith tradition: Beliefs, practices, congregational involvement
2. *Spirituality:* Personal faith, transcendent values, practices within and/or outside religion (e.g., through prayer, meditation, nature, creative arts, service/activism). Include cultural influences (e.g., indigenous spiritual beliefs and practices)

- What role do religion and/or spirituality play in your life?
  - Importance in daily living; shared in couple/family practices?
  - In dealing with life challenges?
  - In the past? In family of origin?
  - Desire for greater spiritual dimension in life?
- How are couple or family religious/spiritual differences handled and accepted?

Explore religious/spiritual sources of distress:

- Is there couple or family conflict or cutoff over spiritual matters (e.g., with interfaith marriage and/or conversion; marriage and family standards; divorce, abortion or end-of-life decisions)?
- Have religious/spiritual convictions contributed to suffering (e.g., concerns about sin, punishment, afterlife) or been experienced as oppressive, harmful (e.g., sexist or heterosexist dogma, devaluation, abuse, or condemnation)?
- Have adversity, trauma, or injustice wounded the spirit?
- Has a spiritual void or cutoff from spiritual roots increased suffering or isolation?

Identify spiritual resources (religious and/or nonreligious):

- How do you find spiritual nourishment, connection, strength, meaning, inspiration? How might current, past, or potential spiritual resources support personal and relational well-being, healing, and resilience? Consider:
  - Personal faith
  - Relationship with God, Higher Power, Universal Spirit, Creator
  - Contemplative practices (e.g., prayer, meditation, rituals)
  - Faith community—connection, involvement (worship, activities), support
  - Spiritual guidance, counsel (by clergy, pastoral counselor, chaplain)
  - Communion with nature
  - Creative arts, music, literature (expression, appreciation)
  - Service to others, activism

---

instance, if identifying as Catholic has ongoing significance, such as in deeply held convictions. If a religious upbringing has not been followed, how has that affected relationships with one's family of origin? Is a Jewish identity expressed in religious observance or experienced more in secular humanism and cultural connections (Meyerstein, 2006)? How have current problems or crises affected one's spirituality?

Where relevant to presenting concerns, such as strong guilt and self-blame, it might be important to explore how one's Christian faith helps or hinders; for instance, is it associated with a loving Christ or with sin and punishment? Is one's image of God benevolent or vengeful? (See Elliott, Chapter 17, this volume, for useful inquiry.) Are there other positive aspects of one's faith that might be drawn on as a resource?

With cultural diversity, interfaith marriage, and spiritual pluralism within families becoming increasingly common, it is important to learn how couples and family members, from their own distinct sociocultural backgrounds, attempt to blend meaningful beliefs and practices in their personal and relational lives. With Native Americans and non-European immigrants, it is important to explore how traditional or indigenous faith beliefs and practices can be respected and integrated with Western medical or psychiatric treatment, and in a holistic approach to therapeutic practice (Falicov, 1998; Moodley & West, 2005; see Falicov [Chapter 8] and Kamya [Chapter 15], this volume).

## Addressing Spiritual Sources of Distress

It is important to address the clinical complexities of religion and spirituality: not only supporting the potential for healing, but also recognizing and countering any destructive impact (Elliott Griffith & Griffith, 2002; Helmeke & Bischof, 2002). For some clients, religious traditions have become outmoded or fail to support their psychosocial and spiritual well-being. Those who feel oppressed or harmed by religious dogma might be encouraged to find alternate constructions and practices consonant with transcendent beliefs and values without rejecting spirituality altogether.

It is crucial to explore how religious ideations or experiences may have had a dispiriting effect, fostering guilt, shame, or worthlessness. One young woman, who had been sexually abused as a child, realized in therapy that the focus on sin and damnation in the church she attended made her feel worse about herself. Her therapist asked her more about the spiritual resources she valued and encouraged her to visit other congregations to find one that better met her needs.

Issues may emerge in meaning-making and causal attributions around problems For instance, one husband believed that the infertility problem he and his wife were suffering was God's punishment for his infidelity. In work with gay, lesbian, bisexual, and transgender individuals, a spiritual source of distress may become apparent as the therapist explores concerns (Haldeman, 2004; see Walsh, Chapter 1, this volume). For instance, adolescent depression, self-harm, and suicide attempts may involve spiritual conflicts for youth who experience gender identity confusion, fear family and religious condemnation, or suffer peer harassment (Rosario, Yali, Hunter, & Viorst-Gwadz, 2006; Yahouse & Tan, 2005).

In couple and family relationships, religious precepts may be used to justify demeaning or abusive treatment of wives and children (Whipple, 1987). One fundamentalist Christian woman told her therapist that her husband was right to beat her when she challenged his authority. She expressed the belief that "a woman of God" and a proper wife must be submissive, and that this was hard for her. Her husband agreed that this was her problem. Family therapists have an ethical responsibility to challenge injustice, abuse of power, and harmful behavior, even if it is supported by interwoven cultural and religious traditions (Kimball & Knudson-Martin, 2002; McGoldrick, Giordano, & Garcia-Preto, 2005). We can help families draw on the transcendent values of every faith for relational justice, compassion, and mutual respect, as well as the dignity and worth of all human beings.

Clinicians also need to attend to psychological, relational, and spiritual wounds caused by the sexual abuse of young boys and girls by Catholic priests (Pargament, Murray-Swank, & Mahoney, in press). The failure of church hierarchy to deal effectively with pedophilia in its midst has also alienated many parishioners from their faith. Therapists can be instrumental in the healing process of survivors and their families and in reporting and accountability to prevent further abuse (see Perry & Rolland, Chapter 20, this volume).

## TAPPING SPIRITUAL RESOURCES FOR HEALING AND RESILIENCE

Suffering, and often the injustice or senselessness of it, are ultimately spiritual issues (see Wright, Chapter 3, this volume). Adversity and suffering have vastly different meanings in various religious traditions, and each faith, through its teachings, calls forth resilience (see Wolin, Wolin, Ranganathan, Saymah, & Zeyada, Chapter 5, this volume). *Resilience* is the ability to overcome adversity, strengthened and more resourceful (Walsh, 2003). It is an active process of endurance, self-righting, and growth out of crisis or persistent life challenges. Some survivors of traumatic experiences become trapped in their suffering or blocked from growth by anger or blame.

Studies of resilience and posttraumatic growth (Tedeschi & Calhoun, 2004) find that spiritual resources such as personal faith, contemplative practices, or congregational support—help people to heal from painful wounds, take charge of their lives, and go on to live and love fully.

Robert Coles (1997) coined the term *moral energy* as a source of courage, a life-sustaining force of conviction that lifts us above adversity. In studying children in hardship or brutalizing conditions, Coles found many who transcended their experience: They valued compassion, fairness, and decency, and showed a generous spirit despite having received very little. In Werner and Smith's (2001) longitudinal study of resilience of at-risk youth in poor multiethnic families, faith was an important protective factor from childhood through adulthood. Religion—Buddhist, Catholic, Mormon, Jehovah's Witness, and others—strengthened them through adversity by providing a sense of purpose, mission, and salvation. Many credited involvement in a highly structured religious group. Follow-up studies found that resilience could be developed and lives transformed at any point in life. A crisis often opened a spiritual dimension previously untapped.

*Family resilience* involves key processes that enable the family system to rally in times of crisis: buffer stress, reduce the risk of dysfunction, and support optimal adaptation for all members (Walsh, 2003, 2006). Family belief systems come to the fore in times of adversity and suffering. Cultural and religious beliefs are the primary source of these shared convictions, which are transmitted through ongoing transactions. Powerful beliefs for resilience—meaning-making, hope, courage, perseverance, and transcendence—are all enhanced by spirituality (Walsh, 2008). As family members pull together and support one another, the family is better able to solve problems and meet future challenges. Sharing spiritual values and practices can strengthen these vital bonds.

The paradox of resilience is that the worst of times can also bring out our best. A crisis can lead to transformation and growth in unforeseen directions. It can be an epiphany, heightening realization of the significance of loved ones or sparking a reappraisal of life priorities for greater meaning and fulfillment. In the midst of suffering, as we search more deeply within ourselves and reach out to others, the hardship endured opens ways for the spirit to grow. In turn, spiritual beliefs and practices strengthen the ability to withstand and transcend adversity. Faith supports efforts to master the possible to accept that which is beyond control. What matters most is being able to give meaning to a precarious situation, having faith that there is some greater purpose or force at work, and finding solace and strength in these outlooks. In therapy, contemplative questions can facilitate exploration and enhancement of such perspectives.

Spiritual distress or an inability to invest life with meaning impedes coping and mastery. The Vietnamese term for posttraumatic stress disorder is "spiritual sadness." From sources in family history, culture, and spirituality, we can help clients invest in traditions, practices, and faith communities. For many, new spiritual pathways can offer a larger vision of humanity and meaningful connections that inspire their resilience.

## Health and Mental Health Benefits of Faith

Our beliefs are powerful influences in health and illness; they can block or facilitate well-being. Medical studies find abundant evidence that faith, prayer, and spiritual rituals can strengthen health and healing by triggering emotions that influence physiological systems (Koenig et al., 2001; Hill & Pargament, 2003). For instance, older persons with strong religious beliefs tend to be more satisfied with their lives and to have lower blood pressure, reducing the risk of heart disease. Both depression and alcohol abuse are reduced by prayer. Those who find strength and comfort in religious beliefs survive major surgery at a significantly higher rate than those lacking faith. Having faith appears to be physiologically soothing; a calmer mind lowers the risk of cardiac arrhythmia. Studies find that faith—the solace and hopefulness in one's outlook—appears to be even more important than frequency of participation in religious services or overall religious activity. Although faith can make a difference, caution is required not to attribute failures to recover from a serious condition to insufficient spiritual purity.

Studies document the significant influence of meditation in reducing stress and blood pressure, improving sleep and mental alertness, managing chronic pain, raising self-esteem, and lowering reactivity in relationships (Grossman, Niemann, Schmidt, & Walach, 2004; Kabat-Zinn, 2003). A review of medical studies on the efficacy of prayer (Dossey, 1993) found that the most beneficial prayers are not directly petitiory but are "Thy will be done" prayers. Contemplative practices positively impact the immune, cardiovascular, and neurological systems, thereby improving health. Religious rituals, such as communal singing or chanting, stimulate endocrine or immune responses to facilitate healing. Some clinicians have adopted the practice of praying for clients who are suffering. However, it is crucial to respect the preferences of nonbelievers and those whose faith differs from our own.

## Facing Death and Recovering from Loss

Facing death and the loss of a loved one are the most painful of all life's challenges (Walsh & McGoldrick, 2004; see Walsh, Chapter 4, this volume). In every culture, faith traditions have developed to address questions about the meaning of life and what happens after death. Although religious approaches to death and loss vary widely, family and community bonds are central in easing this passage and facilitating adaptation for survivors. Clinicians need to consider religious aspects of individual and family distress, such as beliefs about sin and punishment in afterlife. Religious condemnation of suicide and stigma with HIV-AIDS fosters shame and secrecy, contributing to the anguish of families.

The end of life offers gifts to those who face it openly with courage and compassion. A "spiritual life review" can facilitate reflection, a holistic integration, and coming to terms with life as it has been lived (Helmeke, 2006). More than any other human experiences, death and loss put us in touch with what most matters in our lives. One client, a health care professional who lost his partner to AIDS, was both devastated and transformed by their experience. As he wrote to his family, "Words like 'soul' or 'spirit' disappeared with medical training. I've been given a blessing by the illness and the death: An appreciation of the soul, an understanding of the spirit."

It is important to understand varying conceptions of death and afterlife, and how they concern or comfort the dying and the bereaved. For Native Americans and those with Eastern spiritual traditions, the ability to deal with death flows from the larger context in which they understand life; that human beings are an integral part of the natural world. Those with a Western mastery and problem-solving orientation often have more difficulty when there is nothing that can be done to *stop* death; a sense of helplessness and despair contributes to conflict or avoidance of contact and blocks soulful communication. Therapists can help family members facing death and loss by encouraging their full presence and participation in the dying process, drawing on their spiritual beliefs and practices to assist them (see Walsh, Chapter 4, this volume). Religious and moral concerns need to be addressed when they face agonizing end-of-life decisions.

In the wake of traumatic loss and major disasters, spiritual resources play a critical role in recovery, resilience, and posttraumatic growth (Koenig, 2006; Walsh, 2007). Therapists, as well as family members, may feel overwhelmed and helpless at such times. It is most important to offer compassion for our clients' suffering and to help them draw comfort and strength from each other, their community, and their faith.

### Addiction Recovery and Prevention

Researchers have found ample evidence of the role of spiritual beliefs and practices in recovering from addictions and in preventing substance abuse and relapse (Koenig et al., 2001). An emphasis on spirituality is a key component in 12-step recovery programs, such as Alcoholics Anonymous (Minnick, 1997), which can be a valuable adjunct to couple or family therapy (Berenson, 1990). Beyond offering fellowship and group support, these programs address spiritual issues concerning identity, integrity, an inner life, and interdependence. The steps promote a spiritual awakening that prepares individuals and family members to practice the principles for abstinence and greater well-being in all aspects of their lives. One study of African American and Latino inner-city participants in a 12-step program for drug addiction (Green, Fullilove, & Fullilove, 1998) found that persons in drug recovery often undergo intense spiritual journeys as they embrace a Higher Power through the program. Often, this spiritual awakening sparks life-altering transformations along with abstinence. The connection with a Higher Power through prayer and meditation also facilitates reflection that sustains them through difficult times. The serenity prayer, at the heart of recovery movements, can be very helpful to anyone facing difficult circumstances: "May I have the serenity to accept the things I cannot change, the courage to change the things I can, and the wisdom to know the difference."

## Overcoming Barriers of Poverty and Racism

Religious faith and congregational support help people to survive and transcend impoverished conditions, barriers of racism, and other adversity. It has been especially important for African American and Latino families (see Boyd-Franklin & Lockwood [Chapter 7] and Falicov [Chapter 8], this volume). In *Bread and Spirit*, Harry Aponte (1994) urges therapists to attend to spiritual as well as practical needs of poor families. He encourages therapists to go beyond theory and technique to reach for meaning and purpose in people's lives: ·

> Therapy can be an enemy or a friend to spirit. The technology of therapy has attempted to replace tradition, ritual, and customs. Therapy has also masqueraded as spirit. However, just as medication can only succeed when it cooperates with the healing powers of the body, therapy only works when it joins with the indigenous forces of culture and faith in people's lives. (p. 8)

In the midst of despair, there still survives a spirit of love, courage, and hope, although often muted. Aponte believes that we, as therapists, can make a difference by recognizing that potential and joining in a revitalization of family and community spirit (see Aponte, Chapter 6, this volume).

## Reconnecting with Family Spiritual Roots

Therapists trained to look to family-of-origin history for sources of current difficulties need to search also for hidden resources. Discovering the strength of religious roots can be valuable in therapeutic work, especially when experiences of oppression or forced migration have shattered a coherent sense of identity and severed vital linkages with ancestors and cultural heritage (see Kamya, Chapter 15, this volume).

For instance, many African Americans are descendants of Muslims brought from West Africa as slaves, but they often are unaware of this heritage. Because the practice of African religions was suppressed and punished, the practice of Islam was often done in secret and passed down surreptitiously in oral history or by family members imitating behaviors without knowing their source. Mahmoud (2005) has found that, in doing genograms with African Americans in clinical practice, a story might surface of distant relatives who always prayed facing east, refused to eat pork, gave their children "funny" (non-Christian) names, and didn't allow them to be baptized. Restoring vital bonds with a family's religious heritage can be healing and empowering.

## Facilitating Forgiveness and Reconciliation

The value of compassion, forgiveness, and reconciliation is central to the teachings of all major religions (Rye et al., 2000). In the Hindu Bhagavad Gita it is said: If you want to see the brave, look at those who can forgive. Research supports Biblical teachings that unforgiveness wounds the mind, the body, and the spirit of the person who suffered harm. With evidence of physiological and psychological benefits for those who forgive, several individual therapy approaches have been advanced (McCullough, Pargament, & Thoresen, 2000; Worthington, 2006). The role of forgiveness in marital and family therapy is receiving increased attention (Fincham, Hall, & Beach, 2006; Legaree, Turner, & Lollis, 2007). Hargrave (1994) has developed a relational model to facilitate forgiveness and reconciliation in couple and family relationships (see Hargrave [Chapter 16] and Fishbane [Chapter 9], this volume).

Broader systemic applications hold enormous potential. Collective multifaith initiatives for restorative justice in the legal system aim for the reintegration and empowerment of both victims and offenders, with their dignity and humanity restored. The Truth and Reconciliation Commission, initiated in South Africa, has been a model adapted in many other conflict regions to transcend widespread violence and suffering and to transform relationships.

## Use of Contemplative Practices

Contemplative practices are becoming widely used to enhance the work of therapy (Germer, Siegel, & Fulton, 2005). Meditation offers a way to find clarity and tranquility. It can empty the mind of distracting "noise," ease suffering, and rid the body of tension and pain (Kabat-Zinn, 2003). Becoming mindful in still and focused concentration can lead to more deliberate action. Although meditation is most widely used with individual clients for their own physical and psychological well-being, it can have valuable interpersonal benefits for relationship enhancement and transformation, conflict resolution, and reconciliation (Baer, 2003; Barnes et al., 2007; Carson, Carson, Gil, & Baucom, 2004).

The Vietnamese Buddhist teacher Thich Nhat Hahn (2004) has developed mindfulness practices in promoting peace and nonviolence among groups in conflict. For instance, he has been holding a series of retreats for Israeli and Palestinian participants. Initially, they practice mindfulness exercises in separate groups to calm intense reactivity and misperceptions. When they are brought together, they are then better able to gain compassion for each other's suffering and humanity. These steps enable them to take actions toward a just peace.

Meditation can enhance couple and family therapy in various ways, as a resource to the therapist and as a resource to clients as part of the therapeutic process. First, therapists' own practice of meditation outside therapy can increase therapeutic rapport, focus, and effectiveness. Contemplative practices can deepen clinicians' awareness and wisdom, enabling therapists to be more open, attentive, and responsive to clients, and to remain clear and calm in the midst of their turmoil. Meditation also heightens creative processes and openness to new possibilities that arise in the therapeutic encounter. Instead of pushing for change, therapists find greater ease and success as the process flows more naturally. Regular practice also eases therapist compassion fatigue and prevents work-related burnout (see Barrett, Chapter 14, this volume).

Second, therapists can encourage clients, outside sessions, to practice meditation and/or other contemplative and integrative approaches, such as focused deep breathing exercises or yoga. This may be especially helpful for those who are anxious, depressed, or dispirited by mental or physical suffering. The form of meditation used should fit with each client's spiritual beliefs, preferences, and comfort. Although many of these approaches have come from Buddhist and Hindu traditions, they can complement many faith orientations and are widely used by secular persons. People of all faiths practice some form of meditation; it may involve recitation, chanting, or prayer beads. Some might prefer listening to music or reading poetry in a contemplative atmosphere, or perhaps finding tranquility in an early morning walk. Shared meditative experiences with loved ones foster authentic and empathic communication, reduce defensive reactivity, and can deepen couple and family bonds.

Meditation can be used more directly with clients to enhance therapy in and between sessions (Germer, Siegel, & Fulton, 2005). Therapists can provide a quiet place for them to meditate before or after sessions, or can devote several minutes for silent meditation together at the start or end of a session, or after a difficult or upsetting discussion. In the therapeutic process, therapists' contemplative questions with couples can facilitate reflection and draw attention away from petty annoyances toward more meaningful dialogue. Therapists can lead interactive exercises with couples or family members to facilitate more genuine and empathic communication, mutual understanding, and compassion for relational wounds (see Gale, Chapter 13, this volume). Therapists might also encourage clients to meditate before stressful encounters with family members, or as a part of coaching work to bring about relationship changes in family-of-origin relationships. Nhat Hahn (2003) has developed a number of practices for couple and parent–child relationships, and for deeper connection with families of origin, ancestors, and cultural roots. He has even designed a "Peace Treaty" for warring parties to sign at the end of their work.

Despite concerns by some that highly vulnerable clients might experience dissociation, Bell (1998) contends that meditation supports integration and wholeness: clients' clearer knowledge and acceptance of themselves and deeper bonds with others. Deep breathing exercises connect mind, body, and spirit as they reduce anxiety. At the same time, therapists are cautioned to proceed slowly and prepare clients for whom difficult or painful memories and feelings may emerge, such as survivors of trauma. Therapists can help them to hold such experiences in a safe, bounded, and centered way that fosters their transformation (see Barrett, Chapter 14, this volume). A therapist might use guided imagery, for instance, suggesting that a vulnerable client visualize a caring person and interaction from childhood, hold that moment in mind, then describe that experience, such as the secure and comforting feeling of being cradled in the arms of a grandmother.

### Use of Rituals

Through sacred ceremonies and rituals, stories and music, meditation and communion, we find connection with our deepest spiritual core and with all that is outside ourselves. As a Hopi proverb goes: "Work hard, keep the ceremonies, live peaceably, and unite your hearts." Rituals can ease passage through transitions and unfamiliar situations; in times of crisis, they can script our actions and responses, as funeral rites do. Rituals can summon courage through the darkest times.

Ingrid Betancourt, held captive for six years in a Colombian jungle, drew on her Roman Catholic faith for her survival. She found solace, sanity, and stability in daily spiritual practices: talking to God, praying, and meditating. Recalling her father saying the rosary, she made a crude rosary of buttons from a jacket and a lanyard her captors used to strap a rifle. Unsure if 10 beads were the correct number, she used 15 "just in case." She said, "That's the magic of all things. You can have the dark side of man but you can also plug yourself into light and be an enormous light to others. And I think that's what being spiritual means." (quoted in Erlanger, 2008, p. A6).

Imber-Black, Roberts, and Whiting (2003) have developed principles and guidelines for using rituals in family therapy (see Imber-Black [Chapter 12] and Roberts [Chapter 19], this volume). Therapists can encourage family members to draw on spiritual rituals that have been meaningful in their past. We can also help clients transform empty rituals into meaningful ones, create new rites, or bridge formal religious differences in an expression of spirituality that is both more personal and transcendent.

## Encouraging Service to Others and Activism

Suffering can open the spirit to compassion for the suffering of others. In therapy, we can listen for those transcending moments, expressions of concern for others; we can fan the sparks of desire to reach beyond personal struggle or tragedy to take action to benefit others (Aldarondo, 2007). One combat veteran, drinking heavily, was tormented by his role in the deaths of five children and his inability to bring back their lives. His military chaplain asked him, "Do you think you might find five children in need, whose lives you might help to save?"

Often social advocacy requires courage, initiative, and perseverance, which therapists can encourage. These efforts circle back in healing ways for clients. Perry and Rolland (see Chapter 20, this volume) suggest ways to bring spiritually inspired activism into clinical practice and our broader role in building coalitions to address larger systemic "counterspiritualities."

## Responsiveness to Spiritual Diversity

As societies become increasingly diverse, therapists have more contact with many faiths and the need to develop a spiritual pluralism, with knowledge and respect for varied beliefs and practices (Richards & Bergin, 2000). Therapeutic approaches and services need to be sensitive and responsive to this spiritual diversity. As therapists, particularly when from the dominant cultural group, we must be cautious not to take our own values as the norm or be judgmental toward differences in beliefs and practices. Instead, we must seek to understand their meaning and function in our clients' lives.

Cultural traditions and spiritual beliefs need to be integrated in a holistic approach to mental health and health care. When one Hmong family from Southeast Asia brought their young daughter to a hospital emergency room with seizure, a cross-cultural crisis ensued (Fadiman, 1997). The family members wanted the daughter's distress alleviated, but they didn't want to stop her seizures, which they believed to be sacred trance states signifying positive connection with the spirit world. As they put it, "The spirit catches you and you fall down." The well-intentioned medical staff obtained a court-ordered removal of the girl from her parents in order to treat her seizures. However, this only heightened her distress and alienated the parents, who refused further treatment after her return home, resulting in tragedy. If the health care professionals had tried to understand and work with the spiritual beliefs of the family, instead of taking an adversarial approach, the tragedy might well have been averted.

With growing ethnic, racial, and religious diversity *within* families, therapists can help partners, parents, or extended family members understand better and respect one another's beliefs and practices. To resolve conflicts and repair cutoffs, we can help clients to avoid polarization or to shift from a stance of moral superiority or righteousness to an acceptance of different spiritual pathways.

When therapists are of the same faith as clients, it can be easier to form a natural rapport. However, one can easily overidentify with the client, see only positive or negative influences of religion, or be hesitant to question beliefs that are assumed to be fundamental. If we share the same religious background with clients, they may assume that we judge them according to official doctrine.

Therapists who are more secular than clients or not of the same faith need to be respectful of differences, particularly with highly religious families (Delaney, Miller, & Bisono, 2007). Therapists may not have deep knowledge about the many varied spiritual orientations of clients, and may not be trained to offer religious counseling. Yet our practice can be informed by the emerging literature, as noted above. As McGoldrick and her colleagues (2005) stress, culturally sensitive practice begins with awareness of the profound influence of core beliefs and an openness to learn from our clients. The varied ways in which most individuals, couples, and families mix and reshape particular beliefs and practices within and across faiths (as discussed in Chapter 1, this volume) means that therapists need to guard against stereotyped assumptions and generalizations. We must learn from our clients about their own spiritual journey, their needs and preferences, how they may have been wounded, and how they have found healing. We need to be openhearted in listening to and exploring religious and spiritual questions and beliefs that have profound implications for their lives. Most importantly, we need to encourage their efforts to open and expand spiritual pathways to meet current challenges and experience personal and relational growth.

## A Leap of Faith: The Spiritual Essence of Therapy

At its best, the very process of psychotherapy becomes a spiritual wellspring for healing and resilience. As the family therapy field has matured, we have increasingly come to see that the value of our endeavor is found less in therapist strategies and techniques, and more in the quality of our collaborative relationship with clients. A resilience-oriented approach to therapy is forged through this "courageous engagement" (Waters & Lawrence, 1993). We seek to understand our clients as heroes who have been challenged on their own life journeys, to tap into their yearnings for meaning and purpose, and to facilitate a holistic sense of wellness. Becvar (1996) stresses the need to walk a path with heart, following hopes and dreams while enriching the soul.

As therapists, we, as well as our clients, need courage to address moral dilemmas; to question constraining beliefs or destructive actions; to support clients' attempts to move from despair and reach for their hopes and dreams, and to learn from their mistakes and act on their best intentions. When our clients lose hope, our faith in their potential can restore their faith. When we believe in their worth, our clients are better able to rise to meet their challenges with confidence and competence. Valuing human connection, we help our clients to seek reconciliation to heal wounded relationships and encourage them to forge more meaningful personal and spiritual bonds. These are essentially spiritual endeavors (Aponte, 2002).

In these times, we must challenge the constraints of managed care and manualized treatments, as well as cultural pressures for quick solutions to problems, to meet our clients' needs for more soulful conversations about life and death, love and loss, trauma and recovery, meaning and purpose. Yet, even when therapy must be brief, when we are mindfully present, open, respectful, curious, and compassionate, we can have deep, meaningful connections with our clients and support their processes for healing, transformation, and growth. Many of us can recall a single encounter in our lives that catalyzed our reflection and action in more purposeful directions. Such power and potential are there, within the individuals, couples, and families we see, to be activated in the therapeutic encounter and, with our encouragement, to be nourished through spiritual resources in their lives.

As I've come to work less from my head and more from my spiritual core, I know less than I used to, but I trust more my leap of faith, with conviction in my clients' potential. I believe it has made me a better therapist. As Mary Jo Barrett and Kaethe Weingarten have found in their therapeutic work (see Chapters 14 and 18, respectively, this volume), this deeper level of work is not only transformative for our clients but can also be restorative for therapists.

## Exploring Our Own Spiritual Roots and Branches

When we recognize spirituality as a significant dimension in human experience, it requires all us, as therapists, to take stock of our own spiritual orientation (including atheist, agnostic, or secular humanist perspectives) and its influence in our therapeutic work. Our current faith beliefs and practices, as well as our cultural and family traditions and their legacies, operate in many ways, whether intentionally or unwittingly. If we hold a narrow, rigid view of spirituality as limited to formal, institutionalized religion, we may not appreciate the many possibilities for spiritual experience. If our own childhood exposure to religion was largely negative or devoid of spiritual meaning, it may block us from realizing its potential as a source of strength and comfort for clients in distress. Therapists and trainees benefit from deepening knowledge of their family traditions and reflection on their own spiritual journeys (see Roberts, Chapter 19, this volume). Such self-awareness increases our comfort in approaching clients' spiritual distress, and our resources for healing and growth.

## My Personal Spiritual Journey

It was not surprising for me to be drawn to explore spirituality since it was a core issue in my family of origin. Like many families, religion was a complicated matter in our lives, rife with secret keeping, conflict, and cutoffs. My mother had been cut off from her family after leaving the Catholic Church and then converting to Judaism when she married my father. Just before my mother's death, when I was 27 and eager to know her better, she shared the secret she had held from even my father: She had been a nun for 17 years. She died before I could ask her the many questions I was left with. Through my own family-of-origin work, I reconnected with her family and learned more about my Catholic roots.

Naming is often a way of making connections across the generations and in the joining of families by marriage. In my own family, naming became a way for my mother to weave together the disparate threads of her life and identity. Her mother, a devout French Canadian Catholic, named her and her brother Mary and Joseph. She had hoped that her favored son would become a priest, but Joe left the seminary to marry his sweetheart. Hoping to win her mother's approval, my mother not only took his place, entering the convent, she even took his name: Sister Josephine. When she eventually left the religious order to lead a "normal" life, she held on to that part of her identity by becoming Mary Jo. When she married my father and converted to Judaism (at his mother's strong request), she became known as Jo. To bridge the religious divide and to win the approval of her new mother-in-law, she named me after my father's maternal grandmother, Frimid. (Ironically, my Jewish grandmother turned to Christian Science readings in her last years of life.)

Only when I reached adulthood did I learn that my name Froma (like Frimid), derives from the Jewish name Fruma, meaning *pious* or *spiritual*. (No one had ever mentioned the meaning to me.) My name would have had significance for my mother. Although she chose a secular life, she remained a deeply spiritual person. She studied Judaism and made sure I went through Sunday school to Confirmation. A gifted musician, she became the temple organist.

My mother was even elected B'nai Brith president. However, someone in the congregation then attacked her, contending that it was not proper for her to hold such a position—that she was not *really* a Jew. She was devastated. She and my father withdrew from formal religion altogether for the rest of their lives. I left for college and disengaged from Judaism myself for many years, feeling I didn't quite belong anywhere, much as my mother must have felt. My father found a spiritual connection through the Masonic lodge, yet, true to his Jewish faith, never took a Christian vow.

I had always had friends of many faiths and ethnic backgrounds. At college, I had my first experience of anti-Semitism, when my (Christian) friends were all invited to pledge sororities but I was blackballed. (I had not applied to the Jewish houses, not wanting to be segregated.) People in groups that have experienced the stigma of bias and discrimination, such as Jews, may absorb the larger society's prejudices and become conflicted about their own religious identity. Such tensions led me to distance myself from my Jewish roots for some time. Yet my crisis experience became transformative. I found an apartment on my own and focused on my studies; that deep concentration awakened my passion for learning. I also gained a broader perspective on the social world. I became involved in the growing civil rights movement and, at graduation, went into the Peace Corps. I was fortunate to serve in Morocco, where I gained a deep appreciation for the Moroccan blend of Islam with ancient Berber spiritual traditions, lived out in everyday life with strong kinship bonds and an openhearted generosity extended to all, rich or poor, friend or stranger.

Music has a deep spiritual resonance for me as well, as a bond with both my mother and my daughter. My mother, a gifted musician and esteemed piano teacher, was not only the organist at our temple but, with a multifaith command of the great hymns and religious music, she also played at holidays for several Christian congregations in our community. Music, whether sacred or secular, was a transcendent spiritual experience for her, as it became for me as I went with her on those many occasions, inheriting her passion for all forms of music. Most uplifting for me has been singing great choral works—from Bach's Mass in B Minor to Brahms's Requiem. My daughter and I also share this bond: When stressed out, we close our eyes and listen to Celtic songs, Senegalese rhythms, or other deeply moving world music.

## The Therapeutic Interface

Our own spiritual journey can influence our therapeutic work in unexpected ways. Two decades ago, I worked with a family in the aftermath of the father's sudden death in an auto accident. The father had been a minister, as beloved by his congregation as he was by his family. Within months of the death, the mother had moved with three of her four children to a new community to start a new life. When they came a while later for help with adolescent separation issues, we worked together to address the many ramifications of their painful, unresolved loss. I described our "successful" work in presentations on loss. Then, one day, a divinity student in my loss course asked a simple question about the family: "What happened to their spirituality after the father's death?" I was stunned. I replied honestly that I didn't know. I had never asked. And no family member had ever mentioned it.

Moreover, the oldest daughter, age 17 at her father's death, had run off to live on a commune with a cult leader, severing all contact with her family. Although the mother and I worked successfully over time to restore their relationship, never did we explore the possible spiritual meaning of the daughter's attachment to the cult and its charismatic leader, as a replacement for her father, the spiritual leader of her family and community.

How had I not considered the spiritual dimension of family loss, especially in a case in which the father had been a Christian minister and the family's life had been centered on the church community? In many presentations of the case, no clinical colleague or student had ever raised the subject. It seemed that all consciousness of spirituality had been erased by my clinical training. It was a divinity student, trained to attend to the spiritual, who could see this hidden dimension. In later reflection, I believe that my unease at that time with my own complicated spiritual identity contributed, outside of my awareness, to my blindness to the family's spiritual pain. As I have come to embrace my own spiritual complexities, I find my sight is greatly improved, as is comfort in exploring the spiritual dimension in my clients' lives.

In my role as a therapist, if asked about my religion, I generally say that I have Jewish and Christian roots, and that I have deep interest in the many faith traditions in the world, seeing all as spiritual pathways for meaning and connection. I add that I am also interested in the varied ways many people choose and combine faith beliefs and practices to fit their lives, as well as the ways that more secular people find spiritual meaning and nourishment. When working with clients, if I think that briefly sharing some aspect of my spiritual journey might be helpful to them, I may do so as it relates to their dilemma or might inspire them on their own spiritual paths. Any disclosure must be done with exquisite sensitivity to its appropriateness, care not to proselytize, and with potential value in work toward client aims.

I see my own spiritual journey as a lifelong process of exploration, hopefully with deepening and expanding awareness and connection. My bookshelves are chock full of books calling out to be read and reread. Although I don't fit neatly into any one religious category, I identify most strongly with my Jewish religious and cultural roots. Yet, like both my parents, I've stitched together strands of many faith traditions into a deeply personal spirituality. I feel an affinity toward many aspects of Christian, Buddhist, Islamic, and Native American traditions. Rather than seeing these in conflict, I experience them as offering many valuable ways of approaching the spirit, and all sharing values of love, humility, generosity, and compassion. Each helps us grapple with such universal questions as "Where have we come from? Why are we here? and Where are we going?" We may turn to different faiths, or to secular humanism, to seek answers. What matters most is the journey itself; we find meaning in the quest, even when the answers are elusive and when each answer opens a new mystery.

The healing art of therapy has much in common with a spiritual journey. The Native American scholar Vine Deloria (1994) urges us to follow this spiritual path not only for our own well-being but also for the sake of the generations to come: "The future of humankind lies waiting for those who will come to understand their lives and take up their responsibilities to all living things" (p. 272).

## CONCLUSION

Buddhism counsels us to assume a beginner's mind. This chapter, like the others in this volume, is offered not from a position of expertise but toward a multifaith perspective, opening our therapeutic practice to this vital dimension of experience. It is important for therapists to gain appreciation for the spiritual diversity in our society. Experiences that acquaint us with religious/ spiritual beliefs and practices that differ from our own traditions, such as visiting varied faith communities, can deepen our understanding of others and strengthen our sense of connectedness. Many readings cited throughout this volume broaden our knowledge of the diverse beliefs and practices that clients may bring. A beginning understanding of core convictions can serve to prevent ignorance, faulty assumptions, or stereotyped views from interfering with therapeutic rapport. It can also inspire deeper exploration of our own faith traditions, as well as new spiritual possibilities for resilience and growth in our practices and our personal lives.

As Pargament (2007) cautions, spiritual resources are not simply another problem-solving tool or set of therapeutic techniques. Instead, they are embedded in a larger worldview and facilitate the spiritual journey of an individual, couple, or family. They are resources for living and struggling with life's challenges. They can enable our clients and ourselves to tap reservoirs of hope, meaning, connection, and inspiration.

## REFERENCES

Aldarondo, E . (Ed.). (2007). *Advancing social justice through clinical practice.* Mahwah, NJ: Erlbaum.

American Psychiatric Association. (1994). *Diagnostic and statistical manual of mental disorders* (4th ed.). Washington, DC: Author.

Anderson, D. A., & Worthen, D. (1997). Exploring a fourth dimension: Spirituality as a resource for the couple therapist. *Journal of Marital and Family Therapy, 23*, 2–12.

Aponte, H. (1994). *Bread and spirit: Therapy with the new poor.* New York: Norton.

Aponte, H. (2002). Spirituality: The heart of therapy. *Journal of Family Psychotherapy, 13*(1–2), 13–27.

Baer, R. A. (2003). Mindfulness training as a clinical intervention: A conceptual and empirical review. *Clinical Psychology: Science and Practice, 10*, 125–143.

Barnes, S., Brown, K. W., Krusemark, E., Campbell, W. K., & Rogge, R. D. (2007). The role of mindfulness in romantic relationship satisfaction and responses to relationship stress. *Journal of Marital and Family Therapy, 33*(4), 482–500.

Bateson, G. (1979). *Mind and nature: A necessary unity.* New York: Dutton.

Baucom, D. H. (2001). Religion and the science of relationships: Is a happy marriage possible? *Journal of Family Psychology, 15*(4), 652–656.

Becvar, D. (1996). *Soul healing: A spiritual orientation in counseling and therapy.* New York: Basic Books.

Bell, L. G. (1998). Start with meditation. In T. Nelson & T. Trepper (Eds.), *101 interventions in family therapy* (Vol. 2, pp. 52–56). New York: Haworth Press.

Berenson, D. (1990). A systemic view of spirituality: God and twelve-step programs as resources in family therapy. *Journal of Strategic and Systemic Therapies, 9,* 59–70.

Boszormenyi-Nagy, I. (1987). *Foundations of contextual family therapy.* New York: Brunner/Mazel.

Butler, M. H., & Harper, J. M. (1994). The divine triangle: God in the marital system of religious couples. *Family Process, 33,* 277–286.

Carlson, T. D., & Erickson, M. J. (Eds.). (2002). *Spirituality and family therapy.* Binghamton, NY: Haworth Press.

Carson, J. W., Carson, K. M., Gil, K. M., & Baucom, D. H. (2004). Mindfulness-based relationship enhancement. *Behavior Therapy, 35,* 471–494.

Coles, R. (1997). *The moral intelligence of children.* New York: Random House.

Daneshpour, M. (1998). Muslim families and family therapy. *Journal of Marital and Family Therapy, 24,* 355–368.

Delaney, H. D., Miller, W. R., & Bisono, A. M. (2007). Religiosity and spirituality among psychologists: A survey of clinician members of the American Psychological Association. *Professional Psychology: Research and Practice, 38*(5), 538–546.

Deloria, V., Jr. (1994). *God is red: A native view of religion* (2nd ed.). Golden, CO: Fulcrum.

Doehring, C. (2006). *The practice of pastoral care: A postmodern approach.* Louisville, KY: Westminster John Knox Press.

Doherty, W. J. (1995). *Soul searching: Why psychotherapy must promote moral responsibility.* New York: Basic Books.

Dossey, L. (1993). *Healing words: The power of prayer and the practice of medicine.* San Francisco: Harper.

Einstein, A. (1931). Religion and science. In A. M. Drummond & R. H. Wagner (Eds.), *Problems and opinions* (pp. 355–358). New York: Century.

Eliade, M., Trask, W., & Doniger, W. (2004). *Shamanism: Archaic techniques of ecstasy* (rev. ed.). Princeton, NJ: Princeton University Press.

Elliott Griffith, M., & Griffith, J. (2002). Addressing spirituality in its clinical complexities: Its potential for healing, its potential for harm. *Journal of Family Psychotherapy, 13*(1–2), 167–194.

Erlanger, S. (2008, July 11). Freed Colombian grapples with recalling and releasing pain, and with resuming life. *New York Times,* A6.

Fadiman, A. (1997). *The spirit catches you and you fall down.* San Francisco: Ferrer.

Falicov, C. (1998). *Latino families in therapy.* New York: Guilford Press.

Fincham, F., Hall, J., & Beach, S. (2006). Forgiveness in marriage: Current status and future directions. *Family Relations, 55*(4), 415–427.

Fishbane, M. D. (1998). I, thou and we: A dialogical approach to couples therapy. *Journal of Marital and Family Therapy, 24,* 41–58.

Frankl, V. (1955). *The doctor and the soul.* New York: Knopf.

Freud, S. (1961). The future of an illusion. In J. Strachey (Ed. & Trans.), *The standard edition of the complete psychological works of Sigmund Freud* (Vol. 21, pp. 1–56). London: Hogarth Press. (Original work published 1927)

Gallup, G. H., Jr., & Lindsay, D. M. (1999). *Surveying the religious landscape: Trends in U.S. beliefs.* Harrisburg, PA: Morehouse.

Germer, C. K., Siegel, R. D., & Fulton, P. R. (Eds.). (2005). *Mindfulness and psychotherapy.* New York: Guilford Press.

Green, L. L., Fullilove, M. T., & Fullilove, R. E. (1998). Stories of spiritual awakening: The nature of spirituality in recovery. *Journal of Substance Abuse Treatment, 15,* 325–331.

Griffith, J., & Elliott Griffith, M. (2002). *Encountering the sacred in psychotherapy.* New York: Guilford Press.

Grossman, P., Niemann, L., Schmidt, S., & Walach, H. (2004). Mindfulness-based stress reduction and health benefits: A meta-analysis. *Journal of Psychosomatic Research, 57,* 35–43.

Haldeman, D. C. (2004). When sexual and religious orientations collide: Considerations in working with conflicted same-sex attracted male clients. *Counseling Psychologist, 32*(5), 691–715.

Hargrave, T. (1994). *Families and forgiveness.* New York: Brunner/Mazel.

Helmeke, K. (2006). "My spiritual life": Conducting a spiritual life review with the elderly. In K. Helmeke & K. Sori (Eds.), *The therapist's notebook for integrating spirituality in counseling: Homework, handouts, and activities for use in psychotherapy* (pp. 113–123). Binghamton, NY: Haworth Press.

Helmeke, K. B., & Bischof, G. H. (2002). Recognizing and raising spiritual and religious issues in therapy: Guidelines for the timid. *Journal of Family Psychotherapy, 13*(1–2), 195–214.

Helmeke, K. B., & Sori, K. (2006) *The therapist's notebook for integrating spirituality in counseling: Homework, handouts, and activities for use in psychotherapy: Vols. 1 and 2.* Binghamton, NY: Haworth Press.

Hill, M., & Mamalakis, P. (2001). Family therapists and religious communities: Negotiating dual relationships. *Family Relations, 50*(3), 199–208.

Hill, P. C., & Pargament, K. I. (2003). Advances in the conceptualization and measurement of religion and spirituality: Implications for physical and mental health research. *American Psychologist, 58*(1), 64–74.

Hodge, D. R. (2005a). *Spiritual assessment: Handbook for helping professionals.* Botsford, CT: North American Association of Christians in Social Work.

Hodge, D. R. (2005b). Spiritual assessment in marital and family therapy: A methodological framework for selecting from among six qualitative assessment tools. *Journal of Marital and Family Therapy, 31*(4), 341–356.

Imber-Black, E., Roberts, J., & Whiting, R. (Eds.). (2003). *Rituals in families and family therapy* (2nd ed.). New York: Norton.

Joanides, C. J. (1996). Collaborative family therapy with religious family systems. *Journal of Family Psychotherapy, 7*, 19–35.

Jung, C. G. (1933). *Modern man in search of a soul.* New York: Harcourt Brace.

Jung, C. G. (1958). *Psychology and religion: West and East.* New York: Pantheon.

Kabat-Zinn, J. (2003). Mindfulness-based interventions in context: Past, present, and future. *Clinical Psychology: Science and Practice, 10*(2), 144–156.

Kimball, L. S., & Knudson-Martin, C. (2002). A cultural trinity: Spirituality, religion, and gender in clinical practice. *Journal of Family Psychotherapy, 13*(1–2), 145–166.

Koenig, H. G. (2005). *Faith and mental health: Religious resources for healing.* Conshohacken, PA: Templeton Foundation Press.

Koenig, H. G. (2006). *In the wake of disaster: Religious responses to terrorism and catastrophe.* Conshohacken, PA: Templeton Press.

Koenig, H. G. (2007). *Spirituality in patient care* (2nd ed.). Conshohacken, PA: Templeton Press.

Koenig, H. G., McCullough, M. E., & Larson, D. W. (Eds.). (2001). *Handbook of religion and health.* New York: Oxford University Press.

Legaree, T.-A., Turner, J., & Lollis, S. (2007). Forgiveness and therapy: A critical review of conceptualizations, practices, and values found in the literature. *Journal of Marital and Family Therapy, 33*(2), 192–213.

Lambert, N. M., & Dollahite, D. C. (2006). How religiosity helps couples prevent, resolve, and overcome marital conflict. *Family Relations, 55*, 439–449.

Mahmoud, V. (2005). African American Muslim families. In M. McGoldrick, J. Giordano, & Garcia-Preto, N. (Eds.), *Ethnicity and family therapy* (3rd ed., pp. 138–150). New York: Guilford Press.

Marks, L. (2004). Sacred practices in highly religious families: Christian, Jewish, Mormon, and Muslim perspectives. *Family Process, 43*(2), 217–231.

McCullough, M. E., Pargament, K. I., & Thoresen, C. E. (2000). The psychology of forgiveness: History, conceptual issues, and overview. In M. E. McCullough, K. I. Pargament, & C. E. Thoresen, (Eds.), *Forgiveness: Theory, research, and practice* (pp. 1–16). New York: Guilford Press.

McGoldrick, M., Gerson, R., & Petry, S. (2007). *Genograms: Assessment and intervention* (3rd ed.). New York: Norton.

McGoldrick, M., Giordano, J., & Garcia-Preto, N. (Eds.). (2005). *Ethnicity and family therapy* (3rd ed.). New York: Guilford Press.

McRae, S., & Walker, K. (2007). *An evaluation of family-to-family ties: A review of Family Mentorship in Action.* Saskatoon, Canada: University of Saskatoon Institute for Social Research.

Meyerstein, I. (2006). Spiritually sensitive counseling with Jewish clients and families. In K. Helmeke & K. Sori (Eds.), *The therapist's notebook for integrating spirituality in counseling: Homework, handouts, and activities for use in psychotherapy* (pp. 113–123). Binghamton, NY: Haworth Press.

Minnick, A. M. (1997). *Twelve-step programs: Contemporary American quest for meaning and spiritual renewal.* New York: Praeger.

Moodley, R., & West, W. (2005). *Integrating traditional healing practices into counseling and psychotherapy.* Thousand Oaks, CA: Sage.

Nhat Hahn, T. (2003). *Creating true peace: Ending violence in yourself, your family, your community, and your world.* New York: Free Press.

Nhat Hahn, T. (2004). *Peace begins here: Palestinians and Israelis listening to each other.* Berkeley, CA: Parallax Press.

Pargament, K. I. (2007). *Spiritually integrated psychotherapy.* New York: Guilford Press.

Pargament, K. I., Murray-Swank, N., & Mahoney, A. (in press). Problem and solution: The spiritual dimension of clergy sexual abuse and its impact on survivors. *Journal of Child Sexual Abuse.*

Prest, L. A., & Keller, J. F. (1993). Spirituality and family therapy: Spiritual beliefs, myths, and metaphors. *Journal of Marital and Family Therapy, 19,* 137–148.

Richards, P. S., & Bergin, A. E. (Eds.). (2000). *Handbook of psychotherapy and religious diversity.* Washington, DC: American Psychological Association.

Rosario, M., Yali, A. M., Hunter, J., & Viorst-Gwadz, M. (2006). Religion and health among lesbian, gay, and bi-sexual youths: An empirical investigation and theoretical explanation. In A. M. Omoto & H. S. Kurtzman (Eds.), *Sexual orientation and mental health: Examining identity development in lesbian, gay, and bisexual people* (pp. 117–140). Washington, DC: American Psychological Association.

Rye, M. S., Pargament, K. I., Ali, M. A., Beck, G. L., Dorff, E. N., Hallisey, C., et al. (2000). Religious perspectives on forgiveness. In M. E. McCullough, K. I. Pargament, & C. E. Thoreson (Eds.), *Forgiveness: Theory, research, and practice.* New York: Guilford Press.

Satir, V. (1988). *Peoplemaking.* Palo Alto, CA: Science and Behavior. (Original work published 1972)

Simpkinson, C., & Simpkinson, A. (1999). Simply the best. *Common Boundary: Exploring Psychology, Spirituality, and Creativity, 17*(1), 32–37.

Stander, V., Piercy, F., MacKinnon, D., & Helmeke, K. (1994). Spirituality, religion, and family therapy: Competing or complementary worlds? *American Journal of Family Therapy, 22,* 27–41.

Stanley, S., Markman, H., Prado, L., Olmos-Gallo, P. A., Tonelli, I., St. Peters, M., et al. (2001). Community-based premarital prevention: Clergy and lay leaders on the front lines. *Family Relations, 50*(1), 67–76.

Tedeschi, R. G., & Calhoun, L. G. (2004). Post-traumatic growth: Conceptual foundations and empirical evidence. *Psychological Inquiry, 15,* 1–18.

Walsh, F. (1999). *Spiritual resources in family therapy* (1st ed.). New York: Guilford Press.

Walsh, F. (2003). *Normal family processes: Growing diversity and complexity* (3rd ed.). New York: Guilford Press.

Walsh, F. (2006). *Strengthening family resilience* (2nd ed.). New York: Guilford Press.

Walsh, F. (2007). Traumatic loss and major disaster: Strengthening family and community resilience. *Family Process, 46*(2), 207–227.

Walsh, F. (2008). Spirituality, healing, and resilience. In M. McGoldrick & K. Hardy (Eds.), *Re-visioning family therapy: Race, culture, and gender in clinical practice* (2nd ed., pp. 61–75). New York: Guilford Press.

Walsh, F., & McGoldrick, M. (Eds.). (2004). *Living beyond loss: Death in the family* (2nd ed.). New York: Norton.

Waters, D., & Lawrence, E. (1993). *Competence, courage, and change.* New York: Norton.

Weaver, A. J., Koenig, H. G., & Larson, D. B. (1997). Marriage and family therapists and the clergy: A need for clinical collaboration, training, and research. *Journal of Marital and Family Therapy, 23*, 13–25.

Weil, A. (1994). *Spontaneous healing.* New York: Knopf.

Wendel, R. D. (2003). Lived religion and family therapy: What does spirituality have to do with it? *Family Process, 42*, 165–181.

Werner, E. E., & Smith, R. S. (2001). *Journeys from childhood to midlife: Risk, resilience, and recovery.* Ithaca, NY: Cornell University Press.

Whipple, V. (1987). Counseling battered women from fundamentalist churches. *Journal of Marital and Family Therapy, 13*, 251–258.

Worthington, E. L., Jr. (2006). *Forgiveness and reconciliation: Theory and application.* New York: Routledge.

Wright, L., Watson, W. L., & Bell, J. M. (1996). *Beliefs: The heart of healing in families and illness.* New York: Basic Books.

Yahouse, M. A., & Tan, E. S. N. (2005). Addressing religious conflicts in adolescents who experience sexual identity confusion. *Professional Psychology: Research and Practice, 36*(5), 530–536.

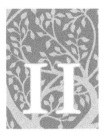

# SPIRITUAL RESOURCES
# IN FAMILIES
*Tapping the Wellsprings*

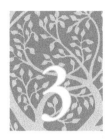

# Spirituality, Suffering, and Beliefs
## *The Soul of Healing with Families*

### LORRAINE M. WRIGHT

I first experienced suffering from illness in my childhood. My grandmother, who lived with us, suffered severe chronic pain from rheumatoid arthritis. I felt the demoralizing effects of suffering, whether it was observing my grandmother's suffering or as I suffered with her. I also learned that her chronic pain controlled all of our lives, how well my brother and I would behave on any given day, how much my grandmother was able to "mother," and how we children became more compassionate because of having a pain sufferer in the family. My grandmother was the center of our family, but the chronic pain she suffered ultimately ruled all our lives. The disease severely disfigured her hands, caused her knees to be swollen much of the time, resulted in her walking with a severe limp, and dictated how well she was able to live her life on any given day. But those disfigured hands made us apple pie, weeded our garden, and lifted numerous cups of tea while we exchanged stories of our lives with her. However, I do not recall as a child hearing *her* stories of suffering with chronic pain. Perhaps I did not listen. Perhaps these stories were not told.

I now have several questions that I would eagerly ask of her. What meaning and purpose did my grandmother give to this life of chronic pain? What did she believe was the best treatment or healing for her pain? What did she believe helped to soften her suffering? What made it worse? What made it better? What help or hindrance were her spiritual/religious beliefs? What invited her to reconnect with her Roman Catholic faith in her later years? Did she pray for relief of pain or to endure the pain? Did she pray at all? What did she believe health professionals did to help or hinder her healing? Which was worse: emotional, physical, or spiritual suffering? I wonder whether these kinds of conversations would have been healing for *both* my grandmother and me.

As a family therapist/nurse educator working predominantly with families experiencing serious illness, I have had the privilege of engaging in numerous therapeutic conversations about experiences of illness suffering. These conversations invariably include family members' descriptions of suffering, the meaning they give to their suffering, their wonder about the spiritual nature of their suffering, and their beliefs about their illness experience. I have become a passionate observer of and participant in the healing effect that occurs in the biopsychosocial–spiritual structure of family members and myself when suffering is softened.

## SPIRITUALITY, SUFFERING, AND BELIEFS: THE TRINITY MODEL

A new trinity has emerged in my practice with families experiencing serious illness: spirituality, suffering, and beliefs. I have found it impossible to think about spirituality without thinking about suffering and beliefs. And I have found it equally impossible to think about suffering without talking about spirituality and beliefs. These three notions are thoroughly intertwined and interrelated. Therefore, I named this interconnection "the trinity model" (Wright, 2005). I discuss each of these concepts separately in order to justifiably bring them together later.

### *Spirituality*

The influence of family members' spiritual and religious beliefs on their illness experience has been one of the most neglected areas in family work. However, family therapists have woken up to this neglected aspect of spirit in human experience. Increasing numbers of articles have appeared in professional journals, and the book in which this chapter appears was one of the first to signal this awakening of the ever-present spiritual aspects in our privileged work with families.

My own clinical experiences with families have taught me that the experience of suffering from illness becomes transposed to one of spirituality as family members try to make meaning out of their suffering and distress. To understand how family members offer compassion and what efforts they make to alleviate suffering, it is imperative that therapists explore religious and spiritual beliefs in clinical work with families. It is through the medium of therapeutic conversations about beliefs, suffering, and spirituality that hope and healing with families becomes possible.

The most significant learning about suffering that I have gleaned in my clinical work with families over 30 years is that a discourse about suffering invariably opens up a discourse about spirituality if we, families and therapists, are open to it. Suffering invites and leads us into the spiritual domain. A shift to and emphasis on spirituality is frequently the most profound response to suffering from illness. If family therapists are to be helpful, we must acknowledge that suffering and the meaning attributed to it are ultimately spiritual issues.

Colleagues and students alike have offered their unsolicited observations on the "spiritual" aspects of my therapy for several years. I found these observations fascinating, because I had not put any direct or intended emphasis about spiritual issues in family work. Only rarely did I mention my own spiritual and religious beliefs as a Christian and, specifically, as a practicing Mormon. I reflected that somehow I must have changed from my early years as a therapist, because this feedback was news of a difference. One very curious observation came when a valued colleague told me that he would describe my clinical work as "secular theology." This comment perturbed me for some time. He elaborated and suggested what he believed to be the most powerful aspect of my clinical work with families: the notion of "reverencing" that occurred between families/clients and myself. In those moments of reverencing, there is profound awe and respect for the individuals seated in front of you. It is not a linear phenomenon in these moments. I feel that same reverencing from family members being given back to me. In these moments of reverencing in clinical work something very special happens between the therapist and the family; it is something felt by all—a deep emotional connection. I know and have felt these moments in therapy, both in the therapy room and from behind the one-way mirror as a supervisor or team member. During these times, I have witnessed the most profound changes in family members' thinking, behavior, illness experience, and, most importantly, in the softening of suffering. In these instances, I have felt an emotion that seems to arise only when there is reverencing. This emotion I submit is pure love. I have come to understand and recognize moments of reverencing as the spiritual care practices of my clinical work that perhaps invite colleagues and students to comment that they observe a "spiritual" aspect to my work with families. I hope this is so, because I believe it makes a quantum difference to the healing process when reverencing occurs.

The quiet intervention of prayer is also receiving more attention in clinical work with families and in my own practice. Dossey (1993) reviewed numerous medical studies examining the efficacy of prayer in producing physical changes. For example, he suggested that the ritual of prayer may trigger emotions that, in turn, may lead to changes in health by positively impacting the immune and cardiovascular systems.

Dossey summoned health professionals to recognize the many nonphysiological reasons that persons and families heal from illness. Over the past few years, I have on occasion adopted the practice of praying for, although not with, clients and families with whom I work. As Dossey (1993) suggested, if a health professional believes that prayer works, not to use it is analogous to withholding a potent medication or surgical procedure: "Both prayer and belief are nonlocal manifestations of consciousness, because both can operate at a distance, sometimes outside the patient's awareness. Both affirm that 'it's not all physical,' and both can be used adjunctively with other forms of therapy" (p. 141). In praying for our clients, we perhaps also heighten our connection with them, and our investment in their recovery and well-being.

In a clinical case analysis of the ways in which nurses open space to spirituality, my colleague and I identified four practices (McLeod & Wright, 2001). These included (1) opening space for the gift of listening, (2) maintaining curiosity and openness to surprise, (3) inviting reflection on spiritual/religious beliefs, and (4) invoking metaphor. These practices were embedded in the therapeutic conversations that evolved among the nurse, the family, and the clinical team.

## Beliefs

What one believes about illness contributes dramatically to how one experiences an illness. No two people and no two families have the same experience with the same disease, whether it is the common cold or multiple sclerosis. Some families view illness as a sign that they are sinful, and disease as a punishment for ungodly living. Other families believe that being ill is a natural physical sign that the ill member should slow down and take care of him- or herself, and no longer neglect his or her health. There are also many beliefs about how family members should behave when illness enters a family. At no time are family and individual beliefs more affirmed, challenged, or threatened than when illness emerges (Wright & Bell, in press).

These beliefs may be influenced by the stage in the family life cycle of the individual, the family, and the illness. How family members experience an illness depends on both the beliefs that they have embraced prior to the illness experience and the beliefs that evolve through the experience of the illness. The beliefs that family members hold are often reconstructed after the experience of an illness (i.e., blueprints are revised); conversely, family members' beliefs influence and shape the processes and outcomes of illness. For example, how family members treat even the common cold depends on their beliefs concerning how they "caught" the cold in the first place. If one believes that colds are related to experiences of loss, one will probably treat one's cold differently than if one believes a cold is due to inadequate rest and working long hours. The person who believes the best remedy for a cold is to rest, drink plenty of fluid, and take vitamin C will probably follow that regimen. If the treatment remedy does not work, will the person's belief about the etiology be maintained? Will there be more openness to other treatment remedies? Many factors influence what people consider treatment options when their original beliefs about the etiology and the cure of an illness have been challenged.

The core beliefs that I found most useful to uncover and explore with families about their illness experience include the following:

- Beliefs about suffering.
- Beliefs about etiology/cause of illness.
- Beliefs about diagnosis of illness.
- Beliefs about healing and treatment.
- Beliefs about prognosis/outcome.
- Beliefs about mastery/control and influence on illness.
- Beliefs about the place of illness in our lives and relationships.
- Beliefs about spirituality and religion.
- Beliefs about the role of family members.
- Beliefs about the role of health care professionals (Wright & Bell, in press).

Family therapists bring their own strong personal and professional beliefs about families and illness to the clinical domain. Their beliefs influence how they view, assess, and—most importantly—care for and intervene with families. For example, a family therapist's beliefs about etiology may influence how a family is received, perceived, and treated. A therapist who believes alcoholism is a consequence of irresponsibility and personal weakness will likely respond differently to a family experiencing alcoholism than to a family experiencing the effects of a congenital heart defect, an illness over which a health professional may believe the individual or family has no control. The core beliefs of family therapists that affect relationships with families are their beliefs about illness, about families, about change, and about their own role as therapists in the lives of family members.

## Suffering

The simple desire to comfort and to care for others in times of illness is an honorable and sufficient foundation from which to engage in therapeutic conversations that are conducive to opening discussion about suffering and spirituality. The alleviation or diminishment of suffering has always been the cornerstone of caring. But what *is* suffering? I conceptualize suffering as physical, emotional, or spiritual anguish, pain, or distress. Experiences of suffering can include serious illness that alters one's life and relationships forever; forced exclusion from everyday life; heartache and heartbreak; and interference with love relationships.

Beliefs of patients and family members are involved in both the experience of suffering and in making inferences about suffering. Certain beliefs may conserve or maintain an illness; others may exacerbate symptoms; still others alleviate or diminish suffering (Wright et al., 1996). When therapists invite persons to reflect on their beliefs, those persons often become more open to consider other possibilities.

In an eloquent and illuminating description of his illness experiences, Frank (1995) offers his idea of how persons make meaning of their suffering. He asserts that people tell stories of their illnesses to make sense of their suffering, and that when they turn their diseases into stories, they find healing. From my own clinical practice and research with families plus the contribution of other colleagues to this area, I have come to believe strongly that talking about the illness experience has the potential to be healing.

I believe that my goal and obligation when working with families is to soften emotional, physical, and spiritual suffering.

## Acknowledging Suffering and the Sufferer

One beginning effort to soften suffering is to acknowledge that suffering exists. Suffering *is* the illness experience, whether it is short and intense or prolonged and pervasive. Suffering is part of our human existence—from stories of Job to stories of Holocaust victims to stories of illness. The deliberate and clear acknowledgment of suffering by therapists frequently opens the door for the disclosure of clients' other fears or worries not previously expressed, for example, the worry of a caregiver that should her health fail, who would care for her spouse? We have also been impressed that acknowledgment of suffering can even occur and invite healing in busy health care units, where there is limited contact with families (Wright & Leahey, 1999).

## Inviting, Listening to, and Witnessing Stories of Illness Suffering

Inviting, listening to, and witnessing stories of illness and suffering provide a powerful validation of a profound human experience. Health professionals are in a privileged position to hear and affirm illness narratives. By acknowledging illness narratives, we engage in the essential ethical practice of recognizing the ill person as the "suffering other" (Frank, 1994). In my clinical practice, I also want to open possibilities, through therapeutic conversations, for recognizing the ill person and other family members as the heroic other, the joyful other, the giving other, the receiving other, the compassionate other, the passionate other, and the strengthened other.

Positive responses and reduction in emotional and physical suffering have convinced me of the necessity to invite family members to tell their stories of illness. In our professional encounters with families, we move beyond social conversations about the illness to purposeful therapeutic conversations (Tapp, 1997). We direct the conversation in a manner that we hope will give voice to the human experiences of suffering and symptoms, as well as courage, hope, growth, and love.

By providing a context for the sharing among family members of their illness experiences, intense emotions are legitimized. I have had many family members tell me that having someone listen to their illness stories, ask questions about their stories, acknowledge their suffering, and commend them for their courage in the face of suffering has enabled them to gain a new and sometimes renewed appreciation of their strengths and ability to cope. Through this acknowledging, witnessing, listening, and commending (Bohn, Wright, & Moules, 2003; Hougher Limacher & Wright, 2003; Moules, 2002), the family's resilience is often rediscovered with very positive outcomes. In many instances, these positive outcomes have included the alleviation of physical symptoms and familial conflict, as well as emotional and/or spiritual suffering: One of our most difficult duties as human beings is to listen to the voices of those who suffer.

## Challenging Our Own Constraining Beliefs

Health professionals' beliefs can hinder or enhance the possibilities for softening of suffering (Levac et al., 1998; Moules, 2002; Wright, Bell, Watson, & Tapp, 1995). One belief frequently offered by health professionals to those with illness is that "life could be worse." This belief frequently enhances suffering due to its lack of sensitivity to another's suffering. We need to recognize that each person's suffering is unique and connected to his or her beliefs. What we believe enhances or softens our suffering, and we as health professionals can inadvertently trivialize suffering through our own constraining beliefs.

### Creating a Healing Environment

The ultimate desired outcome is to create a healing environment for family members that relieves their suffering from illness experiences. Remen (1993) eloquently offered the notion that healing is different from curing: "Healing is a process we're all involved in all the time. . . . Sometimes people heal physically, and they don't heal emotionally, or mentally, or spiritually. And sometimes people heal emotionally, and they don't heal physically" (p. 344).

Frank (1995) offers the powerful metaphor that ill people are more than victims of disease or medical patients—they are wounded storytellers. He argues that people tell stories to make sense of their suffering; when they turn their diseases into stories, they find healing. This coincides with the strong belief in our North American health care culture that eliciting, discussing, and expressing one's illness story and accompanying emotions can be very healing. In my clinical practice, family members have often remarked how they appreciated the opportunity to talk about their illness experiences, and the healing effect these conversations had on their lives and relationships.

The capacity of health professionals to be "witnesses" to the stories of suffering of patients and families is central to providing care; it is frequently the genesis of healing.

### Inviting Reflections about Suffering

To alter existing beliefs, family therapists need to invite family members to reflect about their constraining beliefs (Wright et al., 1996). Through these reflections, a person begins to entertain more facilitating beliefs that lead him or her out of a state of confusion, struggle, or suffering. For example, beliefs about hope and optimism in the illness experience have generally not been addressed by the dominant medical system. Consequently, the appeal of alternative or complementary healing approaches becomes very understandable. Many persons with illness find these approaches more positive than the conventional medical approach, because complementary healing approaches do not shy away from some of the big questions surrounding illness: Why has this illness happened to me? Why do people get sick despite living well? Why do some people die "before their time"?

## Offering Compassion

Compassion, or the Latin root *pati cum*, literally means "to suffer with." The Latin root of *patient* means "one who suffers." So offering compassion is an interactional phenonemon in the context of clinical practice. Based on some fascinating recent research, offering compassion and love seems to affect all of our human systems (e.g., emotions, brain activity, and spirituality; Post & Neimark, 2007). New brain imaging studies show the lighting up of certain areas of the brain during acts of compassion, whereas other studies link compassion and spirituality (Post & Neimark, 2007).

## CLINICAL EXAMPLE: "WHERE WILL I GO *AFTER* I DIE?"

I offer the following clinical example to illustrate the interrelatedness of the trinity of spirituality, suffering, and beliefs, specifically, the trinity model, and its application in clinical practice (Wright, 2005).

This family consists of a 63-year-old English Canadian husband and his 62-year-old French Canadian wife. They have two grown children living elsewhere. The husband experienced a myocardial infarction 6 months prior to this session. The family had been seen for two sessions prior to my being invited for a consultation. The couple had made good progress in these two sessions and reported to me that talking in therapy about how the illness had impacted their marriage had helped to bring forth a lot of worries and fears that each was experiencing. Consequently, they reported that they were now talking more at home, having breakfast together for the first time in many years, and feeling understood by each other.

When I work with families in which one spouse has experienced a heart attack, I routinely ask the nonaffected partner if he or she worries about the spouse having another heart attack. In this case, the wife responded, "Yes, all the time." When I ask the husband if he worries about having another coronary, he confirms that he *does not* worry about dying from a heart attack. The most fascinating aspect of this therapeutic inquiry occurrs when the wife discloses her belief that *she* is going to have a heart attack. She also discloses that she has been on antidepressant medication for 20 years because of her fear of dying. In this verbatim transcript of my clinical work with this family, a significant distinction is made. (LMW indicates Dr. Lorraine Wright; W indicates wife; H indicates husband.)

LMW: So when you say (*addresses wife*) that you have a fear of dying, what do you mean by that?

W: I don't know where I'm going to go, that's the fear. I'm afraid. I don't know where I'm going to go, I don't know why, I mean. I don't know if it's the religion, or the school, I mean it's the way I was brought up.

LMW: So you're saying that the biggest worry around that for you is not how you're going to die, is it? But, where you're going to go after you die?

W: Exactly.

LMW: I see.

W: Exactly.

This is a fascinating and most important distinction and self-disclosure. This dear woman clarifies that it's not her fear of dying that is most troublesome but rather her fear of where she's going to go *after* she dies. Further clarification of this belief then ensues.

W: If you're good, then you're going to heaven, and if you're bad, you're going to hell. So it was always on my mind, everything was a sin, so I grew up like that and I was afraid of everything, and it's still on my mind today.

LMW: Hmmm.

W: So to me, I always see the clock (*gestures a pendulum*) and if you're good (*gestures to one side*) and if you're bad (*gestures to the other side*), and there's no middle. I don't know where I'm going to go.

LMW: So when you evaluate your life today, [wife's name], would you say . . .

W: Well, I was bad sometimes, like everybody else . . .

LMW: Sure . . .

W: But then many times or most of the times, but uh . . .

LMW: But when you evaluate your life now and you look at your life, do you feel good about how you've lived your life?

W: Yes, sure . . .

LMW: Do you think, uh . . .

W: Sure, I wouldn't change my life, even though we went through a lot, I mean, with family and everything, but I wouldn't change my life anyway.

LMW: I wonder, I mean, I know quite a bit about Catholicism, but maybe you can help me more. Do you believe that you will be judged for the way you've lived your life here?

W: By God, you mean?

LMW: By God.

W: Exactly, yes.

LMW: And so, if God were to judge you today, do you think He would be happy with you . . .

W: I don't know.

LMW: . . . or not happy?

W: This is what I'm asking myself, you see.

LMW: Ah . . . and what do you say to yourself?

W: We all know in my family I'm afraid to die, even my children. I kept telling them, really so many times a month, I'm afraid, I'm not afraid to be sick or something, it's to die . . .

LMW: It's to die being fearful how you will be judged.

After this significant disclosure and further clarification of her beliefs, I make a beginning effort to challenge this constraining belief. I do this by asking a question that I routinely ask in my practice: a hypothetical facilitating belief question (Wright & Bell, in press). This question offers or embeds a facilitating belief and is an indirect way of challenging or altering a constraining belief. The question always begins, "If you were to believe . . . " The question invites this woman to consider an alternative facilitating belief, one that suggests altering her beliefs may give rise to new stories and new behaviors.

LMW: This might seem like a very strange question, but I'm going to ask it anyway. If you were to believe, eh, if you were to believe for even ten minutes today that God was very pleased with you, at how you've lived your life as a wife, as a mother, as a person . . .

W: That would change everything.

LMW: What difference would that make in your life?

W: It would change everything for me.

LMW: Can you tell me what it would change? What would be a couple of things that would change for you?

W: First of all, I wouldn't be scared anymore, and then, I would say, well, if I die tomorrow, well, I die tomorrow, then I know where I would go. God knows when.

LMW: And if you weren't scared anymore, how would you live your life differently, do you think? What would be different for you?

W: Well, I would be more, um, calm . . .

LMW: More calm . . .

W: Definitely, because it's all inside, it's working on me all the time and, uh, I wouldn't live that stress that I live all the time and . . . if you understand what I mean?

LMW: Yes, I do—if you could believe, I just want to really make sure I've got this—if you could believe even just for 10 minutes that God was pleased with you, that you had lived a good life, that He would judge you, eh, very well, then you said that would make all the difference in the world for you . . .

W: Exactly, yes, definitely.

LMW: . . . that you would be more calm, and you would be more . . .

W: I wouldn't be on anybody's nerves like I am on account of death—something to do with it, too.

LMW: Yes. Wow, that's incredible, eh?

Here is a woman who has suffered terribly for many years with the belief that she will have a heart attack *and* an even more troubling belief that she doesn't know how she will be judged when she dies. Consequently, she does not know where she will go after death.

In this next transcript, an amazing revelation comes forth. This woman has considered discontinuing all of her antidepressant medication. Of course, I'm curious to learn, if she believed she was going to heaven, would she need less medication? Her responses are astonishing, and her beliefs begin to change right in front of me within our evolving therapeutic conversation. Her response is even more amazing as she completes my sentence for me and knows exactly the connection that I am hypothesizing.

LMW: I don't know, maybe this is a crazy idea, but I'm wondering, um, do you think that if you could believe that you were going to heaven, do you think there's any connection there; that you would need . . .

W: . . . less pills?

LMW: That you need less pills, yes.

W: Sure, definitely.

LMW: Wow. So maybe this idea, eh, that if you have the courage, and are more positive . . .

W: Yes, just like a lightning (*points to head, light bulb?*), hey?

LMW: You start thinking that "yes, I am a good person, I will, eh, probably be judged very well, eh, by God, and, um, be able to go to heaven." And I want you to know I have those same religious beliefs about heaven . . .

W: You do?

LMW: . . . and hell, and that will we be judged, and I hope I do okay too, eh, but I don't worry about it all the time like you do. That must be a terrible thing.

W: Oh, it is terrible, sometimes I used to say to [her husband], it's terrible, you don't know what I feel inside, it's like I could scream.

LMW: Yes . . .

W: Some days I used to say, "I would prefer to die," but still I said, "I don't want to die."

LMW: So you think there could be a connection there. So, as you would come off the pills, maybe then you would be getting more courage about believing, eh, more positively about yourself.

W: Exactly.

At the end of this session, I offer my impressions and commendations to this family. I offer what I believe I have learned from this couple, particularly from this open, courageous woman. I also relate to her how I would like to tell her story to others.

LMW: I want to tell you a couple of my impressions and a couple of things that I've learned from you today. The first thing I have learned is that you've been married 38 years, and the thing that you've really taught me today is that even after 38 years of marriage, marriage can get better, it doesn't have to get worse, eh?

W and H: Yes, yes.

W: I'm so happy about that.

LMW: That you would probably say, I'm guessing, that you would say your marriage maybe is perhaps the best it has ever been, would you go that far?

W: Exactly, yes.

LMW: One of the best . . .

W: For me, yes.

LMW: . . . one of the best periods in your marriage . . .

H: Oh, the best period for us.

LMW: . . . period in your marriage.

H and W: Definitely, yes.

LMW: See, that is incredible, I think. After 38 years, it's even getting better. This is one thing I've really learned today, that we should never give up hope on marriages. That they can even get better, even after many, many years of marriage. The other thing that I've learned today that was very helpful to me is this notion that illness doesn't always have to be a terrible thing in a family, that illness sometimes can be scary, it can be a terrible thing, but some very good positive things can come out of it. Your marriage is stronger, you've come together, you've united more, and that's a very wonderful thing. The other thing (*addresses wife*), when I go back to Calgary, my students will be asking me, "What did you learn?" I'm going to think about you, and you know the story I would like to tell—can I tell you?—is the story about a woman who believed for many, many years—eh, I feel very touched by this story . . . but—a woman who believed for many years that maybe she was going to be judged very harshly by God, eh? That she wasn't sure if she would go to heaven or hell, and yet through her own courage, eh, she made a connection that maybe if she could give up this medication, there was connection there that maybe she didn't have to be on medication any more, if she could begin to have more ideas and better beliefs about herself. That she was a good person and a good wife, and a good mother. And as she started to just think about that a little bit, and allow herself that idea, she also came up with the idea that maybe she could give up her antidepressant medication of 20 years! That is a remarkable story that I would like to be able to tell.

It is my hope that this transcript of my clinical work demonstrates the interconnection between spirituality, suffering, and beliefs. I also trust that this illustrates the phenomenon of reverencing between this courageous woman and me. As our conversation evolved, I believe that we experienced increasing awe, respect, and a deep emotional and spiritual connection. As we said good-bye to one another, she told me that she had not wanted to come to the session that day, but was very grateful that she did. She also spontaneously hugged me as we bid each other good-bye. And I hugged her back.

## CONCLUDING REFLECTIONS

The depth of people's suffering is distinguished by each person's unique experience. I have ached, cried, and lamented when I have suffered for others, but it is only my own suffering that I have experienced firsthand. Experiences of suffering cannot be compared, but unfortunately comparisons *are* made about which suffering we believe is the most horrific. Our most important role as therapists is to be listeners and witnesses to others' suffering. We must acknowledge suffering and the sufferer; ask questions that challenge any constraining beliefs that may be exacerbating family members' suffering; and encourage more facilitating beliefs, possibilities, and opportunities for healing and hope through our questions and commendations.

Through this exchange between family members and therapists about suffering, a domain of spirituality is encountered. This journey into spirituality manifests itself in the offering of reverencing, compassion, and love between and among family members and therapists. Likewise, these efforts to soften suffering cross the border into healing—healing that is reserved not only for family members but also for therapists. As Frank (1995) suggests, the primary lesson that the ill have to offer us is the "pedagogy of suffering." Through this highly privileged exchange, spirituality, suffering, and beliefs become the new trinity and the soul of healing in our clinical work with families.

## REFERENCES

Bohn, U., Wright, L. M., & Moules, N. J. (2003). A family systems nursing interview following a myocardial infarction: The power of commendations. *Journal of Family Nursing, 9*(2), 151–165.

Dossey, L. (1993). *Healing words: The power of prayer and the practice of medicine*. San Francisco: Harper.

Frank, A. W. (1994). Interrupted stories, interrupted lives. *Second Opinion, 20*(1), 11–18.

Frank, A. W. (1995). *The wounded storyteller: Body, illness and ethics*. Chicago: University of Chicago Press.

Hougher Limacher, L., & Wright, L. M. (2003). Commendations: Listening to the silent side of a family intervention. *Journal of Family Nursing, 9*(2), 130–135.

Levac, A. M., McLean, S., Wright, L. M., Bell, J. M., "Ann," & "Fred." (1998). A "Reader's Theatre" intervention to managing grief: Post-therapy reflections by a family and a clinical team. *Journal of Marital and Family Therapy, 24*(1), 81–94.

McLeod, D. L., & Wright, L. M. (2001). Conversations of spirituality: Spirituality in family systems nursing—making the case with four clinical vignettes. *Journal of Family Nursing, 7*(4), 391–415.

Moules, N. J. (2002). Nursing on paper: Therapeutic letters in nursing practice. *Nursing Inquiry, 9*(2), 104–113.

Post, S., & Neimark, J. (2007). *Why good things happen to good people*. New York: Broadway Books.

Remen, R. N. (1993). Wholeness. In B. Moyers (Ed.), *Healing and the mind* (pp. 343–363). New York: Doubleday.

Tapp, D. M. (1997). *Exploring therapeutic conversations between nurses and families experiencing ischemic heart disease*. Unpublished doctoral dissertation, University of Calgary, Alberta, Canada.

Wright, L. M. (2005). *Spirituality, suffering, and illness: Ideas for healing*. Philadelphia: Davis.

Wright, L. M., Bell, J. M., Watson, W. L., & Tapp, D. (1995). The influence of the beliefs of nurses: A clinical example of a post-myocardial-infarction couple. *Journal of Family Nursing, 1*, 238–256.

Wright, L. M., & Leahey, M. (1999). Maximizing time, minimizing suffering: The 15 minute (or less) family interview. *Journal of Family Nursing, 5*(3), 259–273.

Wright, L. M., & Bell, J. M. (in press). *Beliefs and Illness: A model for healing*. Calgary, Canada: 4th Floor Press.

# Spiritual Resources in Family Adaptation to Death and Loss

## FROMA WALSH

> Perhaps they are not stars in the sky, but rather
> openings where our loved ones shine down to let us
> know they are happy.
> —NATIVE AMERICAN SAYING

Throughout the world and across millennia, spiritual beliefs and practices have provided solace and support to individuals, families, and their communities in times of death and loss. The theologian Paul Tillich (1952) has noted that the anxiety of fate and death is the most basic, universal, and inescapable of life's dilemmas. Some anthropologists have even claimed that religion was invented, above all else, to help people accept death, not as a final ending, but rather as a transition to continuing life in another realm. As Malinowski (1965) stated: "Death, which of all human events is the most upsetting and disorganizing to [human] calculations, is the main source of religious beliefs" (p. 71).

Spirituality involves streams of experience that flow through all aspects of life, intertwined with cultural influences. Faith beliefs and practices come to the fore in dealing with life's end and the loss of loved ones. They offer comfort, hope, support, and connection. They address the very meaning of life and death, as well as the mystery of afterlife. They provide guidance in how surviving family members can honor the deceased, mourn their loss, and continue life passage. In some cases, spiritual distress concerning death can contribute to prolonged suffering and to relational conflict or estrangement. Yet mental health professionals have tended to neglect this vital dimension in their therapeutic approach. This chapter examines the profound significance of spirituality with death and loss, and offers case illustrations and guidelines for including the spiritual dimension in clinical practice.

## INTERTWINING OF RELIGION AND CULTURE

Although death and loss are universal, all cultures and religions approach the end of life and mourning processes in their own ways. Most cultures are fortunate in having a worldview that helps individuals, families, and communities to face the inescapable fact of death, including the rhythms of life and an abiding faith in some continuity beyond death. Many cultures provide rich traditions, rituals, and ceremonies to help them prepare for and deal with this major transition.

Religions and cultures over the ages have also recognized the significant impact of loss and the expression of grief by survivors. In ancient Mesopotamia, tiny vials holding tears were buried with the deceased. Before Roman times, Etruscan ceramic jars containing the ashes of the deceased were decorated with sculptures of weeping mourners (usually women). A Jewish proverb holds that just as soap cleanses the body, tears cleanse the soul. In Judaism, grief is considered a natural part of being human—the more we push grief away or hold it back, the less fully able we are to embrace love. Judaism teaches that in a world where everything that comes to be also passes away, respect for the grieving process allows us to honor that reality more fully and keep our hearts open and available to love again. In choosing the joy and richness of a life full of love, we must become comfortable with the grief that accompanies love.

Many religious customs surrounding death are rooted in early paganism or superstition in the ancient world and the Middle Ages. The Jewish practice of covering the mirrors in a house of mourning originated in the belief that the spirit of the dead hovers in the home and, confused by its own image, may take up permanent residence. This custom is still widely practiced, but its meaning has been transformed: to banish vanity at times of grief, when people should focus not on their physical image but on inner, spiritual dimensions of life (Kertzer & Hoffman, 1996).

In 20th-century North America, with the advent of modern medicine, hospitals, and nursing homes, death became institutionalized and removed from natural life. Most family members no longer died at home, surrounded by loved ones. Anglo-American culture tended to deny and to minimize the impact of death and grief (Becker, 1973). The dominant society, even today, urges the bereaved to get over loss quickly: to put it behind them, regain control of emotions, and get "closure."

Western belief systems and medical ethos have heightened the dilemma of acceptance of death in their emphasis on mastery over destiny and in treatments to "conquer" death. The end of life is often approached with dread, in terms of loss of control, failure of treatments, lack of will, or insufficient spiritual purity. By contrast, Eastern and indigenous spiritual traditions approach death not only in terms of the human life cycle but also as a natural part of the larger life cycle of all living beings, the earth, and the cosmos. Buddhism teaches that in accepting death we discover life (Rinpoche, 1994).

For Buddhists, as death approaches, relatives, friends, and/or monks gather and assist the dying process by chanting Buddhist *sutra*. The dying and loved ones are encouraged to relate with warmth and caring to what is happening rather than struggling against it or distancing in fear. It is considered preferable to tell the dying the truth, so that they have the opportunity to put affairs in order, say their good-byes, and repair past hurts or injustices. Although difficult for close friends, partners, and family members, this time is considered the greatest opportunity to communicate caring, love, and trust, with no hypocrisy or lies to please, as happens at other times in life. Speaking the ultimate truth is experienced as extremely beautiful. Relating with the dying person in this way conveys a shared acknowledgment that death is approaching, and that those who are important want to be fully present through this time. Despite leaving family, friends, and favorite surroundings, the continuity of significant relationships is unbroken by death. This demonstration of love and connection offers tremendous comfort and inspiration to the dying person and to survivors (His Holiness the Dalai Lama, 2002; Nhat Hahn, 2002).

Immigrants often turn to their traditional cultural and spiritual connections as they face death and loss. For instance, the waves of Polish immigrants that settled in Chicago over the past century fueled construction of neighborhood Catholic churches and several large cathedrals, even though residents were poor. The church, regarded as the center of the community, holds most importance at death; as one woman remarked to her hospice chaplain: "I want to die under my own bells."

Those from Eastern and indigenous cultures who are facing death and loss may turn to various forms of spiritualism concurrently with Western medicine and formal religion. It is crucial to inquire about traditional spiritual beliefs and practices that pertain to death and loss, such as ancient Asian customs of ancestor worship, African healing rituals (Somé, 1994; see Kamya, Chapter 15, this volume), and *espiritismo* for many Latin Americans (see Falicov, Chapter 8, this volume). Family members may believe that spirits who protect or harm can prevent or cause death, and can be influenced by good or evil deeds. Sudden death and life-threatening illness may be seen and treated as possession by spirits. Crystals, incense, candles, or special potions may be used to ward off death. Visitations by spirits of the deceased are common in many cultures, so they should not be presumed to be pathological delusion. The Mexican Day of the Dead celebrates the annual reunion of loved ones with the deceased at the grave site, decorated and lit with candles "to show the way" of return. The enjoyment of shared food and company co-mingles sadness with joy and comfort in feeling the presence of the departed.

We must be cautious not to superimpose our society's dominant Judeo-Christian European template of values on other faith beliefs and practices. Deloria (1994) tells of attending the burial of a Sioux Indian in a Christian cemetery:

> After the body was in the grave . . . an old woman stepped forward and put an orange on the grave. The Episcopal priest who had conducted the service rushed over and took the orange away, saying, "When do you think the departed will come and eat this orange?" One of the Sioux men standing there said, "When the soul comes to smell the flowers!" No one said anything after that. (p. 171)

In contemporary North American society, with growing spiritual diversity *within* families (see Walsh, Chapter 1, this volume), conflicting approaches to death and bereavement are likely to arise. Many people have left the religious affiliation of their family of origin; with death and loss they may feel spiritually bereft as well. Some seek new spiritual paths or blend traditions; many create their own meaningful observance (see Imber-Black, Chapter 12, this volume). Those who are religious may expect that for a "good" death and spiritual afterlife, all prescribed rituals from their tradition must be followed, such as last rites, "proper" burial, or cremation ceremonies. Such matters can be highly contentious in families and lead to cutoffs, especially if not discussed and planned in advance. This is a common dilemma in interfaith marriages, as in the following case.

> Rachel, who was Jewish, faced unexpected challenges with her husband's death. An Ethiopian immigrant, he had left the Orthodox Church of his upbringing and regarded himself as a secular humanist. As he was dying, his desire was for a simple memorial service and burial where his wife could one day be buried at his side. His siblings, who had

not been close in recent years or involved during his illness, suddenly appeared at his death, insisting that he must have a traditional funeral presided over by an Orthodox priest or else he would go to hell. Knowing he did not share that belief and would not have wanted that, Rachel challenged their strong pressure, while respecting their faith and concern. She sought out the interfaith chaplain who had married them at the college where they had met as students. Now retired, he was most pleased to conduct the service in the campus interfaith chapel.

Arranging burial was more challenging. Rachel was shocked to learn that only Jews could be buried at the Jewish cemetery near their home. Fortunately, she found another Jewish cemetery in a nearby community that had an interfaith section in a lovely hillside setting. She found it comforting, and knew that her husband would have been content, that the arch at the entrance bore the words BEIT OLAM, which has the same meaning in Hebrew and in his native language, Amharic: "at home in the world."

As families approach the end of life, therapists can facilitate discussion and mediate conflict to help family members understand and honor the wishes of a dying or deceased member. We can help them to avoid polarization and to respect and accept varied spiritual pathways at times of death and loss.

## RELIGIOUS BELIEFS
## ABOUT DEATH, LOSS, AND AFTERLIFE

Surveys have found that most Americans strongly affirm beliefs in God, miracles, and life after death (Gallup & Lindsey, 1999). One-third report that a profound spiritual experience has dramatically altered their lives, often at times of loss or threatened loss. Many believe that God intends for them to seek greater purpose in life out of a painful loss. Others find solace in the belief that death and loss are part of God's plan and greater wisdom, which may be beyond human comprehension. Some find strength in the belief that "God only gives us what we can handle," yet others may be offended or feel that their loss was trivialized when well-intentioned relatives, friends, or therapists offer such inspirational homilies to cheer them up.

### Death and Dying

For most people, whether or not they are religious, death and dying bring to the fore existential questions about the meaning and significance of life

(Yalom, 2008). These are, in essence, spiritual concerns and should not be neglected in therapy. In approaching death, those who believe that their lives belong to God are less likely to worry about having completed their lifework. They are much more likely to express concern about not being forgiven by God, dying when they are "cut off from God," or not having a blessing from a family or clergy member (Gallup & Lindsay, 1999). Although some faiths hold strong beliefs in miracles and curing, most acknowledge a point at which the acceptance of God's will is embraced.

Religious views weigh heavily on life-and-death decisions. Personal attitudes of Americans about abortion, euthanasia, and the death penalty vary within and across religions. Viewpoints are influenced by personal situations and reflect a blend of principle and pragmatism (Pew Forum on Religion and Public Life, 2008; see Walsh, Chapter 1, this volume). Most religious conservatives support human life on matters of abortion and euthanasia, strongly opposing both practices, yet they support capital punishment for convicted murderers (although the Catholic Church strongly opposes it). Younger people tend to be more liberal in these beliefs than their elders, often fueling intergenerational tensions within families.

For individuals and couples with diverse sexual orientation, issues are likely to surface around religious death rites in denominations that condemn homosexuality or don't allow burial of same-sex partners together. Painful legal dilemmas concern the rights of a bereaved life partner for survivor benefits and for legal status with nonbiological children raised together. Extended family members may step in at such times, generating conflict and complications. Family therapists or counselors can play a valuable mediating role. It is most helpful to be proactive, facilitating advance discussion, planning, and preparation of legal documents.

Religious beliefs can also complicate adaptation to loss due to stigmatized deaths, such as from HIV-AIDS. The HIV-AIDS epidemic over recent decades has had a profound impact for gay men, their loved ones, and the gay community as they have confronted suffering, untimely death, and issues of mortality. Many individuals and their families have hidden the illness or cause of death in fear of social and religious condemnation. In the face of these challenges, many have turned to more personal spirituality and faith as they engage in existential meaning-making processes (Miller, 2005a, 2005b).

Suicide is morally condemned by Jewish, Christian, and Islamic religions (Domino & Miller, 1992). The early Catholic Church forbade suicide to curtail the impulse to martyrdom. This prohibition was eventually codified in dogma stating that the deceased's soul was eternally condemned to hell, and for this reason the body could not be buried in consecrated grounds. Jewish tradition also withheld burial rituals from those who committed suicide. Islam holds that one who commits suicide will have to reexperience, over and over, the suicidal act.

End-of-life decision-making attitudes have been changing in recent years. More than two-thirds of all Americans now support the legalization of physician-assisted dying in some form. Since Oregon's Death with Dignity Act (see *www.oregon.gov/dhs*), a growing number of ethicists and mental health and health care associations have adopted policies supporting the right of mentally competent, terminally ill persons to exercise some decision-making choice for a peaceful and dignified death (see, e.g., American Public Health Association *www.apha.org/legislative/policy/policysearch/index.cfm*). They also urge the use of terms such as "aid in dying" or "patient-directed dying" rather than "suicide" or "physician-assisted suicide," which connotes mental illness and stigma, and is inappropriate, disrespectful, and distressing for terminally ill individuals and their loved ones.

Although scriptures and theology are generally interpreted as opposing euthanasia, most Protestants, Catholics, and Jews do support it, particularly when a physician agrees and it involves withholding heroic measures to sustain life if death is imminent and the quality of life is very poor. Those who are most religious tend to oppose any actions to hasten death. Yet, increasingly, medical and technological life-support interventions raise profound questions about just what a "natural" death is in our times. Individuals and families confront agonizing dilemmas: whether and when to prolong or to end life. Because such decisions and dissension among family members can haunt survivors and sever relationships, advance planning and discussion sessions are valuable and should include the dying person's wishes whenever possible. Beyond medical, legal, and relational issues, for many these are also profound spiritual matters that require thoughtful consideration in each case.

## Belief in Afterlife

Belief in a spiritual afterlife, offering transcendence over death, has been a core principle of most religious systems over the ages and across cultures (Spilka, Hood, Hunsberger, & Gorsuch, 2003). The belief in immortality in the ancient world has been documented in tombs and burial artifacts found in such places as Mesopotamia and China, the pyramids of Egypt, and pre-Inca cultures in South America. Elaborate rituals and offerings honored the deceased and ensured safe passage to the next world. In ancient Egypt and Peru, even pets were mummified and buried by the side of their masters to provide companionship in the life beyond.

The vast majority of Americans believe in an afterlife of some sort: 81% believe in heaven and nearly 70% believe in hell (Gallup, 2008). Most people believe they will be called before God on Judgment Day to answer for their sins. Seventy-five percent rate their own chances of going to heaven as good to excellent (even though a few of them aren't sure of its existence!).

Most Americans believe in angels; 50% believe in the devil; 33% believe in ghosts. Most envision some kind of journey in the afterlife and believe that their own experience will be positive. Over 15% report having had near-death experiences, often with vivid descriptions of their passage (Gallup & Lindsay, 1999). Most believe the soul resides in a spirit world for all eternity and find solace in the belief that when their time comes, they will join ancestors and be reunited with loved ones. Many believe they can be in contact with the deceased or receive visits from spirits, particularly in times of need, to offer reassurance to the bereft, or when a serious wrong has not been addressed. For believers, the spirits live on in the minds, hearts, dreams, and stories of loved ones. They can haunt as ghosts or become guardian angels and guiding spirits, inspiring best efforts and actions.

The vast majority of Americans link their actions on earth with the quality of their afterlife. The most common influences cited are everything one did in his or her life (84%); having had a spiritual awakening (69%); spiritual state at the time of death (78%); rituals at the time of death (23%); and rituals after death (20%). Evangelical and Pentecostal Christians are more inclined toward beliefs in the supernatural and in channeling, which allows a spirit temporarily to assume control of a human being during a trance state.

In Judaism, beliefs focus on attaining immortality through one's descendants, deeds, and achievements, and through the continuance of the Jewish people. Emphasis is placed on social consciousness and actions in this lifetime to repair the world (*tikkun olam*), improve conditions, and attend to injustices. Although the details of a spiritual afterlife are a matter of speculation, it is believed that these ideals serve to illuminate the dark path (Lamm, 2000).

Indian tribal religions approach death without fear, viewing human beings within the larger context as an integral part of the natural world (Deloria, 1994). Native Americans abhorred the common Yankee practice of hanging wrongdoers, believing that it blocked the ability of the soul to be released from the body in its last breaths. In death, as their souls enter the spirit world, they contribute their bodies to become the dust that nourishes the plants and animals, which in turn feed people during their lifetime. Because the individual, family, and community are seen as intertwined, death, although saddening, is a transitional event in a much larger life cycle and cosmic unity.

Nearly one-third of Americans believes in reincarnation; another 20% believe in the possibility. The recent rise in this belief reflects growing interest in Eastern religions among mainstream Americans, as well as increasing numbers of Hindus and Buddhists. In reincarnation, it is believed that after death, the soul or spirit may be reborn and inhabit other bodies (or life forms) in successive lives on earth before reaching *nirvana*, the highest spiritual attainment on the path of enlightenment.

In Eastern religions, as in many early cultures, death and rebirth have been considered essential elements of the never-ending life cycle (Obeyesekere, 2002). Hindus and Buddhists believe in *karma*, a natural chain of cause and effect. In reincarnation, one's present and future lives are determined by good or bad deeds in past and present lives (see Wolin, Taylor, Wolin, Ranganathan, Saymah, & Zeyada, Chapter 5, this volume).

The doctrine of reincarnation, while applying after death, refers very much to practices in this life. The *Tibetan Book of the Dead*, traditionally read aloud to the dying to help them attain liberation, in fact, offers practical advice to the living (Rinpoche, 1994). Beyond entrance into a state of luminosity, what happens after death is not discussed, because such questions are not considered useful in seeking reality in the here and now. A story is told about a man who asks a Zen master what to expect in the afterlife. He replies, "I do not know." The man queries, "How can that be? You are a Zen master!" His reply: "Yes, but I'm not a dead Zen master."

## HELPING FAMILIES WITH DEATH AND LOSS: TAPPING SPIRITUAL RESOURCES

Coming to terms with death and loss is the most difficult challenge couples and families must confront in their life course. As Robert Lifton (1975, p. vii) has noted, "There is no love without loss. And there is no moving beyond loss without some experience of mourning." The death of one's "soul mate" or "kindred spirit," a child, or a parent of young children is an especially profound loss that leaves a deep void.

### *Family Systems Approach*

Death shakes the foundations of family life and leaves no member unaffected. From a family systems perspective, death is a transactional process involving those who die, their survivors, and those who came before in the multigenerational life cycle. It involves multiple losses including each unique relationship with various members; the position in the family (only son, eldest child); role functions (matriarch, breadwinner); and hopes and dreams for the future. The death of a family member has an impact on the functioning of the family unit, with immediate and long-term reverberations for every member and all relationships. In turn, how the family handles loss can facilitate or hinder the adaptation of all (Walsh & McGoldrick, 2004).

Adaptation to loss does not mean resolution in terms of some complete "getting over it" or "closure." Recovery is best understood as a gradual process, spiraling over time, rather than an outcome. Unattended sorrow may persist (Levine, 2005). Responses vary widely; what is healthy or pathological must be considered in the context of individual coping styles, relationships to the deceased, family processes, legacies of past loss, and cultural norms. A family systems approach to practice facilitates the ability of family members to make meaning of their loss experience, to share their grief, to reorganize functional and relational patterns, to reconstruct their lives, and to love fully beyond loss.

### Continuing Bonds

Death ends a life but not a relationship. Traditional psychiatric views of mourning stressed the need to detach from or let go of the deceased loved one. Bereavement specialists now recognize that adaptive mourning processes involve the transformation of the relationship from physical presence to continuing bonds through spiritual connections (Neimeyer, 2001). These can be expressed in prayers, memories, dreams, deeds, and legacies. Rituals and storytelling are powerful way of honoring and sustaining bonds with the deceased, just as they have preserved connections with ancestors in indigenous cultures from the Australian Aborigines to Native American and African tribal groups.

### Loss in the Family Life Cycle

Deaths that are untimely, sudden, and/or violent can shatter core beliefs, such as "a normal life course," predictability, security, and basic trust (Walsh, 2007). The untimely death of "a good person" or an "innocent" child often is viewed as unjust and can affect the spiritual life of bereaved persons (Doka, 2002). Some draw closer to their faith, whereas others question or turn away from it. It is important for clinicians to explore and to normalize varied reactions. Some may question the existence of a loving God or become angry at God for an experienced injustice. Such responses are usually transient and need not result in permanent estrangement from cherished religious traditions (Gallup & Lindsay, 1999). However they can bring great anguish and precipitate a family or marital crisis.

> One couple was referred for counseling when their first baby died shortly after birth. The couple and entire extended family had greatly anticipated this child, who would have been the first son of the first son in a Greek Orthodox family. When the therapist asked the couple if their faith was some comfort to them, the wife tearfully said she now went alone to church, since her husband refused to go. He pounded his fist on the table, shouting, "I want no more of the church! I'm too angry at God!" As the therapist gently explored the meaning of the loss for him, he sobbed, "I believe that when something happens there's always a reason. I just can't fathom what the reason is here. We did everything right, by the book. I don't blame the doctors or the hospital; God took our son. And it's not fair—I don't mean for myself, but to my son. He never had a chance at life."

It is crucial to be compassionate with those who have experienced such a devastating loss, to understand the shockwaves rippling through the extended family, and to appreciate the struggle to make meaning of the experience. Consultation with a hospital chaplain can be helpful to address profound spiritual distress.

Spirituality involves dynamic processes that ebb and flow, changing in meaning and significance over the life course. Many who have viewed religion as unimportant in their lives find that it surfaces with unexpected intensity with death and loss. Some may become preoccupied with their sins, worrying about their salvation. Others try to bargain with God, promising to mend their ways if a loved one's life is saved. Still others who have accepted an interfaith marriage or lack of religious training for children may fear that a dying spouse or child one will not go to heaven. In such situations, spiritual distress may complicate recovery from loss, as in the following case.

> Kristin was referred for therapy by her mother-in-law, who was concerned about her inconsolable grief after the stillbirth of her second child. She had withdrawn from her husband and was taking her 4-year-old son daily to the grave. The counselor's exploration revealed Kristin's deep spiritual distress and guilt. Raised in a devout Catholic family, she had drifted away; similarly, her husband had not followed his family's observance of Judaism. Deeply in love, they had married in a civil ceremony with no religious rites. When they had their first child, they simply chose not to bring him up in either faith. However, the stillbirth of the second child struck Kristin, unexpectedly, as God's punishment for not having baptized her son. She had not told her husband or in-

laws of her concerns, fearing they would be upset by her religious convictions. It was important to combine individual and couple sessions to
involve both partners for mutual support, open communication, and
decision making regarding religious upbringing for their son and any
future children. They were also referred for consultation with a pastoral
counselor who specialized in interfaith issues.

The spiritual dimension of death and loss for children and adolescents
is often neglected. Even a young child who does not yet fully comprehend
death may pray for a critically ill grandparent, parent, sibling, or pet, and
imagine their spirit at death going to heaven (Biank & Sori, 2006). When
well-intentioned families try to protect children from the reality of death,
it can produce more anxiety, confusion, and upset. In the following case,
tapping the spiritual dimension of a mother's death brought relief for her
husband and small sons:

> Jim sought counseling for help with Brian and Kevin, ages 3 and 5,
> several months after their mother's death. Although the boys had been
> aware that their mother had been ill and hospitalized, Jim had not
> wanted to upset them by telling them she had died, and he didn't
> take them to the funeral. When they asked about her, be began taking
> them weekly to the cemetery to visit her grave, where he told them she
> was sleeping. As winter approached, the boys were increasingly anxious
> about their mother's well-being in the cold ground. The father was at a
> loss as to how to help them with her death.
>
> The therapist explored Jim's faith beliefs concerning what happens
> with death. He replied that, as a Christian, he believed in heaven and
> pictured his wife there, lovely and serene after the ordeal of her cancer.
> When asked if the boys had any notion of heaven, Jim reflected that,
> from saying prayers together, they imagined heaven as a beautiful place
> where Jesus lived with God, and where angels looked down to protect
> them. The therapist asked if it might comfort the boys more to think of
> their mother, not sleeping in the cold ground, but in heaven.
>
> Often, when the spiritual dimension is opened, clients who have
> been blocked are able to handle difficult situations with surprising wis-
> dom and clarity. When the boys were brought into the session, the
> father told them with great tenderness about their mother's death and
> how her spirit was now at peace forever in heaven. The boys were sad
> that she wouldn't be coming back but relieved to know she wouldn't
> suffer any more. They talked about heaven, that beautiful place where
> she would be with Jesus and the angels, and where she would watch
> over them through their lives. Jim assured them that they could still
> take flowers to her grave to honor and remember her.

Parents need to follow up such conversations and let children know that they can raise any questions or concerns that may arise. Artwork is helpful for children to express ideas and feelings about abstract notions of "spirit" and heaven (Biank & Sori, 2006), as well as memories of their relationship and ways to continue their bond.

In middle to later life, family members increasingly face the deaths of parents, siblings, friends, and other loved ones, as well as their own mortality. Not surprisingly, spirituality—in faith, prayer, and active congregational participation—gains importance for most people. Studies of widowhood find spirituality to be a strong, positive influence in successful adaptation (Glick, Weiss, & Parkes, 1974). As one widow described her abiding faith in God, "When I felt like life wasn't worth living anymore, I knew God loved me and would help me come through." One widower, who had never been "a churchgoer," found that his grief and loneliness were eased by reading passages in the Bible every evening, particularly the Psalms. Involvement in faith communities is especially valued by widow(er)s and those with limited kin or social contact. Most congregations support resilience through participation in activities such as choir singing, prayer groups, suppers, and social gatherings, as well as community service. Faith-based support groups help the bereaved find strength by assisting each other.

Over time, across the family life cycle, losses and their meanings are transformed and integrated with other life experience, particularly with other losses and new life. Naming a baby for a deceased relative, a Jewish custom, carries forth the spirit and memory of one who was loved and lost. When a past loss has been especially painful and unmourned, it may resurface around a recent or threatened loss, intensifying the emotional response and blocking adaptation (Walsh & McGoldrick, 2004).

> Roger, going through the breakup of his second marriage, began dreaming nightly of his beloved first wife Eve, who had died after a grueling battle with cancer. With friends urging him to move on and start a new life, he had plunged into remarriage without grieving his loss, then found himself unable to love again. The therapist encouraged him to visit Eve's grave—which he had not done since the funeral. There he meditated and talked to God about his love for her, seeking inspiration for a way to honor her and also go on with his life.

We need to counter the social pressure for immediate "closure" and emotional cutoff to approach mourning processes as an integral part in closing a chapter in the book of life that extends over the generations, from the past and into the future.

# SPIRITUAL RESOURCES IN COPING, ADAPTATION, AND RESILIENCE

In facing death and loss, a family support system, shared spiritual beliefs and practices, and a faith community can facilitate coping, adaptation, and resilience. Spiritual beliefs can foster a coherent worldview, meaning making, and a balanced sense of control and acceptance (Neimeyer, 2001; Pargament, 2007). The solace and hopefulness of strong faith are even more important than frequency of participation in religious services or activities. At the same time, caution is advised not to attribute failures to recover from illness to insufficient faith. As many clergy note, even the most pious saints died.

## Psychosocial–Spiritual Healing and Resilience

Families over the ages have turned to spiritual resources to cope with the precariousness of life and the disruptions wrought by death. Studies confirm that faith can facilitate family adaptation to loss (Greef & Joubert, 2007) and help parents to recover from the death of a child (Gilbert, 1992). Research suggests that beyond simply being religious, what matters most is being able to give meaning to a precarious situation, having faith that there is some greater purpose or force at work, and finding solace and strength in these outlooks (Koenig, McCullough, & Larson, 2001).

Healing involves a gathering of resources within the person, the family, and the community. Medical treatments may fail to cure a disease or to "defeat" death, but therapeutic efforts can foster psychosocial–spiritual healing at life's end and for survivors in the wake of loss. Therapy best fosters this healing impact by activating relational and spiritual lifelines (Walsh, 2006) for the relief of suffering, meaningful connection, and renewal of life passage for survivors.

## The Power of Prayer, Meditation, and Rituals

In facing death and loss, most people of all faiths turn to prayer or meditation for comfort and guidance. We've lost awareness of the frequency of childhood death in the past, revealed in the common nightly prayer, " . . . if I should die before I wake, I pray the Lord my soul to take." Half of all older adults say they want their doctors to pray with them as they face death (Gallup & Lindsay, 1999). As death approaches, meditation can ease anxiety, pain, and suffering as it offers a way to seek clarity and tranquility. Shared prayer or meditative experiences with loved ones can foster genuine and empathic communication at life's end, reduce emotional reactivity, and deepen couple and family bonds (see Gale, Chapter 13, this volume).

Religious rites and rituals connect individuals with their families and communities, and guide them through the passage of death and loss (Imber-Black, Roberts, & Whiting, 2003; see Imber-Black, Chapter 12, this volume). In the midst of shock and grief, they script and facilitate death and mourning processes through funeral, burial, and cremation rites, and prescribed ritual observances over the following months. The Catholic *wake* and Jewish practice of *shivva* bring friends and community members together to share memories of the deceased and to comfort the bereaved family. Rituals also connect a particular death and loss with all others as common human experience, offering participants a sense of collective self. For instance, on Yom Kippur, the holiest day of the Jewish year, all members of the congregation gather to grieve recent losses, to commemorate past losses, and to honor the survival of the Jewish people over the centuries.

It can be helpful to encourage a bereaved person to visit the grave and in other ways to reconnect spiritually with a deceased loved one. One couple planted a garden to remember their child and to yield new life with the seasons. One woman, who traveled frequently for her work, found it meaningful to visit a cathedral in each city, where she would light a candle in memory of her mother. Another woman took her fiancé to her father's graveside, to ask for his blessing to marry. One mother, as she was dying, asked her children to take her ashes to Ireland and scatter them on the land of her grandparents. It is never too late to gather for a remembrance:

> On the 20th anniversary of my mother's death, I wanted to find a meaningful way to commemorate her loss with my husband and daughter, who had never known her. A gifted musician, she had been the organist for our congregation and we shared a love of music, both sacred and secular. I thought of the carillon bells of Rockefeller Chapel on my campus at the University of Chicago, and arranged for a simple concert on the evening of the anniversary. We climbed to the carillon organ and to the top of the bell tower, where we listened to the glorious music filling the air. Looking out at the starry sky, I felt her spirit shining down.

### Traumatic Loss, Recovery, and Resilience

Spirituality has been found to be significant in resilience, particularly in healing and positive growth in the wake of traumatic loss (Calhoun & Tedeschi, 2001; Walsh, 2006; 2007; see Walsh [Chapter 2] and Wolin et al. [Chapter 5], this volume). A resilience-oriented practice framework directs

attention to strengths and resources in the midst of suffering and struggle that can be lifelines in recovery and renewal of life passage. Spiritual
resources are especially valuable in the face of epidemics such as HIV-AIDS
(Kamya, 2000) and in the wake of a major disaster (Koenig, 2006).

A team of family therapists from the American Family Therapy Academy shared a resilience approach with mental health professionals in Kosovo, in the aftermath of the "ethnic cleansing" campaign waged by Christian Serbs against Muslim Albanians (Becker, Sargent, & Rolland, 2000).
The deep Islamic faith of families and their spiritual connection with the
deceased were wellsprings for recovery and resilience.

> In one family, the mother heard the gunshots as her husband, two sons, and
> two grandsons were murdered in the yard of their farmhouse. She and her
> surviving family members talked with the consulting family therapy team
> about what kept them strong. The surviving son told them, "We are all
> believers. One of the strengths in our family is from God (Allah). . . . Hav-
> ing something to believe has helped very much." He was asked, "What do
> you do to keep faith strong?" He replied, "I see my mother as the 'spring of
> strength' . . . to see someone who has lost five family members—it gives us
> strength. We must think about the future and what we can accomplish. . . .
> If [my nephew] sees me strong, he will be strong. . . . When he [grows up]
> and helps the family—for him, it will be like seeing his father, grandfather
> and uncles alive again." (Becker et al., 2000, p. 29)

Resilience does not mean invulnerability in the face of loss, nor does it
mean simply bouncing back. Rather, resilience is forged by tapping personal,
relational, cultural, and spiritual resources for coping and mastery, and over
time integrating the full loss and recovery experience—the suffering, struggle, and strengths that were gained—into the fabric of individual, family,
and community life (Walsh, 2006). As loved ones pull together through
painful losses, relationships are strengthened and the family becomes more
resourceful in meeting future challenges.

Some survivors of traumatic loss become trapped in a victim position
or blocked from healing and growth by anger or desire for revenge. Spiritual
resources can be valuable in helping them to connect with their love for
deceased individuals and to find ways to honor their lives.

> Following his son's death from a drug overdose, one father initially was
> consumed by rage and helplessness, and did not want to go on living.
> At his therapist's urging, he visited the grave, where he prayed to God
> for inspiration to guide his path ahead. That night he slept deeply for
> the first time since the death, dreamed of his son's joyful nature, and

awoke "knowing" that his son's spirit would want him to do something positive to honor his memory. With his therapist's encouragement, he turned self-destructive feelings into concerted action with other families and local authorities to stop drug trafficking in their community.

Family therapist David Treadway has noted that it is through the ache of our grief that we connect not only to the one we lost but also to the suffering of the world. Often, a shattering loss inspires loved ones to dedicate their lives to a meaningful pursuit that transcends their loss experience and benefits others (Walsh, 2006; also see Rolland & Perry, Chapter 20, this volume).

One couple was distraught after their beloved 25-year-old daughter, suffering with bipolar disorder, committed suicide. In work with a therapist, their pain, anger, and self-blame were somewhat eased as they gained understanding of the biological influences in their daughter's depression and hopelessness. With the first anniversary of her death, they sought a way to forge something positive from the tragedy to honor her life. They set up a foundation in her memory and mobilized their Jewish congregation to hold an annual conference to increase public education and decrease stigma concerning serious mental illness. Their faith community continued to be a source of comfort and support for them.

Compassion, forgiveness, and reconciliation are central in the teachings of all major religions (Worthington, Berry, & Parrott, 2001). A life-threatening event or terminal illness can spark an epiphany, awakening couples and family members to the preciousness of time and their bonds. Where relationships have been wounded, therapists can foster healing before life's end by helping clients to gain compassion for others' life struggles and suffering, and, depending on their situation and desire, to seek forgiveness and reconciliation (Walsh, 2006; see Fishbane [Chapter 9] and Hargrave, Froeschle, & Castillo [Chapter 16], this volume).

Forgiveness can also facilitate healing from a traumatic loss, as well as catalyze a process for restorative justice, as in the following case of the shooting death of an 18-year-old by another youth:

Mrs. Young, overcome by grief and wanting to help her surviving children recover from the tragic death of their oldest brother, tapped back into her childhood Catholic religious teachings. This led her to decide she needed to forgive the youth who killed her son. As she said: "I struggled to forgive him even more for myself and my family—I know my Bible and what unforgiveness does to those who carry it—it destroys the body, the mind, and the spirit." Although her husband couldn't forgive to the extent she did, he respected her efforts and forged his own pathway in healing through social activism, by taking leadership in community efforts to stop gun violence.

Mario, the youth offender, with the support of his priest and members of his parish, left his gang and affiliated with a Christian group in prison. He sought Mrs. Young's forgiveness and, with her continuing encouragement and the involvement of his parish, made every effort to turn his life around (Walsh, 2006).

The paradox of resilience is that the worst of times can bring out the best in the human spirit. A life-threatening crisis or devastating loss can lead to transformation and growth in unforeseen directions. It often sparks a reordering of life priorities and more meaningful pursuits. In facing death and loss, the endurance of suffering can lead to spiritual growth. In turn, spiritual beliefs and practices strengthen the ability to endure and to transcend loss. Grieving is a journey of the heart and spirit, bringing us to the fullness of life here and now, and in the future, with those who still share life with us.

## Exploring Spirituality in Clinical Assessment and Therapeutic Work

The spiritual dimension of death and loss should be explored in all clinical assessment. Table 4.1 suggests some fruitful lines of inquiry. Particular attention should be focused on (1) ways that religious/spiritual beliefs or experiences may contribute to current distress; and (2) ways that past, current, or potential spiritual resources might be drawn on to ease suffering and foster healing and resilience.

A broad perspective on spirituality is important in practice given the diversity and complexity of beliefs and practices across and within cultures and families. It is important to learn how each family, from its own distinct sociocultural and religious background, blends core principles of family members' faith with their approach to death and loss.

It should be kept in mind that many who do not consider themselves religious find spiritual nourishment and healing pathways through nature, the arts, and social activism. In working with atheists, it is important to respect their nonbelief in God or an afterlife, and to ask about their views of a good death and end-of-life preferences. Recent research with atheists (Smith-Stoner, 2007) suggests a threefold definition of spirituality—including intrapersonal, interpersonal, and natural aspects—in end-of-life

**TABLE 4.1. Assessment of Spiritual Dimension in Family Adaptation to Death and Loss**

The following questions suggest fruitful lines of inquiry into the spiritual dimension of family experience to explore sources of distress and potential therapeutic resources in adaptation to death and loss:

Initial inquiry

- What role does religion play in your life? Do you identify with a particular faith? How important are beliefs and practices? Involvement in a faith community?
- How important is a more personal spirituality in coping with death and loss? In the past? In family of origin?
- If you are not religious, or are agnostic or atheist, in what ways do you find meaning, strength, and connection in your life?

Spiritual/religious sources of distress

- Have religious precepts or beliefs contributed to your suffering? How (e.g., concerning afterlife, sin, damnation, suicide, sexual orientation)?
- Has a spiritual void or past cutoff from religious roots increased your suffering? Have death and loss wounded the spirit? Or alienated you from religion or God? In what ways?
- How are religious differences within a couple or family handled? Is there conflict about end-of-life decisions, death and funeral rites, or burial/cremation? Other matters?
- With interfaith marriage and/or conversion, is there regret, conflict, or estrangement at a time of death and loss?

Potential spiritual/religious resources

How might past, current, or potential religious and/or spiritual resources support healing and resilience in the face of death and loss?

- Personal faith for comfort, strength, courage, and support
- Relationship with God, Higher Power, or connectedness with Life Force, universe
- Belief in afterlife, reunion
- Spiritual practices (e.g., prayer, meditation, rituals; communion with nature)
- Involvement and support in a faith community
- Spiritual guidance by clergy, chaplain, pastoral counselor
- Spiritual connection with loved ones
- Forgiveness and reconciliation of wounded bonds
- Spiritual connections with the deceased
- Spiritual transcendence (e.g., inspiring creative arts or social action)

care. Study participants expressed a deep desire to find meaning in their own lives, to maintain connection with family and friends, and to experience interconnectedness with the natural world through the dying experience. They indicated a strong preference for both evidence-based medical interventions and physician-assisted dying, and did not want caregivers to offer religious prayer or other references to God.

Most people who come for therapeutic help around end-of-life and bereavement concerns are seeking more than symptom reduction, problem solving, or communication skills; they are seeking deeper meaning and connection, a yearning brought to the fore with death and loss. As therapists trained to help families solve problems, we may feel helpless and uneasy when we are powerless to stop death or bring back a loved one. What is most important is to be fully present with those who are dying and those who are bereaved, and to help them tap wellsprings for strength and comfort in their relationships and in their faith.

With death and loss, the dichotomy of therapist–healer/patient–sufferer is blurred, since we all share these inevitable challenges. As we face our own vulnerability and quell our own anxieties, we are better able to attend to the needs of our clients—and our own loved ones. When my father was dying, I was very uncomfortable simply being with him. I kept wanting to *do* something, to run an errand for him, to get a more comfortable pillow, a milkshake. By calming my anxieties, I became better able to be fully present with him, sitting quietly at his bedside, stroking his arm, gazing peacefully out the window at the flowering mimosa tree as the sunlight passed through it each day from dawn to dusk. Those last few weeks of his life became the most precious and intimate times in our relationship, a profoundly spiritual experience that eased his suffering and passage as it forever deepened our bond.

The end of life offers gifts to those who face it openly with courage and compassion, reaching out to one another. In the midst of despair, a spirit of love and hope can be rekindled. In our professional roles, it can be spiritually enriching to care for those who are dying and to accompany those who are bereaved on their healing journey. The very essence of the therapeutic bond at such times can foster personal transformation, wholeness, and connection, for both therapists and the families we are privileged to serve.

The human condition involves vulnerability, suffering, and healing. We are all mortal, grappling with our own death and devastated by the loss of loved ones. Yet, more than any other experience, death and loss can teach us about the meaning of our existence and put us in touch with what matters most in our lives and in our world. The soul is nourished and our humanity is strengthened by living and loving fully, and by approaching death and loss with openness, courage, and compassion.

## REFERENCES

Becker, C., Sargent, J., & Rolland, J. S. (2000). Kosovar Family Professional Education Collaborative. *AFTA Newsletter, 80*, 26–30.

Becker, E. (1973). *The denial of death*. New York: Free Press.

Biank, N., & Sori, C. F. (2006). Integrating spirituality when working with children and families experiencing loss of a parent. In K. Helmeke & C. F. Sori (Eds.), *The therapist's notebook for integrating spirituality in counseling II: More homework, handouts, and activities for use in psychotherapy* (pp. 67–80). Binghamton, NY: Haworth Press.

Calhoun, L. G., & Tedeschi, R. G. (2001). Post-traumatic growth: The positive lessons of loss. In R. Neimeyer (Ed.), *Meaning reconstruction and the experience of loss* (pp. 157–172). Washington, DC: American Psychological Association.

Deloria, V., Jr. (1994). *God is red: A native view of religion* (2nd ed.). Golden, CO: Fulcrum.

Doka, K. (2002). How could God?: Loss and the spiritual assumptive world. In J. Kauffman (Ed.), *Loss of the assumptive world: A theory of traumatic loss* (pp. 49–68). New York: Brunner/Routledge.

Domino, G., & Miller, K. (1992). Religiosity and attitudes toward suicide. *Omega, 25*, 271–282.

Gallup, G., Jr., & Lindsay, D. M. (1999). *Surveying the religious landscape: Trends in U.S. beliefs*. Harrisburg, PA: Morehouse.

Gilbert, K. (1992). Religion as a resource for bereaved parents. *Journal of Religion and Health, 31*, 19–30.

Glick, I. O., Weiss, R. A., & Parkes, C. M. (1974). *The first year of bereavement*. New York: Wiley.

Greef, A. P., & Joubert, A. M. (2007). Spirituality and resilience in families in which a parent has died. *Psychological Reports, 100*(3), 897–900.

His Holiness the Dalai Lama. (2002). *Advice on dying and living a better life* (J. Hopkins, Ed. & Trans.). New York: Atria Books/Simon & Schuster.

Imber-Black, E., Roberts, J., & Whiting, R. (2003). *Rituals in families and family therapy* (2nd ed.). New York: Norton.

Kamya, H. (2000). Bereavement issues and spirituality. In V. J. Lynch (Ed.), *HIV/AIDS at year 2000* (pp. 242–256). Boston: Allyn & Bacon.

Kertzer, M., & Hoffman, L. (1996). *What is a Jew?: A guide to the beliefs, traditions, and practices of Judaism* (rev. ed.). New York: Touchstone.

Koenig, H. (2006). *In the wake of disaster: Religious responses to terrorism and catastrophe*. Philadelphia: Templeton Press.

Koenig, H., McCullough, M. E., & Larson, D. (2001). *Handbook of religion and health*. New York: Oxford University Press.

Lamm, M. (2000). *The Jewish way in death and mourning* (rev. ed.). Middle Village, NY: Jonathan David.

Levine, S. (2005). *Unattended sorrow: Recovering from loss and reviving the heart*. New York: Rodale Books.

Lifton, R. J. (1975). Preface. In A. Mitscherlich & M. Mitcherlich (Eds.), *The inability to mourn*. New York: Grove.

Malinowski, B. (1965). The role of magic and religion. In W. A. Lessa & E. Z. Vogt (Eds.), *A reader in contemporary religion* (pp. 63–72). New York: Harper.

Miller, R. L. (2005a). An appointment with God: AIDS, place, and spirituality. *Journal of Sex Research, 42*(1), 35–45.

Miller, R. L. (2005b). Look what God can do: African American gay men, AIDS and spirituality. *Journal of HIV/AIDS and Social Services, 4*(3), 25–46.

Neimeyer, R. A. (2001). *Meaning reconstruction and loss.* Washington, DC: American Psychological Association.

Nhat Hanh, T. (2002). *No death, no fear.* New York: Penguin Putnam.

Obeyesekere, G. (2002). *Imagining Karma: Ethical transformations in Amerindian, Buddhist, and Greek rebirth.* Berkeley: University of California Press.

Pargament, K. (2007). *Spiritually integrated psychotherapy: Understanding and addressing the sacred.* New York: Guilford Press.

Pew Forum on Religion and Public Life. (2008). *U.S. Religious Landscape Survey.* Retrieved from *www.religions.pewforum.org.*

Rinpoche, S. (1994). *The Tibetan book of living and dying* (P. Gaffney & A. Harvey, Eds.). San Francisco: HarperCollins.

Smith-Stoner, M. (2007). End-of-life preferences for atheists. *Journal of Palliative Medicine, 10*(4), 923–928.

Somé, M. P. (1994). *The healing wisdom of Africa.* New York: Tarcher/Putnam.

Spilka, B., Hood, R. W., Hunsberger, B., & Gorsuch, R. (2003). *The psychology of religion: An empirical approach* (3rd ed.). New York: Guilford Press.

Tillich, P. (1952). *Dynamics of faith.* New York: Harper & Row.

Walsh, F. (2006). *Strengthening family resilience* (2nd ed.). New York: Guilford Press.

Walsh, F. (2007). Traumatic loss and major disasters: Strengthening family and community resilience. *Family Process, 46*(2), 207–227.

Walsh, F., & McGoldrick, M. (2004). *Living beyond loss: Death in the family* (2nd ed.). New York: Norton.

Worthington, E. L., Jr., Berry, J. W., & Parrott, L. (2001). Unforgiveness, forgiveness, religion, and health. In T. G. Plante & A. C. Sherman (Eds.), *Faith and health: Psychological perspectives* (pp. 107–138). New York: Guilford Press.

Yalom, I. (2008). *Staring at the sun: Overcoming the terror of death.* San Francisco: Jossey-Bass.

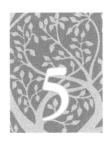

# Religious Perspectives on Resilience

## Buddhism, Christianity, Judaism, Hinduism, and Islam

STEVEN J. WOLIN

*with* WAYNE MULLER

FRED TAYLOR

SYBIL WOLIN

SHANTHI RANGANATHAN

DYAA SAYMAH

HASAN ZEYADA

Joseph Campbell, the noted teacher and commentator on symbols, myths, rituals, and religions once noted that "however the mystic traditions differ, they are in accord in this respect. They call men and women to a deeper awareness of the very act of living itself, and they guide us through trials and traumas from birth to death" (Campbell & Moyers, 1988, p. 8). I (Steven J. Wolin) was attracted to Campbell's remark for the perspective it put on my work as a therapist. It was a clear and important reminder that psychotherapy's roots in the past are relatively shallow and that its scope of influence is narrow. Since ancient times and in places of the world untouched by professional therapy, spiritual teachings, writings, and practices have existed to help people with life's struggles. That many of these live on is testimony to their power and their relevance.

Having devoted over a decade of my life to exploring the topic of resilience (S. J. Wolin & S. Wolin, 1995a, 1995b, 1997; S. J. Wolin & S. Wolin, 1993), I also liked the assumptions that Campbell's remark implied: that spiritual traditions are optimistic. They share the belief that there is a way through "trials and traumas" and that people are capable of finding it. For me, this affirmation of the human capacity for resilience was a welcome contrast to the prevalent concern in therapy with people's vulnerability and psychological damage.

Over time, I found myself wondering what the spiritual traditions could teach me and what guidance, if any, they could offer to my colleagues. I decided to pursue it. I approached adherents of three of the world's great religions—Buddhism, Christianity, and Judaism—and asked them to participate with me in a panel presented at the 1996 annual meeting of the Association for Marriage and Family Therapy in Toronto. I asked each to describe how his or her respective religion viewed the question of resilience. I expressly requested that they limit their remarks to the written texts of their religions and to leave the search for applications to the therapists who attended. My goal was to respect a boundary between religion and therapy while encouraging a dialogue on how the one could enrich the other.

The panel was held over two sessions. Wayne Muller, representing Buddhism, opened the first session. He views resilience as the Buddha-nature, which is in every person. A nameless quality of wholeness, it can contain or bear the weight of whatever one is given. Fred Taylor, representing Christianity, sees the personification of resilience in Jesus, who suffered dreadful pain, isolation, betrayal, and abandonment but never lost the capacity to extend himself in love to others. A core belief of Christianity, Taylor proposes, is that people have the same potential and that they can prevail in overpowering conditions by realizing their promise. Sybil Wolin, representing Judaism, focuses on the Exodus, the biblical account of the Jews' liberation from slavery in Egypt and their journey to Sinai where, at the foot of the mountain, they assemble and receive a divine revelation. She suggests that the Jewish experience in Egypt is meant as a universal symbol of adversity, and the injunction to live with justice and compassion that comes from Sinai is their blueprint for resilience.

The therapists in attendance were invited to reflect on the three talks and to discuss the relevance and applicability of the material to their own work. This chapter distills the major themes that emerged in these conversations, expands the scope to include Hindu and Islamic perspectives, and concludes with my own reflections.

## BUDDHISM (by Wayne Muller)

For the past 22 years, I've spent most of my life in the company of people who suffer. I started by working with teenage runaways and drug addicts in New York. Then I worked with alcoholics, juvenile delinquents, gang members, and people in housing projects. I've also worked with people with AIDS and cancer, and with adults who were abused as children in some painful and intimate way.

As I reflect on my work with the varieties of human suffering, I find it is not the suffering per se that has captured my attention, but rather the grace that seems to be embedded in the sorrow, loss, and grief that life deals us. If we attend with mindful curiosity and deep compassion to the way in which sorrow has been given to each of us, we inevitably begin to probe the nature of sorrow itself—and then, we also uncover what may be born out of that sorrow. We are both broken down and broken open by the unexpected anguish in our life.

One of the things I appreciate about the Buddha is his courage. The story of the Buddha's enlightenment is mythic. The young Siddhartha, after being raised living in a palace, shielded by his protective parents from viewing the outside world, one day took a journey beyond the palace walls. There he encountered an old man, then a sick man, then a corpse, and finally a monk. It was at that moment that Siddhartha realized that suffering is an inevitable part of the human world. He decided to undertake a long process of meditation in order to explore the true nature of this suffering. He vowed to continue his exploration of this truth, whatever the cost, until it was fully revealed to him. Finally, after years of pilgrimage, fasting, and meditation, Siddhartha sat under the Bodhi tree and, as the first star of morning rose in the sky, he became the Buddha—the one who is awake.

After his enlightenment, the Buddha began teaching what he described as the Four Noble Truths. And the first of these is this: The world is filled with suffering. Essentially what he is saying is that if we take birth as a human being, then a certain measure of pain and sorrow will be our legacy. Things that we love will die. Things we hold as precious will be taken from us. People we love and trust will, from time to time, bring us harm, intentionally or unintentionally. Things we believe are permanent and inviolable will dissolve or rust, or fall away. And this is the nature, he said, of all things.

Thus, to be born and to be given sorrow is not a mistake; it is not an injustice; it is not necessarily even a trauma that will induce some subsequent pathology. Sorrow is, in fact, simply one of the legacies of having taken birth as a human being. It is not to be avoided, but rather expected.

The Buddha said that, in any given lifetime, we would be given ten thousand joys and ten thousand sorrows. Sorrow comes in myriad forms—sometimes in the form of hunger or poverty; sometimes in the form of warfare or pestilence, drought or racism, family violence or Nazism or the apartheid system in South Africa. The ways that pain and grief can enter our lives are infinite, but unavoidable, even necessary. Suffering is not necessary in the sense that it's good for us, rather, suffering and joy are like the expansion and contraction of our heart and lungs, like the rhythms of the earth itself, as it moves through the seasons, a natural part of what it means to be alive and awake. Joy and sorrow, in this continual rhythm, are necessary and intimate companions for us.

For those growing up in an alcoholic family, or who are abused or neglected or hurt as children, it was not solely the fault of the abusive family that the child experienced suffering. This particular child may not have been given war, or pestilence, or famine, or poverty, or leukemia; this child received his or her portion of sorrow in the form of family abuse. According to the Buddha, we are given pain because we have taken birth as a human being. The family simply put their peculiar, intimate stamp on the form of that pain. The forms of our sorrow can change; the fact of our sorrow cannot.

The Buddha made a very important and useful distinction between pain and suffering that, as therapists, we miss sometimes in our practice. The Buddha said that pain is inevitable. Pain is part of the deal. The Buddha said that suffering, however, arises from our relationship to the pain that we are given. If I receive some form of harm by my parents when I am quite small, that is pain. Suffering occurs if I believe that I'm toxic, handicapped, defective, and broken because I didn't know what to do with the pain I was given when they were so big and I was so small, if I feel that my trust was betrayed and I conclude from now on that I'll never trust anyone or anything again.

However, at the same time, the Buddha says this: "You are all Buddhas." Each one of us has within us *Buddha-nature*: a nature that is fundamentally perfect and unblemished. There is a light—as in Christianity—an inner light of innate, natural perfection that it not wholly dissimilar from the light Jesus spoke of when he exhorted his followers: *You are the light of the world*. When the Buddha says we each have Buddha-nature, it means we have an inextinguishable fragment of the divine fire which burns in us, regardless of circumstance. Regardless of what we are given or how much difficulty and sorrow we experience, there is something reliable, resilient and true embedded within us, something that will rise up to bear the weight of whatever we are given.

It is this Buddha-nature—this still, small voice, this inner light—that is a nameless quality of wholeness upon which we build our inner home. This inner self, this true nature doesn't break simply because we are given suffering. If that were true, the human race would have expired thousands of years ago, because people have been afflicted with war and famine and pestilence for as long as human beings have been on the earth. A capacity within us remains capable of transcending unspeakable levels of pain and sorrow. I am suggesting that as therapists, as clinicians, as healers, as people who are in the company of those who suffer, we make an alliance (when we begin a therapeutic relationship) with *that unbroken spark of fundamental spirit and divinity.* Sometimes we mistakenly make our alliance with a diagnosis. This error results from a fundamental misunderstanding of the nature of suffering and the nature of healing.

The first question many of us ask when we are given sorrow at any time in our life is "Why me?" Sorrow is the only experience about which we ask this question. If we win the lottery, we don't ask, "Oh, why me? What did *I* do to deserve all this money?" Or if we are tired or happy, we don't go into painful introspection to try to understand why this happiness came to us; or why we feel so tired: "Look at those people over there, they don't look tired. What did I do to deserve it?" The question seems foolish on the surface.

But suffering seems to be something quite different. We take it very personally, as if it has something to do with us. Where do we get this idea? It is relatively simple to discover our development. One of the first things we notice about the world when we're quite small is that whenever we cry, somebody shows up to see what's wrong. And when we smile and make a funny little face, some big person makes a funny face right back at us. Further, when we take our bottle and carom it off the dresser, somebody hands it right back to us. This is pretty cool. The lesson we take from this is: "Basically, I'm in charge of the galaxy as I know it."

This, of course, is how a sense of grandiosity is born. I'm pretty much running the show here. The galaxy responds to my every thought, my every move. But the real problem arises years later; how do I think and feel and behave when someone rapes me? Or what happens when they get drunk and leave me alone for hours, or shout at each other, or bring me great harm? Well, then, I have to figure out: "What did I do that made that happen? I understand the nature of all things—I do *A* and the world does *B*; I smile, they smile. Now, I do *X* and they hit me. I do *Y* and they violate me in some intimate, unspeakable way."

Now I try to figure out what is wrong with me that brought this suffering? "What bad thought did I have that brought this upon me? Or what toxicity, what handicap, what brokenness, what pathology do I have that invited or created this suffering?" Searching for the answer could initiate the pilgrimage for the rest of my life—to discover, diagnose and eradicate whatever I carry in me that makes suffering come to me. But the Buddha says, "Actually, it has nothing to do with you." Even Jesus said, "In the world, you shall have tribulation." Hurt is part of the deal. Perhaps the harm they inflict had more to do with their ignorance or clumsiness than anything we said, or were, or weren't, or did. Perhaps this is simply one way that sorrow comes to us in this lifetime.

If I remain fundamentally convinced that it *is* about me, then I'll spend my life trying to figure out why it happened to me and what is wrong with me because of it. Now, the DSM-IV was written by people, many of them psychologists, who have figured out every conceivable thing that can go wrong with us, which is very impressive. But I would like to suggest that it's fundamentally, unintentionally, and insidiously violent to name someone by what's wrong with them.

You are the light of the world. You are saturated with Buddha-nature. There is a natural, fundamental, innate perfection, a spark of the divine that lies embedded within you that will not be extinguished by your sorrow. And your sorrows are not necessarily pathological.

We don't find "Light of the world" anywhere in the DSM-IV. But how wonderful it would be if the book were large enough to contain both our sorrows and our joys, our pain and our resilience. How wonderful it would be if we didn't have to keep stamping 309.28 in order for therapists to get paid. Because the whole system is driven by diagnosis which, fundamentally, says, "No one gets paid until someone figures out what's wrong with you." I would like to suggest that this system is fundamentally as abusive as the trauma that caused the necessity for this healing relationship.

The Buddha said that the mind is naturally pure and radiant. In the Dzogchen tradition of Buddhism, there is a place called Rigpa, a natural perfection into which we sink. If we watch the sky and we watch the clouds, we can see that as the clouds pass by through the sky, we don't mistake the sky for the clouds. The clouds simply rise and fall away, like all things, like the ten thousand joys and the ten thousand sorrows. Although they may at times obscure our clear perception of the sky, the sky is in no way diminished by the clouds that pass in front of it. In the same way, this relentless Buddha-nature, this luminosity, is in no way diminished or damaged by the painful circumstances of our lives.

Sometimes diagnostic names make us smaller. We need to name ourselves with a name that's large enough to hold both the ten thousand joys and the ten thousand sorrows, to hold this fundamental luminosity. And we need to ally with the deepest name, one that reflects the true nature of that person who is in our company.

There is a Buddhist parable that says, "If you take a tablespoon full of salt and put it into a glass of water and stir it and drink it, the water will taste quite bitter because of the salt. But if you take the same tablespoon of salt and stir it into a large, clear, pure mountain lake and then take a handful of that water and drink it, you won't taste the salt at all." The point of the parable, of course, is that the suffering is not caused by the salt but by the smallness of the container.

What Buddhism and, I would argue, the best of Christianity and Judaism propose is that everything we do in healing should help to make the container larger so that we can hold so much more of the ten thousand joys and the ten thousand sorrows that the Buddha speaks about.

## CHRISTIANITY (by Fred Taylor)

I feel privileged to be a member of this interfaith panel probing how three great religious traditions support the capacity of the human spirit to repair from hardship and suffering. Suffering poses a critical test for theology as well as for psychotherapy. How can men, women, and children today affirm the existence and power of God and their own capacity to receive spiritual empowerment both from God and other people when they find themselves beset and stricken by powers that twist, violate, sicken, and destroy? How do we in the helping professions expand people's resilience—their capacity to endure and grow from suffering?

I have been stimulated both theologically and psychologically by the topic of resilience, as the director of an inner-city social service agency. My organization, For Love of Children (FLOC), works with families, children, and neighborhoods that are typically viewed by mainstream society as "damaged." I find this a troubling diagnosis.

Negatively laden terms such as "dysfunctional," "at risk," and the like blur the connections between family and the social systems surrounding them. Such terms obscure both the possibilities and the problems in these connections. They set up a permanent, uncrossable distance and separate folks into the damaged ones and their fixers. I view traditional philanthropists, who, like myself and FLOC, with our staff of social workers and therapists in that position to the extent that we operate from a perspective that emphasizes deficits, shortcomings, problems, and weaknesses in our clients.

The concept of resilience opens the possibility of a more level playing field, which is far more consistent with my own religious tradition. We are all sinners. We are all challenged. We are all needy. We are all "in recovery" and never leave our vulnerabilities behind. At the same time, we all have within us the capacity for resilience. The proverbial question, whether applied to the individual, the family, or the community, is whether the glass is half empty or half full. A damage mind-set takes one perspective. A resilience mind-set, like the great religious traditions, answers the other way.

Within all the great religious traditions, human beings are characterized by neediness. We are vulnerable to conditions, structures, and forces that threaten us. Response to our neediness can take two basic forms. In the first instance, we can attempt to protect ourselves against vulnerability by establishing a circle of possessions that support and protect us from threat. The Bible warns us against this strategy: "The love of money is the root of all evil" (I Timothy 6:10).

Evil in this instance is not money per se. The threat is the powerful temptation to withhold and hoard our material blessings until we attain a level of security that makes us feel safe. The temptation is fed by the illusion that it is possible to free ourselves from domination by hardship and suffering by dominating our environment. We can never do so perfectly, of course, because we remain vulnerable and hostage to the blows of disease, accident, loss, and death. Paradoxically, chronically withholding people find themselves possessed both by their possessions and by those conditions and powers that threaten to dispossess them. This is the strategy of the closed self, which increases suffering even while it would seek to escape it.

In the second instance, the self may conceivably open out toward others in self-giving, self-expanding love and generosity. This is the response of the open self—openhanded rather than tightfisted. Such an identity is not an abstraction. The Christian tradition is grounded in the story of how Jesus, preeminently and unconditionally, lived out this self-giving identity under concrete conditions in which people find themselves buffeted by destructive conditions and forces. He suffered dreadful pain, isolation, betrayal, abandonment, and death, but his identity with self-expanding love never broke. This is the identity which is at the heart of Christian worship and piety, an identity that has inspired incredible resilience over the ages in inhuman conditions.

Christian piety vests power in the relationship between the believer and a creative, nurturant, and preservative God, a relationship that becomes accessible and believable through the story of Jesus's self-giving life, death, and God's response of resurrection. The story, which Christians refer to as the "Gospel" or "Good News," affirms, celebrates, and evokes in those grasped by faith a radical kind of power that liberates human beings to be who we are meant to be regardless of what has been done to us or what we have done to others.

A powerful exposition of this message is the movie *Dead Man Walking*. The protagonist of this true story is a Catholic nun, Sister Helen Prejean, who takes on a pastoral relationship with a convicted murderer on death row. Two threads run through the story. One is Sister Helen's patient, persistent effort to engage the tightly self-defended, "macho" criminal in preparing for his own impending death. The other is Sister Helen's stressful relationship with the two sets of parents of the teenage couple the prisoner and his partner brutally murdered and sexually abused. The parents can neither understand nor accept Sister Helen's commitment to minister to their children's murderer. They see her actions as a violation of their children's memory and their own grief.

Both relationships—one with the prisoner Matthew, and the other with the victims' parents—push Sister Helen to her psychological and spiritual limits. She is against the death penalty, a position that puts her at odds with the world around her. And Matthew, while welcoming the human contact she offers, resists facing the truth about himself. Only when his final appeal for a stay of execution is denied does his facade begin to crack. He then can no longer push away this servant of God. Step by step, she leads him to acknowledge his brutal deed, not to confirm his condemnation but to free him to accept God's forgiveness.

As the hour of Matthew's death approaches and he has not come close to facing this truth, Sister Helen probes his religious understanding. They talk about Jesus, who died on the cross for sinners. Matthew says that he knows and believes that Jesus died for him, that Jesus will cleanse him of guilt for sinning. Sister Helen replies, "Yes, Matthew, but you have to participate!" Her statement jolts Matthew, and slowly he lets go of his defenses. As he does, a new person emerges, one who is liberated to feel remorse for what he has done with his life and the pain he has caused the victims and their loved ones. Now he is ready to die and to face what he will face beyond death.

This movie, in my judgment, is an ultimate portrayal of the resilience expressed in the familiar Christian revival hymn: "Just as I am, without one plea, O Lamb of God, I come."

The Christian faith, like other great religions, is far too rich to be encapsulated by any number of words, much less a few paragraphs. Nonetheless, there is an authentic congruence between the therapeutic discipline of being as attentive to the surfacing of strengths alongside the surfacing of pain and distress and of holding human sin and God's grace together, with grace, not sin, as the last word.

## JUDAISM (by Sybil Wolin)

The topic of resilience, spirituality, and Judaism brings to mind Roger Kamenetz's (1994) book *The Jew in the Lotus*. In it, he reports an encounter between the Dalai Lama and a group of Jews of varied persuasions, from Orthodox to secular. Students of the Buddhist leader had arranged the meeting in response to his interest in Jewish history. Exiled from his homeland in Tibet and witness to the destruction of ancient Buddhist holy temples and lamaseries by the Chinese, the Dalai Lama wanted to know the secret of Jewish resilience. How, he asked, have Jews preserved their religion for centuries since the heart of their religion, the temple in Jerusalem, was destroyed? How have the Jewish people and Judaism spread to the four corners of the world, finding homes in different countries and diverse cultures, yet maintaining a common identity and core of belief and practices?

As a Jew, I found the book compelling, because it served as a mirror that reflects our enduring capacity for resilience more sharply than our eternal history of victimization. As a psychologist, it gripped me equally for its conceptualization of resilience as a self-conscious achievement that can be reflected upon, understood, taught, and replicated.

Expectably, the Jewish respondents to the Dalai Lama did not offer a single answer or clear prescription for overcoming hardship. Jewish writings suggest many answers, and for each there are many interpretations. What follows is a commentary on the topic through one pair of Jewish eyes. It is based on the Hebrew Bible, the *Haggadah*, or text for the Passover service, and bits of personal experience.

The connection between Jewish spirituality and resilience first occurred to me at a wedding when, at the end of the ceremony, the officiating rabbi placed a glass on the floor and the groom, as tradition directs, crushed it under his heel. The shattering noise of the glass is meant to interrupt the mood of celebration and to introduce a sober yet reassuring observation. On the one hand, the symbolic crushing of the glass conveys that we cannot expect the joys of life to continue endlessly. Even in our moments of greatest happiness, we must not forget that shattering experiences also inevitably occur. On the other hand, we are reminded that we can prevail. Just as the groom symbolically crushes the glass, according to Judaism, an individual has the capacity to break the debilitating hold that hardship imposes. The timing (after vows have been exchanged) suggests the understanding and the wish that marriage be a way for bride and groom to sustain that capacity.

The place reserved for hardship in the Jewish wedding ceremony and woven into other rituals, such as the Passover Seder, also permeates the Hebrew Bible and other Hebrew texts. From its opening pages, with the expulsion of Adam and Eve from the Garden of Eden, the murder of Abel by Cain, and the destruction of the world by God, to its close, with the agonies and protestations of Job and the cynicism of Ecclesiastes, and the destruction of the kingdom according to the prophesy of Jeremiah, the Hebrew Bible is a book of sighs and lamentations. It portrays in vivid detail every imaginable form of human suffering side by side with our enduring capacity to repair.

As Elie Wiesel (cited in Rosenblatt, 1995, p. 44) reflects on the expulsion of Adam and Eve from Eden, "Rejected by God [Adam] drew closer to Eve. Never were the two so united. . . . Expelled from paradise, they did not give in to resignation. In the face of death, they decide to fight by giving life, by conferring a meaning on life."

Naomi Rosenblatt, in her book *Wrestling with Angels*, expands on Wiesel's reflection:

> Our hearts go out to Adam and Eve for their primal loss . . . but they also earn our admiration. As they leave the Garden arm in arm, we see a couple bound together by adversity. . . . [This] is a far cry from the tearful scene depicted in Renaissance paintings. They don't apologize or despair. Their perseverance defies the pessimistic "fall of man" interpretation of their expulsion from the Garden. With their departure, we witness instead the "rise of man" as the first man and woman forge a covenant of love and interdependence dedicated to their mutual survival and growth. (p. 44)

Among the tales of suffering and repair narrated in the Bible, the Exodus stands out as a determining experience in Jewish history, practice, and worship. The story also conveys a characteristic view of resilience in Judaism. The Exodus is the account of the Israelites' journey from slavery in Egypt through the desert and to the foot of Mount Sinai, where the people received a divine revelation that many live by to this day. Its importance to Jews, I believe, derives from the power of the story to represent the claim of hardship on our lives and, in the words of Joseph Campbell, to serve as a "guide through trials and traumas from birth to death" (Campbell & Moyers, 1988, p. 8).

The Exodus drama begins with Joseph, one of Jacob's 12 sons. He was his father's favorite, distinguished for his coat of many colors. His brothers, who were envious, resentful, and angry because of his privileges, conspire to kill him. But one brother, Reuben, halts the plan, and instead the brothers sell Joseph to a band of traders en route to Egypt.

In time, Joseph prospers in Egypt, and his descendants become numerous. Eventually, Pharaoh perceives their growing numbers as a threat and enslaves them. A degrading, misery laden, and life-threatening experience ensues. "The Egyptians ruthlessly imposed upon the Israelites. . . . They made life bitter for them with harsh labor at mortar and bricks and with all sorts of tasks in the field" (Exodus 1:13–14).

The low point is reached when Pharaoh threatens the continuation of Jewish life by decreeing that all firstborn sons of Jewish families be drowned in the Nile. Moses is saved from that fate by his sister Miriam, who arranges to have him brought up in the Egyptian court. As a young man, Moses witnesses an Egyptian taskmaster beating an old Jewish man and is driven to murder. Fleeing to Midian, he becomes an instrument of God, as the appointed leader who challenges Pharaoh's power. With his brother Aaron, Moses leads the people, now a multitude, out of bondage, across the Red Sea and through the desert. When the people reach the foot of Mount Sinai, in thunder and smoke, they receive the word of God, which consists of the Ten Commandments and the law that will govern them thenceforth. The Exodus story ends as the people are about to enter the land of Canaan and establish themselves as a nation with a purpose, a clear identity, and a commitment to live by the law they had been given in the desert.

Every Spring, Jews gather together at Passover for a Seder celebration that revolves around retelling this story. The Seder instructs us about the place of hardship in our individual and collective lives, and the necessity and means of overcoming it. The idea finds expression in many symbols, which mingle the dark and the light, the bitter and the sweet, hardship and resilience. A central symbol of the seder ceremony is the *matzah*, unleavened flat bread without yeast, which the Jews prepared without time for dough to rise when they fled Egypt. Bringing together hardship and resilience, it represents at once the poor man's bread; the bread of affliction; and the bread of freedom, hope, and redemption. The Seder plate displays an egg, a symbol of rebirth and of mourning for the destroyed Temple in Jerusalem. It contains bitter herbs, which remind us of the bitterness our ancestors suffered; parsley, which recalls spring and life; and salt water for dipping, which recalls the people's tears. The entire event recalls an event laden with both terror and promise, destruction and creation, life and death.

A key passage in the Seder service instills participants with a sense of their own resilience and the necessity of exercising it. In each generation, we are to regard ourselves as if we personally had gone out of Egypt. In Hebrew, Egypt is translated as *Mitzrayim. Tzr*, the root of *Mitzrayim*, which translates as narrow, constrained, and inhibited, suggests a meaning that transcends the particularity of Egypt. Everyone, it suggests, in all generations, labors under the burden of one form of slavery or the other. Everyone must struggle to break free, to wander in the desert, and strive to reach physical, spiritual, and emotional independence. Each year the Seder ritual defines the eternal nature of the journey, charts the route, and holds out the hope and promise that we are capable of traveling it. As the *Haggadah* states, the celebration moves us—

. . . from slavery to freedom
from despair to joy
from mourning to celebration
from darkness to light
from enslavement to redemption . . .

Our means for progressing from one end of the journey to the other is outlined in Exodus. In unmistakable terms, the Jews are told how to live down the past, how to shed a slave mentality, and how to forge a new identity as a free people. Rich in the language of "thou shalts," the law rests firmly on a foundation of choice, duty, action, accountability, responsibility, and social and personal conscience.

Clearly this vocabulary has not been a preferred terminology for therapeutic discourse and practice. If heard at all, it is usually at the margins. Perhaps we should ask, in the same spirit as the Dalai Lama, whether it might be worth renewed consideration.

The legislation delivered at Sinai flows backwards into its source. It is a paradox of Judaism that whereas the law and way of life that Moses brought down from the mountain aimed to liberate the people from a slave mentality, it relied upon the experience in Egypt as its primary rationale. In receiving the law, the people learned that slavery would indelibly be etched in the conscience, but from then on would be filtered through the lens of understanding and be given new meaning. "Because you were slaves in Egypt, you know the heart of the stranger." So primary is the idea that it is repeated in varying forms 36 times in the *Torah*, more than any other single thought, defining the Jewish people's identity and naming their purpose.

Biblical law is designed to help keep us from the most likely consequence of our bitter experience—repeating the past and perpetuating its ravages from one generation to the next. The alternative it spells out is to take the experience of Egypt and to turn it inside out. It teaches that we do not need to re-create Egypt wherever we go, that we can learn from our suffering instead. It is a far-reaching moral vision of how to stop the suffering of others: how to be compassionate; to do justice; to treat one another with fairness and dignity; to respect the environment; to honor the dead; to give charity; never to seek revenge or to hold a grudge; to love one's neighbor; to bless one's children; to care for the widow and orphan; to remember that we were made in the divine image and to act accordingly; to create and not to destroy. In this context, *resilience* can be defined as a partnership with the divine to wipe out all forms of slavery and to create a sanctuary on earth, where everyone can be safe and everyone can thrive.

Jewish spirituality does not transport us away from life's troubles. Rather, its wisdom is that we are shaped by our troubles, that over and over again we return to Egypt, but that each time we return, the real possibility of an Exodus exists. Judaism tells us that we are all holy and that all of us are capable of achieving freedom. The religion places a heavy burden on the individual by making resilience a moral obligation, locating its source in the will, and naming action as the channel through which it is expressed. The task is formidable, and the choice is ours. In the words of the Deuteronomist (30:19), "See, I set before you this day life and prosperity, death and adversity. . . . Choose life that you and your seed may live" (Hertz, 1990, pp. 882–883).

## PANEL DISCUSSION

Following these three talks, the panelists discussed with the therapists who attended the relevance of these ideas and their applicability to their own practices. Overall, the remarks highlighted the need for continuing discussion of the place of religion and spirituality in therapy. For the most part, those people in attendance had found meaning in religion and their lives were significantly influenced by it. They described the tension they feel practicing a profession they perceive to be hostile to an essential part of themselves and their life experience. Many expressed frustration at having to exclude religion from their work, especially because it had been so helpful to them personally. Their expressions of appreciation for the talks related to their feeling legitimized by the "official" sanction given by the inclusion of the topic in the program.

For my own part, the interfaith nature of the seminar and the discussion that followed were particularly gratifying. Accustomed to thinking of religion as divisive to the point of untold bloodshed, I was pleased to be in a setting where the theme of healing was the focus, and the points of commonality could emerge. The experience satisfied a human need in me that far surpassed my interest as a therapist.

## ADDITIONAL PERSPECTIVES

Revising this chapter for the second edition of this volume presented the opportunity to expand the scope of spiritual perspectives on resilience to include Hinduism and Islam. These contributions proved quite valuable to understanding the commonalities and differences toward overcoming adversity across five religions.

## HINDUISM (by Shanthi Ranganathan)

*Resilience* is defined in *Webster's* dictionary as a combination of two attributes highly relevant to individual and family responses to adversity: elasticity and buoyancy. *Elasticity* refers to the properties that enable individual and family systems to respond flexibly and maintain patterns of functioning when confronted by serious life challenges. Buoyancy is the ability to recover quickly from a misfortune, trauma, or transitional event causing or calling for adaptational changes in patterns of functioning. There are four concepts in the Hindu religion that contribute to these attributes of elasticity (or flexibility) and buoyancy (or ability to rebound).

*Karmayoga* is the performance of any activity with utmost dedication and commitment, without being attached to the fruits of the action. This principle was first delineated in the Bhagavad Gita (Chapter 4, Verse 18), which states that there is no point in brooding over the fruits of action, because many hidden variables beyond our control determine the results of our actions. Brooding only begets attachment, and attachment leads to the desire to possess, the inability to fulfill one's desires leads to frustration; frustration leads to anger; and anger leads to delusion.

*Karmayoga* focuses on the adherence to duty (*dharma*) while remaining detached from the reward. It involves discharging social obligations as an offering to God. When action is done without attachment to the results, it is liberating. If one acts as an instrument in the hands of the Lord, as a participant in the cosmic activity of Nature, that Karma will not be binding: Karma then becomes karmayoga. Karmayoga gives the individual evenness of mind in gains and losses, and in success and failure. There is no renunciation of action but renunciation of longing for the fruits of action. Karmayoga helps individuals to face conflicts, problems, trials, and tribulations of life without being unduly affected by them. They develop the resilience to carry on with duties, because they have learned the skill of surrendering the fruits of action to the higher power.

*Prarabdha karma* is the sum total of all accumulated actions, including those yet to be done. Hindus believe that every human being has several births. One's karma is the sum of all that an individual has done, is currently doing, and will do. These actions [good and bad] have a cumulative effect. The fruits of the present deeds are carried on to the next birth, and they create past, present, and future experiences, thus making one responsible for his or her own life.

The pain or joy one experiences is the result of prarabhdha karma, where *pra rabdha* means "previously accumulated." The effects may be seen immediately or delayed, in this life or in the next birth. This karma theory provides one the resilience to accept adversities by viewing them as the result of one's own actions in earlier births or in the present one. Individuals assume responsibility for whatever happens to them. In addition to developing the courage to face problems, they also develop the maturity to do good deeds to make this life or the following births more meaningful.

Acceptance of things over which one has no control should not be misinterpreted as fatalism. Rather, it gives the individual the courage to accept negative things and to take appropriate action wherever necessary. Hindus are not disillusioned by their "destiny" but develop the ability to exercise free will to change things over which they have control.

*Rituals and celebrations* are parts of daily routine in Hinduism. Rituals in the form of prayer, yoga, and visiting temples are an integral part of the Hindu culture. Making garlands, preparing tasty food as an offering to God, and reciting songs in praise of the Lord all form part of this routine practice. Added to this, every 2 months there are celebrations in the form of festivals, which are not only religious but also social in content and purpose. During festivals like *Diwali*, new clothes are bought for all people, including those who work for them and their family; relatives are visited and blessings are solicited. Even for death Hindu scriptures give clear prescriptions. There are several rituals around death for a period of 1 year. There is a mourning period, wherein all relatives and friends provide support. A specific day is chosen [either the 16th or the 40th day after the death] when all relatives and friends are invited to the family home, a special lunch is served, and new clothes are worn. A visit to the temple is also mandatory. All rituals such as these allow the bereaved to carry on normal activities without feeling guilty.

For the Hindu, *a personal God* provides great comfort in times of adversity. In difficult situations, when human attempts fail to turn life's troubles around or failure is foreseen, one turns to one's personal God, who has "functional expertise and responsibilities." The Hindu pantheon contains many such helpers. We have *Brahma*, the creator, *Vishnu*, the protector, and *Shiva*, the destroyer, each providing help. Then there are a wide variety of Gods who are specialists. For example, *Ganesh* (or *Ganapthy* or *Vinayak*— commonly known as the elephant God) removes obstacles. *Hanuman*, the monkey God, removes anxiety and fear. *Lord Vaidhyanath*, the doctor God, cures illness. *Lord Balaji of Thirupathi* brings wealth. A Hindu with a health problem takes the required Western or traditional *Aruvedic* treatment and also prays to *Vaidyanath* for a speedy recovery. Others pray to *Hanuman* to remove anxiety. Someone starting a new project seeks the approval of *Ganesh*. Hindus achieve the same feeling of confidence by turning to their personal Gods that Westerners obtain by seeking the help of human specialists. The result of receiving a specialist's guidance is empowerment and assistance, enabling Hindus to overcome their problems. In the famous Meenakshi temple in Madurai, there is a statue of *Jwara deva*—the God of fever. The personal God is intimate with individuals, who see their personal God as a dependable ally. One who prays feels much relieved, because "I have spoken to my God and he will take care of me."

Well-educated Hindus also know the nuances of their personal Gods. For example, while Shiva's job description is the destroyer, a *Shivam* in Sanskrit, also means auspicious, propitious—something good. A synonym for Shiva in Sankara is "the God who does good." A non-Hindu might reasonably ask how the destroyer can also do good. The answer is both/and; Shiva stands not for destruction for its own sake, but for a process of continuous change and renewal. This understanding of Shiva leads to a more well-informed acceptance of the facts of life. Changes are not only inevitable but also desirable. As Alfred Lord Tennyson noted in "The Passing of Arthur":

> The old order changeth, yielding place to new.
> God fulfills himself in many ways.
> Lest one good custom should corrupt the world.

In these lines Tennyson says that even one *good* custom—good for one particular context—has to keep changing when the context itself is changing continuously. No change means no improvement or evolution. Change comes with certain pain. So welcome any pain that leads to change; accept change as a fact of life. Such an understanding leads to greater resilience.

## ISLAM (by Dyaa Saymah and Hasan Zeyada)

Islam plays a vital role in strengthening Muslims' resilience in response to adversity. From our extensive experience in community mental health, we have found that Islamic beliefs, values, practices, and rituals have a significant protective function for victims of trauma and ongoing stresses.

Muslims are taught five core beliefs. First is the belief in one God (Allah). Second is belief in the prophets and messengers of God, including Adam, Abraham, Moses, Jesus, and Mohammed. Third is belief in all the revealed books of God, which are the Torah (Moses), the Psalms (David), the Gospels (Jesus), and the Qur'an. Fourth is the belief in all angels of God. Fifth is the belief in the Day of Judgment and resurrection, and the belief in fate (Qadar; Sarwar, 1998).

Muslims express their beliefs through the practice of rituals, called the Pillars of Islam, through which they stay connected to God and Islamic teachings. The first is *Shehadah*, the declaration of faith in one God and Mohammed as his messenger. The second is the daily performance of the five obligatory prayers. The third requires giving a percentage of personal wealth as charity. The fourth is fasting, for healthy Muslims, during the month of Ramadan. The fifth is the *Hajj*, a pilgrimage to the holy city of Mecca. The core teaching of Islam, as with other religions, is to keep God in mind and to do good things for others at all times. Life in this world is rewarded in the afterlife, which is eternal.

Faith in Islam comes from believing in God and his messenger, the Prophet Mohammad. Such faith helps Muslims give meaning for all life experiences. Furthermore, Muslims believe in fatalism (destiny), which means that everything that happens in life comes from God. This belief enables people to accept whatever happens, whether positive or negative. Good things that happen are a matter of fate; bad things are considered a test from God. Difficulties must be accepted with great patience. An event that seems to be negative may turn out be positive in the long term. Such thinking is vital in helping Muslims to decrease feelings of anger, blame, or revenge.

Muslims believe that God is looking after them and planning their future. They find relief from suffering and the fear of death—a major source of anxiety—by reassurance of the afterlife, as long as they are content in their connectedness with God. Fatalism doesn't mean dependency and passivity. Rather, Islam encourages Muslims to make their utmost effort to achieve good deeds and to avoid harmful actions, guided by Qur'anic teachings. They must accept the consequences of their deeds, as they are a test from God for their strength of faith and their patience.

Islam regards patience as the key prerequisite to buffer individuals and their families against terrible events and traumas they may encounter. Patience involves acceptance, tolerance, and avoidance of anger. Through patience, individuals can control themselves, regulate their emotional reactions, and free their hearts from fear, revenge, and hate. Patience assists in decision making without overreaction. This patience, practiced both in times of crisis and ongoing negative events, and in aggressive or oppressive situations, enhances endurance and suppresses anger.

In times of trouble or tragedy, Muslims initiate positive, constructive actions. If treated well, they respond in kind. If they suffer harm or injustice, they view the matter from a different perspective to consider the positive side and learn a lesson from such experience. This is an important element in resilience.

The practice of Islamic *rituals* supports positive mental health. Ramadan (the month of fasting) and the Pilgrimage to Mecca, in particular, provide opportunities to break away from harmful social habits, to resolve conflicts, and to attain peace of mind. In many cases, substance-dependent individuals give up alcohol and drug use through faithful adherence to religious commitments during Ramadan and through the cleansing of the inner self, devotional awakening, and faithful performance of the Pilgrimage rituals.

During daily prayer rituals, Muslims withdraw from the outside environment to strengthen their relationship with God and to bring peacefulness and calmness to their souls. In times of crisis, stress, or chaos, particularly when important life decisions have to be made, Muslims tend to intensify praying and increase repetition to a higher degree in *Zeker*, or recitation. They believe that in repeatedly mentioning God, their hearts gain tranquility. Such concentration helps to distract from stressful events and negative thinking processes. Prayer works as a meditation practice, relaxing the body and mind, and enabling return to daily routine after a crisis or a stressful situation.

Throughout the month of Ramadan, Muslims refrain from eating and drinking from sunrise to sunset. The ultimate aim is to bring people closer to God and to each other, and to feel compassion for the poor and hungry. Fasting also teaches Muslims to practice control over their needs and desires. Observance of Ramadan increases the practice of other key rituals such as praying (*Zeker*) and charity (*Zakah*). During this month, God urges Muslims to adhere more to forgiveness and reconciliation. They are not allowed to create any conflicts with each other. People tend to resolve their grievances during this period, because fasting is regarded as useless while one has conflicts with others. This enhances tolerance and control over anger, resentment, and aggression. Throughout this month, Islam calls on Muslims to strengthen their social networks through visits to relatives and friends. This increases the potential for social support in times of adversity.

*Hajj*, the Pilgrimage to Mecca, is practiced at least once during the lifetime of Muslims who are physically and financially able. During this annual event, hundreds of thousands of Muslims worldwide gather in Mecca to pray and ask forgiveness from God for vices that they have committed in their lives. During *Hajj*, all economic, racial, and social differences become trivial as all Muslims wear the same simple white garments and practice the same rituals together. Such rituals emphasize the principles of equity among Muslims, and strengthen social networks and support. After completing the *Hajj*, Muslims return to their normal lives, having gained peace of mind and freedom from burdens of guilt, sadness, or anxiety.

Muslims aspire to emulate and learn from the life of the Prophet Mohammed and his followers, especially in response to adversity. Mohammed set an ideal model of patience after he lost beloved ones and vital social networks during difficult times in his life. He began life in conditions of poverty and lost his parents as a child. Yet he overcame these adversities, becoming one of the great leaders in history. In battles on many different fronts, he strove for patience, forgiveness, and reconciliation. Despite all the hardships Mohammed endured, he supported his family and friends and was exemplary in his sacrifice for the sake of the group. His close followers also were exemplary in their strong relationships and limitless support to each other.

The Qur'an, the holy book for Muslims, is filled with wisdom that incorporates important aspects of resilience, including tolerance, forgiveness, and reconciliation. It teaches Muslims constructive ways to cope with crisis, to be patient through stressful situations, and to seek forgiveness and reconciliation with others, even with aggressors. Muslims are encouraged to turn to the Qur'anic verses for guidance on moral conduct, ethical relations, and all personal difficulties they may encounter.

The *family* holds a central place in Islam. The purpose of marriage is to create and to live in an atmosphere of love, harmony, and companionship to fulfill the higher purpose of life. Islamic teachings encourage communication in family relationships based on honesty, transparency, and, above all, respect, especially for parents and elders. The extended family has a genuine concern to contribute to the well-being of all members. In this regard, the Prophet said, "The best among you are those who are best to their families."

In adverse situations, this strong support system is activated. Family cohesion facilitates coping and adaptation. Kin and social support, including emotional, tangible, and informational aspects, are particularly valued in difficult times. When children face difficulties, their parents, older siblings, and extended family members provide support, protection, and guidance to overcome challenges and alleviate suffering.

Islam promotes the collective identity, connectedness, and solidarity of all Muslims. Religious teachings encourage Muslims to gather together daily for prayer at mosques. The ultimate goal is to form a small faith community that practices many forms of social cohesion, including information sharing and providing emotional and practical support. Islam even considers the smile as one of the essential forms of social support. The importance of support and care is stressed for persons in crisis and for those who suffer prolonged adversity or misfortune, particularly older adults, people with special needs, and the poor. Attending to those who are ill or bereaved is a high priority. One of the daily practices in Islam is the offering of *Zakah*, giving money for the poorest people. Because it is a core value that Muslims who are rich should look after the poor, being poor is not viewed in a stigmatizing manner. Rather, those who are fortunate in life are expected to help those who suffer misfortune. In these many ways, Muslims benefit from strong kin relationships and social solidarity as they face adversity, and they are rewarded by God in the afterlife for acts of generosity, kindness, and care. Thus, these essential beliefs and practices in Islam sustain resilience for those who provide assistance, as well as those who suffer.

## CONCLUSIONS

As I had expected, all five religions were rich in insights about resilience. Each acknowledged and respected the capacity for resilience as basic to human nature. This is not to say that any of them saw people as invulnerable—able to escape the hurtful and harmful aftereffects of hardship. On the contrary, Buddhism, Christianity, Judaism, Hinduism, and Islam all know and portray in their teachings the full extent of human frailty and susceptibility to sorrow. The Buddha said that in any given lifetime we would be given ten thousand joys and ten thousand sorrows. The resurrection of Jesus is inextricably connected to his trials, and all Jews carry the indelible scars of slavery. In Hinduism change is inevitable and leads to certain pain. For Muslims, bad things that happen are inevitable and are considered tests from God.

The issue in all religious teachings is not how to avoid hardship and pain but how to live with meaning, joy, gratitude, and awe, while knowing the irrevocable claim that sorrow makes on our lives. All perspectives converged powerfully on this point.

Nevertheless the five religions had sharp distinctions. The three workshop speakers identified a core dimension of their religion that informed its relationship to resilience. For Buddhism, resilience can be viewed as an "inner light" or Buddha-nature, which we come to know through a process of enlightenment as exemplified and taught by the Buddha. By finding our own Buddha-nature we can remain calm in the face of all adversity. In Christian terms, resilience involves the capacity to extend the self in love to others. Compassion and empathy strengthen us as we meet life's challenges. In Judaism, resilience emanates from the will and is expressed in action. Given our free will, we can perform right action and repair the world.

Although there are many similarities among Buddhism, Christianity, and Judaism, the contributions from Islam and Hinduism add several unique elements to the discussion of resilience and religion. Hinduism teaches dedication and commitment to duty, without attachment to reward or outcome in this life, thus strengthening the ability to face any disappointment or trial. The connection to personal Gods that can provide assistance with every trouble gives great solace, assurance, and relief. Finally, in Islam, beliefs in fatalism and in the afterlife also provide solace in times of crisis. Moreover, the teachings of the *Qu'ran*, including ritual observances such as daily communal prayer, and family and social support for those in need, provide great resilience to the entire Muslim community.

I believe that the uniform respect for people's resilience described here across religions is far more essential than their distinctions. My hope is that this resilience perspective will transcend the boundaries between therapeutic schools and be accepted as a fundamental premise in the mental health field as a whole.

## REFERENCES

Campbell, J., with Moyers, B. (1988). *The power of myth: Program I. The hero's adventure* [Video]. (Distributed by Mystic Fire Video, New York/Doubleday, New York)

Hertz, J. H. (Ed.). (1990). *The Pentateuch and Haftorahs.* London: Soncino Press.

Kamenetz, R. (1994). *The Jew in the lotus.* San Francisco: Soncino Press.

Rosenblatt, N. H. (1995). *Wrestling with angels.* New York: Delacorte Press.

Sarwar, G. (1998). *Islam: Beliefs and teachings.* London: Muslim Education Trust.

Wolin, S., & Wolin, S. J. (1995a). Morality in COAS: Revisiting the syndrome of overresponsibility. In S. Abbott (Ed.), *Children of alcoholics: Selected readings.* Rockville, MD: National Association for Children of Alcoholics.

Wolin, S., & Wolin, S. J. (1995b). Resilience among youth growing up in substance-abusing families. *Pediatric Clinics of North America, 42*(2), 415–429.

Wolin, S., & Wolin, S. J. (1997). Shifting paradigms: Taking a paradoxical approach. *Resiliency in Action, 2*(4), 23–28.

Wolin, S. J., & Wolin, S. (1993). *The resilient self: How survivors of troubled families rise above adversity.* New York: Villard Books.

# The Stresses of Poverty
# and the Comfort of Spirituality

## HARRY J. APONTE

Theodora, twice widowed, lived poor. Her son had been killed attempting a robbery. Both her twin daughters, Jeannie and Jeannette, had sickle-cell anemia. Because Jeannette for years had also been ravaged by a cocaine habit, Theodora was raising her daughter's first child. Every weekend Theodora also helped Jeannie with her neurologically impaired son. On top of all that, she personally cared for the godfather of the twins, a widowed, elderly man whose health was fading. Theodora did not deny the difficulties of her life, but she had hope. Her support was the local African American Baptist church. She loved her family, and had her church and her God.

When asked about all her troubles, Theodora answered, "All this goes along with making me stronger" (Aponte, 1994, p. 226). She saw purpose in her personal sacrifice for her family. Now, however, she also faced a moral dilemma of whether to support Jeannie in caring for her addicted sister's youngest daughter. Theodora knew Jeannie did not have the energy to care properly for either her own health or that of her sickly son. She certainly could not also care for her twin's child. Theodora reluctantly but firmly said, "Let [the child] go into the system." For her, Jeannie's health and her obligation to her own children came first. Theodora had her recourse: "We'll pray about it" (Aponte, 1994, p. 236).

## THE CHALLENGE OF POVERTY

Theodora was poor by this society's economic standards, and conscious of the racial stresses. She had more than the ordinary share of personal troubles. Yet she did not feel defeated or bitter. Her self-esteem and emotional strength drew vitality from her faith.

The Theodoras of this world suffer the daily trials and challenges of the rest of society. However, the added burdens of their poverty and minority status often contribute to the following:

1. Loss of a sense of identity and self-worth.
2. Diminished power over everyday living and their future destiny.
3. Separateness from the larger society, and a loss of stable relationships in their personal lives and communities.

Jeannette had surrendered to her addiction. Theodora and Jeannie, facing the same personal, social, and economic circumstances, held onto their hope through their church and faith.

In treating poor minority clients, therapists find daunting social and environmental circumstances that undermine clients' physical and emotional health, as well as family relationships. They encounter the consequent personal "underorganization" of the families (Aponte, 1994, pp. 13–31) that resists the usual psychological interventions. We therapists are left looking for new ways to help with the effects of society's troubles on the most undervalued of our citizens. An underutilized asset with the resource-deprived poor is their spirituality.

Spirituality speaks to the very heart of people's existence: the essential meaning, purpose, and value of life itself. It gives a transcendent significance to every pilgrim's personal and social circumstances (see John Bunyan, 1976). For the disadvantaged, spirituality is a resource that can transcend their personal discouragement, the deprivation of poverty, and oppression by society. In an impersonal environment it can enhance identity and self-worth by giving meaning to a person's struggles. In a disempowering society, it can generate autonomy through the internal gyroscope of a person's convictions. In a disconnected society, it can offer relationship through a transcendent sense of kinship with our every neighbor, through a faith community and, for the believers, a spiritual connection with God.

Spirituality is a fundamental life resource, offering therapists a source of strength, connection, and direction for their clients. It is for therapists to learn how to recognize, speak to, and work with spirituality, a universal component of the human experience. For work with the poor it is a potential beam of light in the darkness of destitution.

## What Is Spirituality?

St. Paul discovered an altar in Athens that the Greeks had dedicated to the "Unknown God" (Acts 17:23). He believed he knew who that God was, but he spoke to the Greeks' pursuit as to a universal human impulse. Consciously or unconsciously, everyone is searching for an overarching meaning and purpose to pain and pleasure, life and death. Everyone has a spirituality. Everyone's life draws on some aspect of spirituality, which in its fullness is composed of morality, a belief system, and a communal sharing with humanity that often relates to a personal God.

Those who live closest to pain, deprivation, and death are often the closest to their spirituality. However, they can also plunge to the depths of hopelessness. The impoverished and marginalized members of society need a therapy that recognizes that *their* lives are worth living and fighting for even in the face of the greatest losses, deprivation, and oppression. Our therapy can take into account the spiritual in their lives—their morals, beliefs, and religious communities, *enfin* their God, within or without a formal religious affiliation, which Pargament speaks of (1996, p. 216)—as the "search for significance" taken explicitly to the level of the "sacred."

As important as it is, spirituality in people is not easily grasped. It comes as a complex and often conflicted bundle of legacies from parents, culture, electronic media, and religious institutions that often do not match and may even contradict each other (Aponte, 1998). Yet that spirituality is hidden in all people's hearts, secretly influencing their lives, while publicly manifested in society under many names and guises.

Spirituality in all of its forms and manifestations shapes the character of the individual, family, and community. For the individual, a stronger spirituality can mean a more internally articulated personal morality and philosophy, and consequently greater personal individuation and internal freedom. For the family, a shared philosophy of life can mean a shared identity and lasting bond. For the community, a common social morality can mean a fraternity of mutual caring. Given the interplay of spirituality at the various levels of the social ecosystem, a healthy spirituality can translate into both the freedom of individual autonomy and social diversity, within the context of the connection of mutual responsibility for the community as a whole. When spirituality is diluted or negated at any level of a society, its life forces of purpose and caring bleed out, and its psychological and social structures weaken.

## The Loss of Spirituality among Poor Minorities

America's poorest and most troubled minorities have suffered the greatest loss of their spiritual roots. Many have lost their cultural and religious traditions in the historical turmoil of this country through slavery, colonization, and territorial dislocation (Aponte, 1994, pp. 1–7). The vitality of their families and communities was sapped when roots of their cultural and spiritual values were suppressed or cut off.

In America today we are in the midst of serious culture wars. At one end of the spectrum, we have the secularist movement, which would prefer to have spiritual and religious expression outside of the public forum, and limited to the privacy of people's personal lives. At the other end of the spectrum are those who view religion and spirituality as integral to all aspects of life, private and public. At the present moment it appears that secularization of public institutions, such as schools, is the prevailing trend. Paradoxically, at the same time, more politicians are identifying themselves as defenders of religious life, because they see the need to reassure the great majority of the population that they, the politicians, recognize the value and importance of religion and spirituality. ("Nearly three-fourths of Americans say their whole approach to life is based on religion" [Paul, 2005, p. 65].) Yet the often contentious cacophony of belief systems and social values in today's fragmented and disjointed society is not fostering cohesion in our society. On the contrary, intolerance among diverse belief and value systems is feeding the culture wars.

Because the more vulnerable members of our society are the more dependent on a healthy society, they also hurt the most when the society at large is hurting. When the moral and spiritual foundations of a society fragment, communities' internal fabric and social supports break down. In this social environment, neighborhoods are vulnerable to whatever socially opportunistic viruses are out there. Committed families become scarcer. The vulnerability of the more severely weakened family ties in poor communities intensifies. The ad hoc pseudofamilies of gangs multiply. The violence increases with the diminution of the sense of family and community that leads to the deadening of kinship love and fraternal empathy. Drugs and alcohol offer an escape from the emptiness, insecurities, angers, fears, and stresses of life. The plague of personal aloneness and worthlessness spreads.

In the face of pain, those who have an active spirituality have a context that can give meaning and hope to the challenges of daily living. In loneliness and discouragement, those who have a spiritual community have a home where they can experience belonging and mutual caring. In helplessness and despair, those who believe in God have the potential of a relationship that to them means strength and love. U.S. and Canadian studies have found that those "who attended religious services regularly . . . had lower rates of depression, panic, and mania" (Cooper, p. 16; Koenig, 1999; Matthews, 1998).

The deprived and disadvantaged need a renewal of spirit that is not dependent upon socioeconomic conditions. In this crucible of society's failure, spirituality offers hope—the ability of the most disadvantaged to transcend the turbulence of life and find meaning in every personal struggle. Spirituality provides emotional support, the motivation to contend, and a transcendent significance to the pain of life. As Frankl has said, people can cope with suffering when that "suffering has meaning" (1963, p. 179).

## SPIRITUALITY IN ACTION

To address more effectively the loss of personal self-worth and power, along with the dilution of family/community ties among poor minorities, therapists need to bridge better the psychological and the spiritual. Clinicians should strive to do the following:

1. Work consciously with the spirituality in people's lives.
2. Build a value base (platform) for their clients' therapy.
3. Pivot the therapy on their clients' life (moral) choices.

### Working Consciously with Spirituality

To work deliberately with the spirituality of the disadvantaged starts with attending to the spiritual aspects of their personal struggles. However, for therapists, understanding and working with spirituality must happen within the borders of good clinical diagnostics and technical interventions. Their task as therapists is to treat spirituality as a facilitator of therapeutic outcome. For therapists, spirituality makes possible a deeper understanding of the potential of the human spirit within the turbulence of the human struggle. It potentially strengthens the will of people to strive, offering them a resource within themselves, as well as the possibility of the support in their families and communities of shared belief, along with the relationship with the transcendent.

The seat of spirituality is in the heart. That also happens to be where therapists are toiling when they touch on clients' attitudes and feelings about themselves and their problems. Helping clients search themselves for self-acceptance, a loving feeling toward a family member, or an optimistic outlook about the solution of a problem is to find hope from within. For those with belief in a personal God, that source of hope may also lie in the presence that abides in the soul. That hope can overcome discouragement from both the world outside and the battered spirit within.

To work consciously with spirituality also calls for working actively with both the people and institutions in which clients' spirituality finds its nurturance. Some family members are potential sources of love and encouragement even if clients at the moment have difficult relationships with them. Even with families that appear fragmented and depleted, the challenge for therapists is to mine the spiritual strength, shared values, and religious practices that exist among family members.

Religion may also provide "family" in the form of a church or other faith community, which can be especially important when people have little family to sustain them. They may discover among fellow worshipers guidance from the clergy, personal support from the brotherhood or sisterhood, and a safe social milieu for their children. A religious fellowship may be the only community that cares about them and is prepared to embrace them just as they are.

There are those who believe that "the only institution with the spiritual message and physical presence to offer" the values poor minority families need is the church (Leland, 1998, p. 22). However, religion may for some people also hold some deeply hidden conflict. In their histories, church and God may come with both positive and negative connotations. They may report memories of solace and support, as well as of disappointment and betrayal. Sadly, often they have done little to resolve and heal the relationship with their faith communities. Therapists can help them revisit, reengage, and rework earlier personal stories to liberate their spirituality.

## Building the Spiritual Platform of Therapy

Attending to the spiritual aspects of clients' personal struggles calls for clinicians' awareness of the spiritual environment they create in their therapy. All therapy rests on a spiritual platform of values and a philosophical outlook that reflects the spirituality of the clinician and the clinician's therapeutic philosophy. Therapists judge what is sick or healthy, and what are worthy or unworthy goals. They determine the merits of a solution not just according to whether it works but also whether it is right or wrong. The values by which they conduct their therapy (Aponte, 1994, pp. 168–185) support or undermine, and contribute to or detract from the spirituality of their clients. The therapy helps to shape people's philosophical perspectives on their problems and, thereby, the spiritual quality of their lives.

Therapists have values ingrained from their respective professions and orientations to therapy. They are not value-neutral. Even when it comes to diagnostic exploration, "There is no way of asking neutral questions," says Michael White (cited in Wylie, 1994, p. 46). Particularly in today's world, therapeutic models and schools come with pretty well-formed convictions about the roles of men and women in marriage, sexual mores in and out of marriage, and Eastern versus Western spirituality. However, therapists often are not even aware of the spirituality their therapeutic approaches bring to bear on clients' issues.

Therapists also carry inside themselves their own *personal* spirituality (Aponte, 2002) that influences their foundational attitudes about: pain and conflict, acceptance and battle, individual effort and the need for relationship. Therapists' personal beliefs about the journey of life affect their views about the value of internal spiritual fulfillment in the face of economic and social adversity, about whether the experience of suffering is a sign of spiritual failure or an opportunity for growth and change, and about whether love is or is not necessary for emotional healing.

Do therapists believe that people can change themselves even if they cannot change life's circumstances? The conviction that people can change their attitudes about themselves and about life even if they cannot alter what is happening to them can bring hope to the most hopeless. The belief that people can have self-respect and do the right thing no matter how bad their problems may be can affirm the worth of the lives of clients and of those they love.

The belief that hard times can promote change means that, however unwelcome, adversity can be what people need to turn their lives around. Hardship can prompt people to consider changes they never thought they could make. Peck (1978, p. 16) says, "It is only because of problems that we grow mentally and spiritually." Socioeconomically disadvantaged people may in their difficulties discover new hope that can overcome despair about themselves and their lives.

Belief in the restorative potential of relationship means faith in the power of love. Ties to spouses, children, and relatives, as well as to the neighborhood and society, however flawed and complicated, offer the strength and support of human kinship. Religion, with its community of the faithful and the relationship with God, offers the power of the spiritual family. Therapists' beliefs in the healing power of love, whether in their clients' relationships with family, neighbors, or God, can make possible what seemed otherwise impossible.

However, therapists' beliefs are only half of the spiritual equation in the therapeutic relationship. The other half belongs to even the least powerful client. In therapy, clinicians are in a position to lend importance and power to clients' values and religious convictions. With poor minorities in particular, it is critical to negotiate equitably (Aponte, 1985) the spiritual base of the therapy, that is, the morality, worldview, and religious beliefs by which clients engage in solving their particular personal issues. The disadvantaged and disenfranchised of our society often enter therapy protecting their deeply felt vulnerability with a mask of hardness—emotionally disengaged and suspicious. When they can assert their personal worth, values, and identities, it is easier for them to acknowledge flaws and hardships. They can risk the openness of personal vulnerability when they sense that their values are recognized and respected. They have greater control over the definitions of and the solutions to their problems. When they see that the therapist takes seriously their complaints about the social agency's services, their opinions about parental authority and discipline, and their religious perspectives about their source of strength—then they can listen to the therapist's ideas about what they might do differently to help their situation. They are more receptive to crafting a common understanding about the goals and means of the therapy. The personal values and life perspectives that clinicians and clients bring to their co-construction of a spiritual platform give direction and meaning to the therapy.

## Therapy That Pivots on Clients' Life Choices

Viktor Frankl spoke to the ability of the human spirit to overcome the oppressiveness of circumstances through the freewill choices—decisions—that people make.

> Man not only behaves according to what he is, he also becomes what he is according to how he behaves. . . . What he becomes—within the limits of endowment and environment—he has made himself. (1967, p. 47)

Although Frankl was referencing the human spirit's ability to transcend the oppressiveness of the concentration camps by the attitudes and moral decisions people choose, we can reference the oppressiveness of urban ghettoes.

Therapy that pivots on clients' free will is a work grounded in clients' belief that they can direct their own lives. The freedom to choose is where people convert their personal uniqueness into their personal action. It is where they decide, issue by issue, how they will live their lives. For the powerless and the invisible, acting on the freedom to choose is to claim their potential and importance in the face of daunting circumstances.

The power and freedom to make life choices ultimately flow from people's essential moral nature to choose good over bad, better over worse. Free will lends spiritual wings to the psychological effort to overcome personal distress. The exercise of choosing can be action that is an internal decision about attitude or an external one about behavior. The act of choosing itself grants people ownership of themselves at the very moment that their decision can change or affirm the course of their lives.

The choices that clients make about their lives in therapy are steeped in their values, ethics, and beliefs—in a word, in the *morality* of their spirituality. For the poor and the marginal, these moral decisions are an exercise in human freedom and self-determination. They can choose reality or denial, active struggle or passivity, self-betterment or despair. In that personal exercise of free will lies the mystery of their essential self-worth and independence even in the face of oppression and deprivation. By supporting clients' potential to exercise their free will on the basis of their own values, therapy can support clients' personal identity and power. Therapy based on the freedom of clients to decide about the course of their lives calls for therapists to help clients identify options and rationales for the choices they face. By offering the technical resources of the intervention and providing the support of the relationship, therapists bolster their clients' motivation and ability to choose. When therapists help them make choices they can own, clients are better able to accept responsibility for the consequences of their decisions.

By working consciously with spirituality, building by mutually consent a value platform, and centering on clients' free will, clinicians lay the foundation for a therapy grounded in clients' spirituality. This approach to spirituality lends support to clients' freedom and power, while recognizing that, like everyone else's spirituality, clients' spiritual lives are ultimately a mystery, their mystery. Spirituality, with all its power and mystique, is a rich and fertile environment in which persons otherwise impoverished may grow and change.

## AN ILLUSTRATION

The following is an example of a young woman who overcame the worst in life with a boost from her spirituality. A clinician built the following therapeutic effort on the woman's religious experiences.

The spiritual strength of families lives within family members' hearts, as well as in their community life. The spiritual potential for our work with the poor in particular lies in our ability to reach deeply for the personal *significance* of what troubles them, and to access the sources of spirituality lying within them, their families, and their faith communities. In today's environment of brief therapy and managed care, it is especially urgent to make that extra effort to tap into the deepest sources of strength of clients.

For 5 months, a therapist had been working with Tess, a 29-year-old African American woman, and Grace, her 9-year-old daughter. Progress in therapy was slow in coming. This was a family on food stamps, with a mother recovering from years of abusing cocaine. She came for help with her daughter, who, in the last year, had been violent at home and disruptive in school. The therapist requested a consultation.

At the time the consultant met with the family and the therapist, the therapist had not seen the family for a few weeks. In their last session, Tess had been upset and ready to give up on her daughter. Instead, Tess, without Grace in the room, opened up to the therapist about a secret pain inside herself. She revealed that when she was Grace's age, she had been repeatedly abused sexually by her father. To her continued distress, her mother had not acknowledged the abuse even after Tess's revelation to her. Tess had been living with this secret shame. Early in life she had smothered the pain with cocaine, but even now she held the hurt hidden within herself. In the therapy she had refused any work on herself, and after this talk with her therapist was still undecided about getting help for herself.

In the consultation, Tess stated that what she wanted help with at that moment was to recapture the love that she and Grace had lost in the last year. However, in talking about Grace, she added that they had gotten along better in the last few weeks, since Tess had returned to church. Her church attendance was news to the therapist. The consultant asked her to expand on what happened with church. Tess described a powerful spiritual experience, with a history.

The story that unfolded was that following the molestation by her father, Tess gradually sank into cocaine abuse. She subsequently became pregnant and gave birth to Grace. She raised Grace alone but with difficulty, because she was strung out so much of the time. A few years ago, she had become pregnant again and had given birth to a "cocaine baby." Three months later, while Tess was high, the child died of sudden infant death syndrome. Tess became distraught with guilt. At the funeral, a Baptist minister whom an aunt had brought to the services sought out Tess. At the minister's invitation, she commenced praying at home and attending church. It was enough to motivate her to stop her addiction cold turkey. Tess became more attentive to Grace, and life for both herself and Grace improved.

However, over the last year, Tess had stopped going to church, although she did not stop her prayers. She and Grace had begun to battle again, and Grace's behavior had deteriorated. Several times, Grace hit her grandmother when corrected by her. Grace's anger carried over into school, and she became unmanageable in class. The school insisted that Tess get help for Grace, and Tess began work with her present therapist. However, the therapy was not bringing about the change they sought. Nor had Tess trusted her therapist with her secret until their previous meeting.

Since that last session, the situation with Grace had continued to decline. Tess became desperate and again returned to church. She spoke of a renewed connection with God. She awakened to how she was being hurtful to Grace—yelling at, hitting, and not listening to her. She then stopped hurting Grace and was able to connect emotionally with her. Grace responded, and her behavior improved rapidly.

The consultant acknowledged and affirmed the significance of Tess's spiritual experience. He then asked where she now wanted to go with therapy. Tess believed she had to decide whether to explore the history and the pain of the incest. It was apparent that Tess was feeling stronger since her return to church. She agreed to bring her hidden pain to therapy even as she continued to work on her relationship with Grace.

How does one explain this spiritual experience of Tess? Whatever the mystery of what happened to Tess spiritually, its psychological effect appeared to be everything her therapist could wish for. Tess holds herself accountable for her behavior with Grace. Also, Tess, who had been shut down, isolated, and angry in her secret shame, can open herself to help from her therapist. Because of her renewed church involvement, she no longer thinks of herself as alone; rather she feels cared about by her God. Consequently, she regards herself as worthy of help. She matters.

Therapy has had and will have a critical place in Tess's change, but the impetus for the depth of this change has come from life outside therapy, from Tess's church and prayer life. Her religion has become one of those healing life forces that Duncan (1997) calls "extratherapeutic factors" and considers so influential on the outcome of therapy. Her spirituality has given Tess a sense of belonging and of being loved, which allows her to trust and be vulnerable in therapy. In her spirituality, Tess has found the motivation and courage to face her demons. The pain of her baby's death gave Tess the original opportunity to discover her spirituality. The recent trouble with

Grace has been the goad that now has urged her back to church. Her therapist has discovered Tess's spirituality, the new source of hope in this woman's life.

## WHOSE SPIRITUALITY?

As a professional, how does the therapist relate to Tess's spirituality? Yes, she needs to stretch herself to understand and to get a feeling for the thinking, direction, and energy that Tess's spirituality lends to her life. However, what about the therapist's values and belief system that interface with Tess's spirituality?

The relevant question here is how to support the spirituality of the disadvantaged who are particularly vulnerable to therapists' influence. Past self-proclaimed "neutral" therapists wanted to believe that they did not communicate political, moral, and religious values. However, therapists today, in their honest desire to help, increasingly feel entitled to promote their values and belief systems.

Many therapists now view their roles as experts on spirituality and values. In his book *Soul Searching*, Doherty (1995) calls for the inclusion of moral discourse in the practice of psychotherapy and the cultivation in therapists of the virtues and skills needed to be "moral consultants to their clients in a pluralistic and morally opaque world" (pp. 7–8; also see Chapter 11, this volume). Like Sigmund Freud, his source of moral authority seems to be science and the field of psychotherapy. Doherty argues that psychotherapists "saw the oppressiveness of cultural norms dressed up as moral principles and could see themselves as agents of emancipation who deconstructed clients' unexamined but powerful moral codes and helped them to make their own decisions" (1995, p. 11). Does he see therapists as liberating clients from the "oppressiveness" of unquestioning faith? His thinking is in line with that of Michael White, who, according to Wylie (1994, p. 44), "deconstructs the dominant authority . . . [and its] culturally determined prescription for the way people *should be*," and in White's own words, is "about opening up possibilities for people to become *other* than who they are" (Wylie, 1994, p. 44; emphasis in original). Wylie continues: "For White, the personal is, and must be, deeply embedded in the political" (p. 44). By Wylie's account, White's therapy rests on his political values.

Emilio Santa Rita (1996) sounds like just such a psychotherapeutic "emancipator" when talking about the "cultural baggage" (p. 325) of a modern American ethnic group whose heritage stems from the Catholicism of the Philippines. He sees as emotionally pathogenic their adherence to their traditional religion's "beliefs on abortion, contraception, and homosexuality [which] contribute to a self-righteous, judgmental stance that is out of place in a pluralistic society with alternative lifestyles" (p. 326). These therapists assert through their therapy philosophical attitudes with serious implications about how people *should* think about and live life.

As noted earlier, Paul (2005) states that three-fourths of Americans base their lives on religion. That statistic is followed with the statement that "32 percent of psychiatrists, 33 percent of clinical psychologists and 46 percent of clinical social workers feel the same" (p. 65). To what extent does psychotherapy potentially place itself between people and their spiritual roots? For ethnic and racial minorities whose cultural heritage and family values are often steeped in their religious beliefs, does therapy assume the posture of critic to their very spiritual identity and religious values? For the power-poor disadvantaged, does therapy become a place to remake their values and religious faith according to the beliefs of the professional psychotherapist?

## *The Clinical Implications of Our Various Belief Systems*

Poor families often find themselves in therapy under some kind of control from courts, schools, and departments of social welfare. They even face control from state-sponsored medical services for welfare clients. They may be ordered into treatment, but even when they voluntarily seek therapy, their health plans usually choose the therapist for them. Many disadvantaged families come into therapy on unsteady cultural and moral foundations and weakly supported community values. Counselors have an inordinate influence and power over such families that depend on the system for survival.

The varieties of philosophies that therapists bring to their work potentially insinuate morality and worldviews that in practical ways can affect therapy's goals, assessment, and interventions. Whether it is ensconced within their politics, therapeutic philosophy, or personal religion, therapists' spirituality skews how they look at their clients' lives. The approach to a client's issues, for example, may reflect a Buddhist outlook that doubts "all fixed assumptions about the nature of things" (Epstein, 1995, p. 62) or, in contrast, the spirituality of St. Francis of Assisi, who says that "realness is whatever corresponds to truth and fact" (Foley, 1949, p. 34). For a victim confronting family denial of sexual abuse, does the objectivity of reality matter? Therapists' views about morality also influence how they handle accountability for the abuse and the role of forgiveness in healing (Aponte, 1998; see also Barrett [Chapter 14] and Hargrave, Froeschle, & Castillo [Chapter 16], this volume). Therapists' divergent philosophies about life translate into fundamentally different approaches to helping families in therapy.

As a consequence, clinicians face the challenge of detecting what values and philosophy are built into their own work. Is it therapy's responsibility to supply families with new and better belief systems? There are those who openly identify their therapy's system of values, as often do Christian therapists, Buddhist-oriented therapists, and feminist therapists. Most therapists, however, do not publicly acknowledge their belief systems. When clinicians, who found their therapeutic approach on a distinct spiritual or political philosophy, let people know the value base of their therapy, their clients have a better chance to judge whether to contract for the therapy being offered. Most clients do not get that chance.

Therapists who are unaware of their therapy's spiritual values are seldom able to lend clients a level of awareness that allows them to exercise control over the values that dominate the therapy. Therapists who know their value biases can choose whether to promote their beliefs with clients. Those working with poor minorities can help clients exercise their right of refusal about the values and belief systems the therapist uses to solve problems. Ideally, with awareness and security about their own spirituality, therapists can empower clients to exercise *their* spirituality in the therapeutic relationship.

### Training Therapists on Their Own and Their Clients' Spirituality

It is clear that if therapists are to work with spirituality, their training must include the study of spirituality in the treatment of emotional and relationship problems (Aponte, 1996). This present volume is just one illustration of the current proliferation of publications on spirituality and therapy. However, there is an added resource, which is the formal and supervised examination of how our own spirituality is manifested in our therapeutic work. Through awareness of our own spirituality, we therapists can gain insight into our client families' ethnic, cultural, and religious belief systems, all of which are "full of possibilities for misunderstanding" (Montalvo & Gutierrez, 1990, p. 35) in therapy.

Practitioners need to be both comfortable and skillful in examining, talking about, and working with spirituality. They need to be able to see and work with the power and potential of clients' spirituality even when they confront clients' ambiguity and conflict about their beliefs, values, and affiliations. They need to be able to disclose their own beliefs when necessary and appropriate. Ultimately therapists will want to potentialize their most vulnerable clients' ability to choose the spirituality that lights clients' own paths to *their* own solutions.

## CONCLUSION

Poor and minority clients often bring to therapy the effects of their hurtful histories and difficult socioeconomic circumstances. These realities are around them and inside them. A therapy that is sensitive to their lives needs to overcome those forces that would erase their identity, diminish their self-worth, or take away their power over their lives. Therapists will, I hope, offer a therapy that connects the disadvantaged to the strength, guidance, and love that is congruent with and that exists within their own culture, belief systems, and religions. At times, therapists will have to offer suggestions of values and perspectives on life that may influence their clients' work with them. They will, I hope, do so with some humility and always with respect for clients' right to choose their own values. Spirituality offers drive, direction, and structure to any clinical effort. Therapists can help their most disadvantaged clients reach into their spiritual resources for the hope to transcend their social and economic circumstances, and live with dignity and self-respect.

## ACKNOWLEDGMENT

Theresa Romeo-Aponte deserves grateful acknowledgment for her contributions to all aspects of this chapter.

## REFERENCES

Aponte, H. J. (1985, September). The negotiation of values in therapy. *Family Process, 24*(3), 323–338.

Aponte, H. J. (1994). *Bread and spirit: Therapy with the new poor.* New York: Norton.

Aponte, H. J. (1996). Political bias, moral values, and spirituality in the training of psychotherapists. *Bulletin of the Menninger Clinic, 60*(4), 488–502.

Aponte, H. J. (1998). Love, the spiritual wellspring of forgiveness: An example of spirituality in therapy. *Journal of Family Therapy, 20*(1), 37–58.

Aponte, H. J. (2002). Spiritually sensitive psychotherapy. In F. Kaslow (Series Ed.) & R. F. Massey & S. D. Massey (Vol. Eds.), *Comprehensive handbook of psychotherapy: Vol. 3. Interpersonal/humanistic/existential* (pp. 279–302). New York: Wiley.

Bunyan, J. (1976). *The pilgrim's progress.* New York: Penguin.

Cooper, G. (2007). Clinician's digest. *Family Therapy Networker, 31*(3), 15–18.

Doherty, W. J. (1995). *Soul searching.* New York: Basic Books.

Duncan, B. L. (1997). Stepping off the throne. *Family Therapy Networker, 21*(4), 22–33.

Epstein, M. (1995). *Thoughts without a thinker.* New York: Basic Books.

Foley, T. (1949). *In the spirit of Saint Francis.* Paterson, NJ: St. Anthony Guild Press.

Frankl, V. E. (1963). *Man's search for meaning.* New York: Washington Square Press.

Frankl, V. E. (1967). *Psychotherapy and existentialism.* New York: Washington Square Press.

Koenig, H. G. (1999). *The healing power of faith.* New York: Simon & Schuster.

Leland, J. (1998, June 1). Savior of the streets. *Newsweek,* pp. 20–25.

Matthews, D. A., with Clark, C. (1998). *The faith factor.* New York: Viking.

Montalvo, B., & Gutierrez, M. J. (1990). Nine assumptions for work with ethnic minority families. In G. W. Saba, B. M. Karrer, & K. V. Hardy (Eds.), *Minorities and family therapy* (pp. 35–52). New York: Haworth Press.

Pargament, K. I. (1996). Religious methods of coping: Resources for the conservation and transformation of significance. In E. P. Shafranske (Ed.), *Religion and the clinical practice of psychology* (pp. 215–239). Washington, DC: American Psychological Association.

Paul, P. (2005). With God as my shrink. *Psychology Today, 38*(3), 62–68.

Peck, M. S. (1978). *The road less traveled.* New York: Simon & Schuster.

Santa Rita, E. (1996). Philipino families. In M. McGoldrick, J. Giordano, & J. K. Pearce (Eds.), *Ethnicity and family therapy* (2nd ed., pp. 324–330). New York: Guilford Press.

Wylie, M. S. (1994). Panning for gold. *Family Therapy Networker, 18*(6), 40–48.

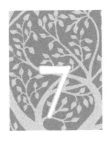

# Spirituality and Religion
## *Implications for Psychotherapy with African American Families*

### NANCY BOYD-FRANKLIN
### TONYA WALKER LOCKWOOD

Spirituality and religion have been essential components of the cultural heritage of African Americans and a major source of strength, resilience, and survival skills. This chapter addresses the incorporation of these issues into the treatment process with African American clients and families—an area that has often been neglected in the clinical literature. Clinical case examples are presented to illustrate the central concepts.

In recent years, the mental health field has begun to address the role of spirituality and religion in psychotherapy (Bergin & Jensen, 1990; Bergin, 1991; Jones, 1994). Surveys have found that two out of three Americans view religion as important in their lives (Gallup & Lindsey, 1999). Yet few therapists address religious or spiritual issues with their clients. Bergin's (1991) explanation is that "such matters have not been incorporated into clinical training as have other modern issues such as gender, ethnicity and race" (p. 396). A number of studies have indicated that this oversight may lead many people to seek counseling from clergy rather than mental health professionals. Bergin (1991) suggests that "perhaps this spiritual humanism would add a valuable dimension to the therapeutic repertoire if it were more clearly expressed and overtly translated into practice" (p. 396).

There have been few attempts to discuss the central role that these issues can play in psychotherapy with specific populations, particularly with African Americans (Boyd-Franklin, 2003; Comas-Díaz & Greene, 1993; Constantine, Lewis, Conner, & Sanchez, 2000; Hines & Boyd-Franklin, 2005; Stevenson, 1990; Wimberly, 1997). Spirituality and religion have long been acknowledged as major strengths within African American families and sources of resiliency and survival skills (Billingsley, 1992; Boyd-Franklin, 2003, 1991; Stevenson, 1990; Hill, 1999). Research has documented the very powerful role of religion and spirituality in the lives of many African American women.

Spirituality and religion are interconnected but hold very different meaning in the lives of African Americans. Many African Americans have an internalized sense of spirituality but are often not part of an organized religion or church (Boyd-Franklin, 2003; Boyd-Franklin & Lockwood, 1999). Watts (1993) found through his research that religion and spirituality are two distinct entities for African American men. *Spirituality* refers to an outlook on life and a personal relationship with God, whereas *religion* refers to church doctrines. African Americans' spiritual power and a belief in something higher than themselves provide a reinforcing function of conviction and fulfillment. This can be a positive factor in the treatment of addictions and alcoholism, and can help to counter resistance (Smith, Buxton, Bilal, & Seymour, 1993).

The African American community is diverse, and clinicians encounter considerable variability on the issue of spirituality and religion. Spirituality or religion/religious orientation may manifest as a deeply ingrained personal belief system, as a formalized set of religious beliefs and institutional practice, or as a combination of both. It would be a serious error for clinicians to stereotype all African Americans as possessing a uniform set of beliefs.

## THE ROLE OF SPIRITUALITY IN THERAPY WITH AFRICAN AMERICAN CLIENTS AND FAMILIES

It is important to recognize that for persons of African descent, the psyche and the spirit are often seen as one (Knox, 1985; Mbiti, 1990; Nobles, 2004). Psychological pain is frequently expressed in spiritual terms (Boyd-Franklin, 2003). Knox (1985) summarizes the most commonly expressed beliefs as "God will solve my problems" (p. 32), "God is punishing me for having sinned" (p. 32), and "God never gives you more than you can carry" (p. 32). These beliefs can be used as a part of "spiritual reframing" with African American clients in therapy (Boyd-Franklin, 2003; Mitchell & Lewter, 1986).

Spirituality often refers to a belief in a "Higher Power" or God. References to prayer and God are ingrained within African American culture: Even individuals who do not consider themselves to be religious incorporate these references into everyday life. For example, a parent told her therapist in a family session that she asked God for help in dealing with her son's increasingly dangerous acting-out behavior. This mother did not attend church, but she reported a deep spirituality and prayed or "talked to God" when she was troubled. It is important that therapists not assume that religious references imply institutional religious or church involvement.

It should also be noted that adolescents and young adults in a stage of rebellion against families who are very religious might engender strong conflicts by forsaking religion and spirituality. These same individuals, however, are very likely to draw on these strong beliefs when they are in trouble, adopting a "crisis intervention" approach to spirituality. It is also not unusual for once-rebellious men and women to return to the church when they have children of their own. Once mental health practitioners are aware of the role that spirituality and religion play in the lives of African American clients, they can utilize this understanding in therapy. These issues become particularly important when one explores the responses to treatment in the African American community.

## RESPONSES TO TREATMENT
## IN THE AFRICAN AMERICAN COMMUNITY

Many clinicians in the mental health field are unaware that attempts by the therapeutic community to be neutral, secular, and "aspiritual" have led to therapy being viewed as "antispiritual" by some members of the African American community, particularly those with strong religious beliefs (Hines & Boyd-Franklin, 2005; Boyd-Franklin, 2003). This is reinforced when therapists who do not know of the deep spiritual roots in African American culture ignore this key component of their clients' core belief systems. In addition, ministers who would otherwise be powerful referral sources may be reluctant to refer troubled congregants to mental health providers because of the profession's reputation for being narrowly secular. (This may be true also of other cultures with strong religious beliefs.)

This issue has particular relevance when it is viewed in the broader context of skepticism about therapy within the African American community. This skepticism has many historical roots within the culture. The legacy of racism and discrimination has compelled many African Americans to view institutions (clinics, hospitals, schools, etc.) with "healthy cultural suspicion" (Hines & Boyd-Franklin, 2005; Boyd-Franklin, 2003), leading to a reluctance to discuss "family business in public." Therapy is considered very public within African American communities, particularly poor communities. Another confounding variable is the view held by many African Americans that therapy is a shameful process and is only for "sick or crazy" people. Although these concerns are not held by African Americans exclusively, the strength of these beliefs within Black communities should not be underestimated.

Given these considerations, it is incumbent on therapists working with African American clients and families to maximize the joining process and facilitate the development of trust. This is particularly true in cross-racial therapy. Therapists who fail to inquire about religion and spirituality may be missing an opportunity to create a therapeutic alliance with African American clients who have a strong belief system. Maximizing the joining process does not mean that the therapist must share clients' beliefs; rather, the therapist shows interest and inquires respectfully about the meaning and significance of spiritual beliefs and practices in each client's life.

In recent years, a number of authors have stressed the importance of incorporating spirituality and religion into the treatment of African American clients (Hines & Boyd-Franklin, 2005; Boyd-Franklin, 2003). Others have emphasized the role of Black churches within these communities (Billingsley, 1992). Therapists without training, however, may be frustrated in trying to incorporate these issues into treatment. This chapter provides useful clinical guidelines and case illustrations.

## THE ROLE OF THE BLACK CHURCH AND THE "CHURCH FAMILY"

Within the Black community, many different denominations and religious groups are represented, including Baptist, African Methodist Episcopal, Jehovah's Witnesses, Church of God in Christ, Seventh-Day Adventist, Pentecostal churches, Apostolic churches, Presbyterian, Lutheran, Episcopal, Roman Catholic, Nation of Islam, and numerous other Islamic sects (Boyd-Franklin, 2003). We focus primarily on the Baptist and African Methodist Episcopal groups, which account for the largest percentage of Black members.

Black churches have long served a multitude of needs in African American communities (Boyd-Franklin, 2003). They have established their own schools and historically have served as the focal point of political activism since the days of slavery, when they were forbidden (Lincoln & Mamiya,

1990). During segregation, they provided what Frazier (1963), in his seminal work, described as "a refuge in a hostile white world" (p. 44), and perhaps the only opportunity for Black men and women to feel respected for their abilities. To this day, they are places where Black people, irrespective of socioeconomic level, can achieve status. In our view, African Americans have used this as a major coping mechanism in handling the often overwhelming pain of racism and discrimination (Boyd-Franklin, 2003). African Americans consistently report higher levels of religious involvement than do White populations in the United States (Chatters, Taylor, & Lincoln, 1999; Constantine, Lewis, Conner, & Sanchez, 2000).

It is important that therapists be aware of meaningful concepts such as "church home" and "church family" (Boyd-Franklin, 2003; Hines & Boyd-Franklin, 2005). The church home is the one the family regularly attends, often for generations. Families who move to a new community often travel a long distance to attend services at their home church. This identification can be so strong that even when individuals go away to school or relocate for a job, they continue to support this church financially. The concept of a church family captures the fundamental role of a Black church as a support network. Often members of the church are considered non-blood-related, extended family members. Church family members often share meals and fellowship before and after services. Church families often resemble extended families, wherein the minister, the minister's spouse, deacons, deaconesses, prayer partners, and "sisters or brothers" in the church function as resources in times of need (Boyd-Franklin, 2003). These church families can be as highly cohesive as close-knit extended families.

When some African American families move, they may be anxious to find a new church home and church family, often providing letters of introduction from their minister. This connection may be extremely important for African American clients isolated from natural support systems. Efforts can be made as a part of the therapeutic process to acquaint or reacquaint clients with these networks of support. This may be particularly useful for single mothers, in that churches can serve valuable socialization and child-rearing functions. Many African American mothers who do not attend church themselves will send their children to services, Sunday school, or social and recreational activities at the church. For many poor families, the "vacation Bible school" substitutes for summer camp and provides constructive activities for children.

The minister is often sought out for counseling by people who would not choose to go for "treatment." Although this courtesy is rarely given, mental health and family service professionals would benefit greatly from meeting with ministers in the communities they serve, given their very powerful leadership position in the African American community. This is helpful from the point of view of community entry, organizational involvement, and as an equal partnership in the community referral network. This connection can counteract the "healthy cultural suspicion" discussed earlier.

One researcher who collected "life stories" from elderly African Americans residing in southwestern Virginia found that the roles of the Black church and religion/spirituality were salient themes for those he interviewed (Nye, 1993). In expanding upon E. Franklin Frazier's classic work (1963), Nye (1993, p. 105) identified six subthemes of the function of the African American church:

1. An *expressive* function, or as an outlet for one's deepest emotions. This was found in the way many respondents couched their deepest concerns in religious terms and references.
2. A *status* function, or religious participation that confers recognition, which may be lacking or denied in the wider, White-dominated world.
3. A *meaning* function, or a source of order and understanding for one's life. This function is particularly important in maintaining continuity.
4. A *refuge* function as a haven in an often hostile world.
5. A *cathartic* function, or as an avenue for the release of pent-up emotions and frustrations felt by an oppressed minority.
6. An *other worldly* orientation function that guides the person to see eventual fulfillment in the next life (Nye, 1993, p. 105).

There are at least two other valuable functions:

7. A *social function*, that is, the opportunity to meet, socialize, and share fellowship with others who share a similar background and interests. This peer involvement can be especially important for adolescents vulnerable to pressures to join gangs, use drugs, or become sexually active.
8. A *child-rearing and socialization function*, which is especially important for single parents. Often churches provide child care during services, in addition to youth activities.

The following case illustrates the process of incorporating spirituality and religion into therapy with an African American family.

Martha was referred by her pastor for home-based family therapy. A 44-year-old African American single parent with six children, Martha resides in a housing project with three of her children: Dominique (age 17), Daniel (age 13), and Roshanda (age 9). The three oldest children (ages 24, 22, and 21) live within walking distance. Martha is a recovering addict who has been drug free for 10 years and still attends Narcotics Anonymous meetings regularly.

Martha has a strong spiritual identity: She proclaims that God revealed himself to her 10 years ago, when she got on her knees to pray that he rid her of her addiction. During the initial interview, she stated that God granted her sobriety in exchange for her service to him every day of her life, and her willingness to spread the gospel of Jesus Christ.

Martha is currently a member of an influential Baptist church in her community. The church is a powerful agency in her life. The pastor also acts as a surrogate father to her children, particularly to her daughter Dominique.

During the first 6 months of treatment, Martha repeatedly used religious metaphors for her life struggles. She was very receptive to spiritual or religious reframes from her two counselors, conveying her feeling that God had brought them to her because she needed help in making new strides in her life.

After the family had been in treatment for approximately 6 months, Martha revealed that she was in crisis and was considering removal of her children from her home because they were threatening her sobriety. Martha complained that the children were violating the rules of the home, such as not informing her where they were or when they would return, and engaging in physical violence with one another and verbal aggression toward her. She found their behavior so stressful that it brought on intense migraine headaches.

Martha stated that she was not willing to allow her children to threaten her gift from God. She believed they must be put out of the house so that she might have the opportunity to become strong again in the commitment to sobriety that enabled her to function as a person and as a mother. She discussed contacting the child welfare agency and asking for their removal. Martha and her counselors brainstormed ideas on how to deal with the crisis in a less drastic manner.

Although Martha had a very supportive family network, its members were consumed by their own interpersonal problems. Martha's support network was extensive and included her prayer partner, friends from church, her pastor, as well as God. With the support of her therapist, Martha called her friends from the church, who responded immediately. Martha's prayer partner and her husband were willing to take the children in for as long as Martha needed. Thus, Martha's children were able to stay within the extended kin network, eliminating the threat of removal by a child welfare agency while Martha had an opportunity to regroup. This experience reaffirmed Martha's faith in God, as well as her trust in her counselors to assist her in her time of crisis. Moreover, Martha was encouraged to call her prayer partner to pray together several times a day. Martha was also encouraged to call her pastor, who knew of her family situation and had been supportive in the past, as well as to attend Narcotics Anonymous meetings daily, so that she could once again feel safe in her sobriety.

This case demonstrates how crucial a client's spirituality and "church family" can be in a time of crisis. Martha was assisted in identifying a resource to which she was already connected that could offer support. The church also fulfilled for Martha the six functions discussed earlier: expression, status, meaning, refuge, cathartics, and other worldly orientation (Nye, 1993).

This case also underscores the value of contacting Black ministers in the community. When the home-based family therapy project began, the directors contacted the local minister and developed a close working relationship. He therefore trusted the project and felt comfortable referring this family. Given the concerns about therapy in the Black community, it is unlikely that this would have occurred without initial outreach.

Integrating spirituality into clinical practice is critical in working with many African American clients. This minimizes attrition and facilitates the joining process between client and clinician. Furthermore, an understanding of spirituality, as well as the religious institutions themselves, can offer great insight into the lives of African American clients. At major life transitions, spiritual resources become especially important, particularly with the loss of a loved one.

## SPIRITUAL ISSUES OF DEATH AND DYING

For members of all cultures and religious groups, death and dying are times when spiritual beliefs and rituals are utilized (Walsh & McGoldrick, 2004; see Walsh, Chapter 4, this volume). This has been particularly true for African Americans given their historical vulnerability to sudden and often violent death. Within the African tradition, life and death are seen as part of a cycle of existence (Nobles, 2004; Mbiti, 1990). Because of the African philosophy of collective unity rather than individualism, times of loss bring the entire extended family, friends, members of the church family, and community together to mourn. A funeral is one of the most important rites of passage in the African American community. It is often held many days after the death to allow extended family members who live at a distance to attend (Boyd-Franklin, Steiner, & Boland, 1995). Funerals in Black churches are frequently cathartic and very emotional experiences. In fact, many Black churches have a nursing corps to help mourners who faint or develop medical symptoms during the service.

The belief in a life after death is also a strong component of the African American tradition. A funeral service is often called a "homegoing," or a "celebration of the life." Music, an active part of all Black church services, expresses these deeply held beliefs. Before and after the service and the burial, family and friends bring food and gather at the home of the deceased. These occasions offer spiritual fellowship, support, shared grief and mourning, as well the joy of a lifetime of memories.

It is striking, however, that after this brief period of mourning, family members are expected to "get on with life," "be strong," and "wipe away the tears." In contrast to the public spiritual catharsis of the church service, the period of mourning is often a very personal, private spiritual time. Because of the pressure to move on, there are often issues of unresolved mourning in African American families, particularly when a series of losses occur in rapid succession. African Americans experiencing this kind of pain frequently express it in spiritual terms, such as "a pain in the soul." In many African American families, when a much-loved family member is lost, a vacuum in the connectedness of family relationships may be experienced. This is particularly true when the deceased held the family together and served as a "switchboard," facilitating family communication (Boyd-Franklin, 2003).

When this type of significant loss has occurred, family members are particularly vulnerable to depression, psychosomatic complaints, and—in children and adolescents—acting-out or conduct-disordered behavior. The following case illustrates how a therapist incorporated spirituality in helping the members of an African American family begin the healing process after multiple deaths and losses.

Jamar, a 14-year-old African American youth, was brought for therapy by his aunt Laverne Smith on the recommendation of his school guidance counselor. In the last year, Jamar's school performance had declined drastically and he was now in danger of failing. His aunt was also concerned because he had been picked up by the police in an incident that was termed "gang violence."

The therapist learned that Jamar's behavioral problems had begun when his mother died from AIDS the previous year. Just 3 months later, his maternal grandmother—who had raised Jamar, his four brothers and sisters, and cared for his mother when she was terminally ill—died of a heart attack. Jamar's aunt reported that he was devastated and withdrew from the family after these losses. In her words, he "went to the streets." Prior to this, Jamar had been highly responsible, helping to care for his mother and younger siblings (ages 11, 9, 5, and 4). His aunt now had custody of all the children but was overwhelmed, particularly by Jamar's behavior. When asked how she coped, she replied that she "prayed to the Lord. . . . From him comes my strength."

The therapist inquired about the family's spiritual and religious beliefs. Ms. Smith replied that the family's "church home" was a large, active Baptist church in the community. She reported that Jamar had been very involved, including participation in the choir and membership on the junior usher board, but had "fallen away from the church" since the deaths of his mother and grandmother. When the therapist attempted to explore these issues with Jamar, he became silent.

In a session about 3 months into therapy, after the therapist had visited the school with Jamar and his aunt, and helped them develop a plan to address his school problems, the therapist met with Jamar alone and again explored his feelings about his losses. He told the therapist that he had been "very angry with God" for taking his mother and his grandmother, and that he had turned away from the church and his family. Jamar's therapist empathized with his loss and helped him to see that his anger was a normal part of the grieving process. For the next few months, Jamar was seen individually, with bimonthly family meetings with his aunt and occasionally with his siblings. His individual sessions were very productive. He gradually opened up and talked more about his anger and how he felt that it was "eating him up."

In one session the therapist explored Jamar's anger at his mother and grandmother for dying and leaving him. An "empty chair" technique was used to allow him to express out loud his anger, sadness, and love to his mother and grandmother. As the anniversary of his mother's death approached, the empty chair was used, and Jamar expressed his anger, sadness, and hurt to God. After both sessions, he burst into tears.

In one family session, with his therapist's help, Jamar told his aunt and brothers and sisters what he had been experiencing. Several of them reported that they had been having these mixed feelings also but had told no one. The therapist helped to normalize the feelings of anger, sadness, loss, and love. It was clear that there was a great deal of unresolved mourning in the family. Jamar, in an important moment of insight, shared with his aunt that this was why he had pulled away from his family and the church and was "running the streets."

The therapist suggested that the entire family might benefit from a ritual of mourning during this anniversary period. With the therapist's help, the family members designed a "memorial service." The aunt suggested inviting their minister and some members of their "church family." As the guest list of people who were important to the family grew, Jamar reluctantly agreed to have the service at the church. He picked the music, his mother's and grandmother's favorite hymns, which he asked a cousin to sing. The therapist attended. The minister led the service, and family members spoke about their memories of the loved ones; Jamar talked about how he had many feelings of love, anger, and loss. When the hymn "Precious Lord" was sung, there was not a dry eye in the congregation.

This ritual, with Jamar and other family members' active involvement, and with the therapist's participation, was very significant for the entire family. Jamar became less angry. Subsequent sessions focused on "healing." His aunt reported that he was home more and studying again. His grades began to improve. Although Jamar still does not attend church, he reports that he has "made his peace with God."

This case illustrates many of the multigenerational issues concerning religion and spirituality in African American families. Jamar's "anger at God" and his rebellion against the family's religious beliefs are typical of many adolescents. The case also demonstrates the ways in which spiritually meaningful rituals can be used as a therapeutic tool to help heal unresolved grief and mourning (see Imber-Black, Chapter 12, this volume).

## GUIDELINES FOR THERAPEUTIC WORK WITH AFRICAN AMERICAN CLIENTS AND FAMILIES

Mental health professionals can benefit from an understanding of the importance of spirituality in the process of change for all communities, but especially for the African American community, in which it is, for many, an already existing strength/resource upon which to build. The following are guidelines for incorporating spirituality or religion into treatment with African American clients.

1. The decision to integrate spirituality into therapy should be contingent on a careful assessment of a client's spiritual or religious worldview and the role or impact that it has on the client's life (Boyd-Franklin, 2003; Constantine et al., 2000; Knox, 1985). Clients frequently reveal such ori-

entation by referring to God as either a source of strength (i.e., "God never gives you more than you can carry") or retribution (i.e., "God is punishing me for having sinned").

2. It is important not to impose a spiritual or religious orientation on clients. Clinicians also should not assume that all African Americans have a religious or spiritual orientation. There is tremendous diversity in the African American community.

3. Clinicians should be aware of the risk of an African American client leaving therapy prematurely because the clinician failed to address that client's spirituality or belief system. It is key that the therapist be able to initiate this type of dialogue and empower clients to discuss their spirituality or belief system as they would any other area of relevance. Otherwise, clients may become confused and doubt that the therapeutic relationship is the appropriate area for spiritual concerns.

4. Clinicians should understand that being in therapy might generate spiritual conflict for African American clients (Boyd-Franklin, 1991). Clients may feel that it goes against their religion, particularly when religious leaders have communicated pejorative views of therapy (i.e., that it is "atheistic"). In addition, individuals themselves may be suspicious of therapy, viewing it as antispiritual or antireligious. In our experience, women in therapy groups have revealed that they had never spoken of spiritual beliefs or conflicts with previous therapists, fearing they would not be interested in this part of their lives (Boyd-Franklin, 1991). For some of these women, psychological scarring results from shame and guilt originating in religion. Therapists' sensitivity to these issues can help clients to experience a release from that pain.

5. Therapists should be aware that in times of crisis the church can be utilized and offers aid to African American families in need. Families may be more receptive to help from a church that is a familiar community resource than to help from an outside agency. In addition, a church can help families that are socially isolated and emotionally cut off from extended family members to reconnect with their "home church," or find a new church that will provide a supportive network.

6. When doing family genograms or ecomaps that include other social systems involved in the client's life, therapists should be careful to assess the role of the "church family" in the lives of African Americans who report a church affiliation (Boyd-Franklin, 2003).

7. Differences in spiritual or religious beliefs may trigger conflict or intergenerational disagreements in African American families. This commonly occurs with conversion to another religion, such as from Christianity to Islam, or from Baptist to Jehovah's Witness. Also, surveys find that African Americans tend to be more accepting of interracial marriages than

of interfaith unions, which can spark family conflict (Gallup & Lindsey, 1999). Tensions often rise around the religious upbringing of children. In such cases, the therapist can bring key family members together to discuss issues in ways that foster mutual understanding and tolerance for different beliefs and practices.

8. Therapists should be aware that psychological symptoms, such as depression, anxiety, psychosomatic illness, and acting-out or conduct-disordered behavior, might mask issues of unresolved grief and loss. Often these losses involve psychological and spiritual pain. If a family member has a strong spiritual or religious orientation, then incorporation of these issues into therapy can help to expedite the healing process.

9. As the first case illustrates, ministers are very powerful figures within Black communities. Clinics, hospitals, and therapists working in these communities should make a special effort to reach out to these leaders. This personal contact helps to build trust and credibility for therapeutic work.

## IMPLICATIONS FOR TRAINING

It is imperative that client needs and dilemmas concerning strong religious or spiritual beliefs be given the same importance in training programs as issues of gender, ethnicity, and race (Bergin, 1991). Therapists must be trained to recognize, assess, and appreciate the diversity of spiritual or religious beliefs that exists within each family, and also be cautioned to not assume that clients hold certain beliefs.

This issue raises a number of ethical concerns in training and therapy. Professional organizations have instructed therapists about their ethical obligation to understand the needs of diverse clients. Religion and spiritual beliefs are vital parts of most cultures. When these issues are ignored in training, therapists are vulnerable to committing ethical abuses by intentionally or unwittingly imposing their own religious/spiritual values and beliefs on clients. Careful training and supervision are necessary to help psychotherapists learn to provide effective therapy with African Americans and clients from other cultural groups that hold strong religious or spiritual values.

## CONCLUSION

It is essential that spirituality be integrated into the coping measures and theories of psychosocial competence (Watts, 1993) and resilience (Walsh,

2006), as well as the theory and practice of psychotherapy. Spirituality is one of the many powerful facets of human life experience, and more than any other throughout time, it has offered hope and solace to those who are suffering.

## REFERENCES

Bergin, A. E. (1991). Values and religious issues in psychotherapy and mental health. *American Psychologist, 46*(4), 394–403.

Bergin, A. E., & Jensen, J. P. (1990). Religiosity of psychotherapists: A national survey. *Psychotherapy, 27,* 3–7.

Billingsley, A. (1992). *Climbing Jacob's ladder: The enduring legacy of African-American families.* New York: Simon & Schuster.

Boyd-Franklin, N. (1991). Recurrent themes in the treatment of African-American women in group psychotherapy. *Women and Therapy, 11*(2), 25–40.

Boyd-Franklin, N. (2003). *Black families in therapy: Understanding the African American experience* (2nd ed.). New York: Guilford Press.

Boyd-Franklin, N., & Lockwood, T. W. (1999). Spirituality and religion: Implications for psychotherapy with African American clients and families. In F. Walsh (Ed.), *Spiritual resources in family therapy* (pp. 90–103). New York: Guilford Press.

Boyd-Franklin, N., Steiner, G. L., & Boland, M. G. (Eds.). (1995). *Children, families, and AIDS/HIV: Psychosocial and therapeutic issues.* New York: Guilford Press.

Chatters, L. M., Taylor, R. J., & Lincoln, K. D. (1999). African American religious participation: A multi-sample comparison. *Journal for the Scientific Study of Religion, 38,* 132–145.

Comas-Díaz, L., & Greene, B. (Eds.). (1993). *Women of color: Integrating ethnic and gender identities in psychotherapy.* New York: Guilford Press.

Constantine, M. G., Lewis, E. L., Conner, L. C., & Sanchez, D. (2000). Addressing spiritual and religious issues in counseling African Americans: Implications for counselor training and practice. *Counseling and Values, 45*(1), 28–39.

Frazier, E. F. (1963). *The Negro church in America.* New York: Schocken Books.

Gallup, G., Jr., & Lindsey, D. M. (1999). *Surveying the religious landscape: Trends in U.S. beliefs.* Princeton, NJ: Princeton Religion Research Center.

Hill, R. (1999). *The strengths of African American families: Twenty-five years later.* Lanham, MD: University Press of America.

Hines, P. M., & Boyd-Franklin, N. (2005). African American families. In M. McGoldrick, J. Giordano, & Nydia Garcia-Preto (Eds.), *Ethnicity and family therapy* (3rd ed., pp. 87–100). New York: Guilford Press.

Jones, S. L. (1994). A constructive relationship for religion with the science and profession of psychology. *American Psychologist, 49,* 184–199.

Knox, D. H. (1985). Spirituality: A tool in the assessment and treatment of Black alcoholics and their families. *Alcoholism Treatment Quarterly, 2*(3/4), 31–44.

Lincoln, C. E., & Mamiya, L. H. (1990). *The Black church in the African American experience*. Durham, NC: Duke University Press.

Mbiti, J. S. (1990). *African religions and philosophy* (2nd ed.). Portsmouth, NH: Heinemann Press.

Mitchell, M. M., & Lewter, N. C. (1986). *Soul theology: The heart of American Black culture*. San Francisco: Harper & Row.

Nobles, W. (2004). African philosophy: Foundations for Black psychology. In R. Jones (Ed.), *Black psychology* (4th ed.). Hampton, VA: Cobb & Henry Press.

Nye, W. (1993). Amazing grace: Religion and identity among elderly Black individuals. *International Journal of Aging and Human Development, 36*(2), 103–114.

Smith, D. E., Buxton, M. E., Bilal, R., & Seymour, R. B. (1993). Cultural points of resistance to the 12-step recovery process. *Journal of Psychoactive Drugs, 25*(1), 97–108.

Stevenson, H. (1990). The role of the African-American church in education about teenage pregnancy. *Counseling and Values, 34*, 131–133.

Walsh, F. (2006). *Strengthening family resilience* (2nd ed.). New York: Guilford Press.

Walsh, F., & McGoldrick, M. (2004). *Living beyond loss: Death in the family* (2nd ed.). New York: Norton.

Watts, R. (1993). Community action through manhood development: A look at concepts and concerns from the frontline. *American Journal of Community Psychology, 21*(3), 333–359.

Wimberly, E. P. (1997). *Counseling African American marriages and families*. Louisville, KY: Westminster John Knox Press.

# Religion and Spiritual Traditions in Immigrant Families

*Significance for Latino Health and Mental Health*

## CELIA JAES FALICOV

We do not own the expertise about the spirit. As therapists, we are not the new priesthood. We all have our own personal philosophical, social, and spiritual perspectives. We have varying degrees of commitment to our values. We have, in effect, our respective "religions." However, the poor come to us sometimes clothed only with their ethnicity, culture, and spirituality. It is not for us to dress them with our apparel.
—HARRY J. APONTE (1994, p. 246)

A journey of migration to a new land and language involves many losses and the challenge not merely to adapt, but to reinvent a life by absorbing new elements without forfeiting old ones. Established religious, spiritual, and healing practices are enduring aspects that resist replacement with the values and beliefs of the dominant host culture. This persistence can help resurrect some aspects of the life immigrants left behind and provide strengths to cope with the multiple changes and social stresses they encounter. Psychotherapists need to be sensitive to the enduring presence of religion, spirituality, and health beliefs among immigrants and to develop respectful curiosity about the use of those resources in psychotherapeutic work.

During cultural, developmental and other life cycle transitions, immigrant families turn more intensively to the comfort and continuity of past traditions, such as prayer and local cures. The human tendency to search for stable meanings in the midst of change by revisiting cultural beliefs and rituals has been called *ideological ethnicity* (Harwood, 1981). This drawing toward one's primary ethnicity can be used as a therapeutic resource to help immigrant families utilize practices that enhance continuity and belonging, while propelling life forward. Even acculturated immigrants, who may have become disdainful or dismissive of indigenous practices or magical beliefs, may tend to tap into their ancestors' core beliefs when times are especially stressful or desperate.

## THE IMMIGRANT'S PARADOX

Recent studies report that the generation of foreign-born immigrants has better health and mental health than that of its children born and raised in the United States. The longer they live here and the higher their acculturation to American society in terms of language, citizenship and self-identification, the more they suffer from medical problems, such as high blood pressure, diabetes, and psychosomatic symptoms, as well as mental health problems, including depression and drug and alcohol abuse. This finding of decreasing physical and mental health with increased acculturation has been dubbed the immigrant's paradox (for a review of these studies, see Organista, 2007).

Migration exposes immigrants and their children born in the United States to poverty, exclusion, and discrimination, all of which pose stress and health risk issues. It appears that people who replace the values of their culture with those of the mainstream do worse than those who manage to retain significant family values. Efforts to assimilate, rather than to increase cultural and social protections, lead to divestment of original cultural assets and social networks, such as those provided by religion and spiritual practices. This loss of significant values and belief systems may in turn impact health negatively.

A key ingredient of resilience in response to migration stresses is the maintenance of dual visions of continuity and change in language, values, and belief systems, a by-product of which is a sense of narrative coherence in the lives of immigrants and their children (Falicov, 2002, 2003). The phenomenon of the immigrant's paradox makes it all the more important to understand and explore the ongoing significance of spiritual and religious traditions, and related health beliefs and practices, in immigrant families.

This chapter addresses two key sets of belief systems that are especially relevant to psychotherapy with immigrants and particularly with Latinos, the largest immigrant group in the United States today. One set of belief systems is focused on health, illness, and traditional healing practices, and the other set concerns religion and spirituality. Despite differences in content, exploration of these two sets of belief systems is relevant for clinical work with immigrant groups from Asia, Africa, and Europe.

## HEALTH AND ILLNESS BELIEFS

Immigrant families often maintain a dual system of beliefs and practices concerning physical and mental problems—the Western medical model, and traditional healing approaches rooted in rural mythologies and indigenous healing practices. Rather than view indigenous healing as an unconventional alternative, it can be seen as having its own spiritual meaning and as playing a complementary role alongside mainstream medical approaches.

The indigenous health beliefs of Latinos can be grouped in two categories: (1) traditional indigenous syndromes based on cultural and spiritual beliefs about causation and healing practices and (2) beliefs in the supernatural, magic, or bewitchment. Southeast Asians, East Indians, and Africans, among others, have their own culturally based illness beliefs, which may include magic and the supernatural in the causation and resolution of physical and emotional ailments. With their underlying spirituality, the healing embedded in these approaches affirms immigrants' connection to their worldviews and may provide a sense of intactness and empowerment in the face of crisis.

### Traditional or Indigenous Syndromes

A *traditional* or *indigenous* syndrome refers to the commonly shared conception of a physical or an emotional problem in a traditional society. Because these conceptions often stem from local cultural beliefs, these illness have been called *culture-bound syndromes* (although, of course, Western mainstream medicine is also culturally grounded in a particular belief system). Indigenous categories are identified with nonmedical labels that summarize observed clusters of symptoms, and they derive from knowledge that is passed on informally from generation to generation. Beliefs in spiritual or supernatural causes and treatment of physical and mental distress are more prevalent among poorer and less educated classes with limited access to mainstream medical diagnosis and treatment but they are also practiced in higher and more educated classes, often secretly.

Traditional or indigenous syndromes are sufficiently distinct from the conventional psychiatric diagnostic classifications that the fourth edition of the *Diagnostic and Statistical Manual of Mental Disorders* (DSM-IV; American Psychiatric Association, 1994) now includes in its Appendix a glossary of *culture-bound syndromes*, including several that are specifically relevant to various ethnic groups. The descriptions help clinicians make a differential diagnosis between culture- bound syndromes and conventional categories, such as anxiety or depression. This formal recognition of culture-bound syndromes also legitimizes the therapist's exploration of these illnesses with clients and their corresponding beliefs of causation and culture-based approaches to cure. Furthermore, with research now confirming the strong connections of body, mind, and spirit, therapists are in an optimal position to explore spiritual aspects of client concerns.

Common culture-bound syndromes among Latinos are *mal de ojo* (evil eye), *susto* or *espanto* (fright), *empacho* (indigestion), *nervios* (nerves), and *ataques de nervios* (nervous attacks) (Harwood, 1981). Underlying these illness experiences are beliefs in the power of strong emotions—one's own or another's envy, anger, fear, and frustration—or of spiritual forces to influence bodily health.

*Susto* or *espanto* (fright) is a syndrome that can affect individuals of all ages. A parent who brings a son to a clinic after a fall from a bicycle may say that the child has lost his appetite or the gleam in his eye; a woman may feel out of control after being frightened by her husband's threats to harm her. The underlying explanation of *susto* or *espanto* is deep fright after a traumatic experience. This explains individuals' symptoms of restlessness, listlessness, weight loss, or lack of motivation (Tseng & McDermott, 1981).

*Mal de ojo* (evil eye) embodies the belief that social relations contain inherent dangers to well-being. Persons with *vista fuerte* (strong vision) can exert a strong power, robbing weaker persons of their ability to act on their own accord. Common motivations are envy or revenge. The victim of *mal de ojo* may experience severe headache, uncontrollable weeping, fretfulness, insomnia, and fever. *Mal de ojo* is thought more commonly to attack women and children, because they are believed to be more vulnerable.

*Empacho* refers to a type of indigestion or gastrointestinal infection that afflicts children and adults and is thought to be caused by a complex interaction between physiological and social factors. Stomach pains are thought to be a symptom of intestinal blockage caused by one being forced to eat against one's will, either by allowing another to override one's personal autonomy or by excessive politeness in accepting food when one is not hungry.

*Nervios* (nerves) not only refers to a general state of distress connected to life's trials and tribulations but it also describes a specific syndrome that includes "brain aches" or headaches, sleep difficulties, trembling, tingling, and *mareos* (a form of dizziness), or simple anxiety and nervousness. A person may be said to be vulnerable to "suffering from nerves."

*Ataque de nervios*, incorrectly dubbed "the Puerto Rican Syndrome," also appears in other Latino groups. A common feature is a sense of being out of control. The symptoms may include dissociative experiences, hyperkinesis, seizure-like or fainting episodes, mutism, hyperventilation, crying spells or shouting. Yet the victim may experience amnesia for what happened during the *ataque*. *Ataques* appear to be more common among women and people in lower socioeconomic levels. Some *ataques* are socially acceptable responses to certain situations, such as when one has witnessed or received news of a shocking family event. An *ataque* may be interpreted as a call for help or a way out of an impossible situation (Guarnaccia, DeLaCancela, & Carillo, 1989).

## Beliefs in Disorders of the Supernatural and Bewitchment

### Magic and Bewitchment

*Mal puesto* or *brujeria* (bewitchment and witchcraft) provide explanations for prolonged disorders that cannot be accounted for by indigenous syndromes and for which traditional healing approaches have not worked. In spite of a declining belief in witchcraft, serious disruptions in social relations are sometimes thought to be the result of various forms of bewitchment. Individuals raised in collectivistic cultures often believe in the power of interpersonal disruptions to create significant psychic damage to all the parties involved, and this damage may be magnified by appealing to magical intervention. Among these interpersonal disruptions are unrequited love, quarrels and breakups among lovers, infidelity, or conflicts among close family members. Following these incidents, it is believed that one of the parties may have hired the services of a sorcerer (*brujo* or *bruja*) to bewitch or to place a hex on the other party. *Mal puesto* is believed to be an explanation for infertility and various forms of mental illness or "insanity," including schizophrenia.

### White and Black Witches

There are elements of cultural syncretism here in notions of magical causation. In pre-Hispanic Mexico, the use of magic was thought to benefit individual health and group survival. But it also had its dark side: It could be used to harm enemies through poisoning, drought, plagues, fatal illnesses, or other forms of harm.

The Spanish Conquest brought a different religion, Roman Catholicism, with its own beliefs and magical practices. The cult of the saints had its own stories of miracles and its own physical sacrifices and punishments to gain favors or concessions. The devil was believed to be the cause of all malignant forces, and witches were thought to have made a pact with the devil.

Both worldviews and conceptions of spiritual influences, the indigenous and the European, operated separately at first, but over time a reciprocal blending of concepts developed. Today, white and black witches are still consulted secretly for a wide variety of problems. White magic is called upon to ward off dangers, alleviate illnesses, locate work, bring success in a new enterprise, provide luck in romance, or recuperate a lost love. Black witches are consulted when one wishes to harm an enemy, defeat a rival, or defend from an evil hex placed by another person (Scheffler, 1983).

Through their wisdom about human relationships, white witches may become the equivalent of local psychotherapists in the ethnic neighborhood. Often, they manage to positively connote every person involved, reassure clients, and create a boundary and a closure to traumatic events. In turn, customers feel better and newly empowered with alternative ways of thinking and behaving (Falicov, 1998).

## Spirituality and Traditional Healing

The world of white and black witches exists, but it is not readily accessible in conversation even among Latinos, let alone with outsiders. More acceptable and somewhat more public is the world of "natural healers," who use herbs and massages but may also prescribe tasks and even talk to spirits. In fact, most markets in Latin American countries have a stand with a person who sells natural herbs, potions, and amulets and will give referrals to medicine men in the community. If one is a trusted customer, then a referral to a white witch may also be provided.

*Curanderismo* is the indigenous method of cure for many of the traditional illnesses described, such as *susto, empacho,* or *mal de ojo. Curanderos,* or traditional healers, may also be consulted for impotence, depression, or alcoholism, even by those who do not profess to believe in traditional illnesses or cures. *Curanderos* are a heterogenous group distinguished by specialties—in specific disorders or particular healing powers. They use a range of

treatments—herbal remedies, inhalation, sweating, massage, incantations—
and a variety of ritual cleansing treatments (Gafner & Duckett, 1992).

*Curanderos, brujos,* and *espiritistas* frequently perform *limpias.* These
important and widely used cleansing rituals require branches of various
plants, eggs, perfumed waters, religious images, dissected animals, and
candles specific to each problem. Rituals take place next to *altares* (altars)
decorated with ritual objects, candles, incense, and images of saints, the
devil (occasionally), or supernatural beings.

Sometimes *curanderos* specialize in certain Western medical treatments
for conditions, such as menstrual cramps or prolapsed uterus, and may have
anatomical charts or other objects found in modern medical offices. Yet
*curanderos,* who have been trained, or mentored, in traditional diagnostic
and healing practices by elder practitioners, do not see themselves in com-
petition with medical providers, particularly with regard to serious health
problems. Clients, too, may see value in using a dual system of health care,
alternatively or together (Applewhite, 1995).

*Curanderos* are skillful at creating a warm and intimate atmosphere,
and they pay tribute to family connectedness by including relatives and asking them to take an active role in decision making about treatment. They
are reassuring and authoritative, and exude confidence in their ability to
diagnose and cure the illness—factors that may contribute to satisfaction
through suggestibility.

Although *curanderos* do not ask or answer many questions, they do allow
for ventilation of fears and hostilities on the client's part. For example, it is
believed that *susto,* if left untreated for some period of time, can lead to "soul
loss," a condition of extreme anxiety, with an inability ever to experience
contentment in life. The cure is a ritualized recapture of the soul and its fast
reentry into the body. But close observation of a *curandero's* healing shows
that much more than a ritual is involved. Tseng and McDermott (1981)
report that a client with *susto* developed a transference-like attachment to
the *curandero.* She expressed a lot of her fears to him and received strong
reassurance both in words and medicine. In addition, she was distracted
from her symptoms by a series of tasks that brought her into social contact,
increased her self-worth, and gave purpose to her days. There is convergence
of therapeutic elements between the *curandero's* practices and mainstream
psychotherapy and psychopharmacology.

*Yerberos,* or herbalists, are especially knowledgeable of traditional remedies and the use of hundreds of plants to treat body and mind. *Yerberos* are
a widely used health resource in Latino communities (Brandon, 1991).

*Espiritismo,* or spiritualism, refers to an invisible world of good and evil
spirits that can attach themselves to human beings, thus influencing behav-

ior. Beliefs in the existence of benevolent and malevolent spirits are embedded deep in the history and living traditions of indigenous peoples in the Americas. Among Puerto Ricans, for example, a belief in spirits has been traced to the Taino Indians, who believed that everything in nature has a spirit. Today, the belief in an enduring spiritual presence of a loved one after death is common among Puerto Rican Americans (Garcia-Preto, 2005; Shapiro, 1994).

Group prayers concentrated on the well-being of one person are thought to gather energy fields that could target positively the sick person's organ or mind. For example, an extended family and network group could get together in a storefront church or *espiritista* shop to pray for the recovery of a relative who has fallen mentally ill, hoping that the energy fields created by the strength of the prayers emanate toward the person's mind, thus helping the person to heal.

Important modern interpretations of spiritualism come from a social justice perspective (Comas-Díaz, 2007). These are primarily based on classic writings by Fanon (1967), who suggested that colonized people live in tension, containing anger that may be released destructively or displaced into magic and spiritual systems. When political action is not possible and self-determination is limited, placing oneself under the protection of benevolent and powerful spirits may help to counteract fear, powerlessness, and lack of agency (Lechner, 1992; Comas-Díaz, 1995). In this context, spiritualism has been thought to act as an adaptive stress-reducing mechanism among Puerto Ricans in the United States.

Many Latinos, such as Puerto Ricans and Cubans, turn to *espiritistas* or spiritualists or mediums who communicate with the spirits and have the power of healing. In *Families of the Slums*, Minuchin, Montalvo, Guerney, Rosman, and Schumer (1967) describe how these indigenous agents "speak" the inner language, a kind of "spiritualese" that is reserved to describe psychological distress. This distress may be seen as originating from supernatural sources rather than one's own inner life. The locus of control is external, and motivation for change may come in the form of a visit by God, hearing a voice from beyond, or seeing a ghost who summons one to return home or to stop drinking. These compelling spiritual experiences may be invoked to "save face," that is, to bring on necessary change without requiring clients to acknowledge responsibility or remorse openly. These authors give an example of a couple that came for consultation. They had couched the wife's infidelity in terms of possession by the spirit of a prostitute. With the problem framed this way, the spouses externalized the problem and joined together in going to an *espiritista*. The spiritualist, working within a cultural framework that endorsed externalization, accepted their explanation.

He assigned them a "task" to bring the estranged husband and wife together cooperatively: They were to take a long trip to dispose of a chicken leg stuck with a nail to exorcise the spirit of the prostitute. The authors comment that a mainstream psychotherapist would have directed the couple to reinternalize their problem, and that this could have rendered the problem unsolvable for the couple.

*Santería* is a religion prevalent among Cubans, some Puerto Ricans, and other Caribbean groups. In worship and ceremonies, it combines deities of the Yoruban or Orichas (Africans from South Nigeria) with Catholic saints. In Cuba this religion is known as *lucumi* and in Brazil, as *macumba. Santeros* are priests or priestesses who function as healers, diviners, and directors of rituals. *Santeros* are very practical and try to resolve concrete problems here on earth, as well as predict through divination the immediate future. They treat *bilingo*, or hex and spirit possession. A *santero*'s "diagnosis" of possession and a client's experience and report of the same may complicate differential diagnosis for psychotherapy practitioners, who may wonder whether the client is psychotic (González-Wippler, 1996). An assessment of developmental aspects of the illness is helpful to this differential diagnosis. Acute and temporary breakdowns linked to interpersonal events might be culturally understood. However, long-term problematic adjustments are not dissimilar to schizophrenia or affective disorders, and should be treated as such.

The notion that the underutilization of conventional health services among immigrants is related to the use of alternative indigenous methods has been called into question by very interesting findings of a large comparative study in a Los Angeles public housing setting. Becerra and Inglehart (1995) found that all groups—Mexican, Chinese, Anglo Americans and African Americans—use alternative practices in addition to, and not in place of, conventional medicine. Alternative remedies were used for minor illnesses and to prevent major ones, but not to treat chronic or life-threatening illnesses. It appears that consistent users of unconventional approaches are also consistent users of conventional medicine, and they appear to be individuals concerned with a high range of self-administered health care.

Thus, health for many immigrants involves a complex interaction of physical, psychological, social, and spiritual factors. Religious beliefs are often expressed along with spiritual and health practices. Latino immigrants are adept at blending beliefs and practices, and they do not insist on theological consistency. It is not uncommon for a person to believe in the Catholicism of Spain; the African cults, as they have become interpreted in the Caribbean; along with more recent conversions to American Protestantism. Within multigenerational families, many varied beliefs and practices may be expressed.

## RELIGIOUS BELIEFS

Religion can serve multiple purposes for many immigrants. Religion can provide internal continuity and transportability of beliefs and practices both in the privacy of one's mind or home and in the public area of the church. In so doing, religious activity can reaffirm ethnicity in a new context as something valued and respected.

Religion also supports immigrants' adaptation to the new country by lending concrete help and community involvement, which includes participation in holidays and festivals (Falicov, 2005, 2007). Finally, religion also maintains long-distance connections. People's ties are reinforced as they help their church monetarily at long distance or seek spiritual guidance and sustenance from a distance or when visiting (Falicov, 2007). In countries that allow for return visits by immigrants, it is common for the first and the second generations to return every year, or every 2 or 3 years, to the original town for religious celebrations, such as the Feast of the Patron Saint in Puebla, Mexico, giving the second generation an opportunity for a significant experience there (Smith, 2002). It is interesting that homeland churches also encourage involvement and loyalty among the children of immigrants. An East Indian church prints a small magazine in English for its expatriates to shed light on their religious preaching and to help them keep in touch with the religious activities of their homeland congregations (Levitt, 2002). Involvement in a faith community in the United States, usually as a continuation of one's religious practices, is significantly associated with sending remittances to the country of origin for immigrants from the Phillipines, Vietnam, and Latin America. One possible explanation that this suggests is a link between religious practices and moral responsibility toward those left behind, such as older parents (Rumbaut, 2002).

Roman Catholicism provides a common denominator of beliefs and values for many Latino groups, in spite of cultural variations in actual practices. Protestant Evangelical and Pentecostal congregations increasingly draw Latino immigrants to their more emotionally expressive and interactive worship services. More than half of Latino Catholics identify themselves as charismatic. While remaining committed to the Catholic Church, many of these immigrants believe in divine healings and speak in tongues, practices that not only are more typical of Protestant Renewalist movements but also fit with indigenous roots that include belief in magic and supernatural experiences.

The impact of religious beliefs and spiritual practices on illness and healing have increasingly received health professionals' attention (Bergin, 1991; Dossey, 1993; Wright, Watson, & Bell, 1996; see Walsh [Chapter 2] and Wright [Chapter 3], this volume). Religious beliefs shape many interpretations and attitudes toward physical and mental illness, cures, and adaptations. These are primarily Christian beliefs in God as supreme being, in life after death, and in the existence of a soul. Beliefs about heaven and hell, sin, guilt, and shame also play a role in meaning making and in causal attributions of responsibility.

Catholicism also encompasses some magical thinking, beliefs in miracles, propitiatory rituals, promises (*promesas*), and prayers. Although small altars to saints are everywhere in the streets of Latin America, immigrants may create home altars with flowers, crucifixes, bottles of holy water, and saints depicted in plastic statuettes or postcards. These practices emphasize the Latino belief in endurance of suffering and denying oneself in exchange for needed favors.

Devotional offerings, daily prayers, masses at home, vows of penance, and even pilgrimages to shrines may be offered to special saints in return for their intercession and commendation. Numerous prayers are offered to the Virgin of Guadalupe, the patron saint of Mexico, who is also revered in Puerto Rico and other parts of Latin America. This deity offers enormous psychological protection, spiritual nourishment, and unity among people. Her portrait, a most powerful icon, hangs in living rooms, and dangles from key chains and over automobile dashboards. She is a perfect fusion of indigenous Aztec and Catholic European elements, the only brown-skinned Catholic saint who validates the promise of Catholicism for indigenous people. Multiple popular meanings and profound love are bestowed upon this Virgin by gang youth, feminists, and social justice activists. The emotional significance of the Virgin of Guadalupe for immigrants is eloquently expressed in the following quote:

> And so *la Virgen {de Guadalupe}* is called upon to cure ills north and south for loved ones or for anyone else who suffers. This gathering in L.A. [to celebrate the day of the Virgin of Guadalupe] might not be as monumental as the festival in Mexico City. But there is an intensity here that matches or maybe even surpasses the devotion back home. Perhaps it is the yearning to remain rooted in a rootless time where one's address can't be changed by twists of the economy or the border patrol. (Martínez, 1996, p. 111)

## RELIGION, SPIRITUALITY, AND PSYCHOTHERAPY WITH IMMIGRANTS

In spite of the widespread importance of religion and spirituality for Latinos and many other immigrant groups, very little has been written about the interaction of religion and psychotherapy for these populations. Church and congregational life are often important parts of a client's ecological niche (Falicov, 1995, 1998, 2005) and can be a great resource for families in therapy. Immigrants commonly attend church in the United States because it provides a place of belonging, a way to meet other immigrants, and a socializing and educational setting for their children and themselves (see also Kamya, Chapter 15, this volume). They often turn to clergy for counsel in times of stress. Sending children to parochial schools and getting involved with church activities and needs can provide an avenue for self-expression and status for men and women who have little opportunity for stimulation or acknowledgment through their jobs or life situations.

Adherence to church doctrine, regular church attendance, and the roles played by clergy and organized religion vary among Latino groups. Therapists should ask whether clients find spiritual solace or any form of support through involvement in a faith community. Mexicans are a devout group for which church attendance and observance of religious holidays and rituals are considered vital (Falicov, 2005a, 2005b). For older Mexicans, the church provides spiritual support in the form of hope or helps individuals face pain and accept suffering. Religious leaders may be important auxiliaries to the treatment process. For many Puerto Ricans, the church is a place for communions, weddings, or funerals. Going to church is not considered necessary, however, to reach God or the supernatural. Puerto Ricans have a special relationship with saints, whom they believe can be personal emissaries to God (Garcia-Preto, 2005). Exposure to other religions has led to the incorporation of other beliefs and rituals for many Latino immigrants.

## The Interweaving of Spiritual Traditions in Life-Cycle Transitions

The interweaving of religion and indigenous traditions among many Latino groups is particularly apparent during important life-cycle transitions, such as birth and marriage or death and bereavement (Falicov, 2005b) Mexicans embrace death, unlike the dominant American culture, which has tended to avoid and minimize it. The Day of the Dead is an annual public fiesta in which folklore, religious litanies, sugar candy skulls, and paper skeletons poke fun at death. Families enjoy festive graveside picnics, leaving food and drink for their deceased loved ones. The event includes a grieving ritual that takes place annually for 4 years after the death of a family member. The family erects at home a portable altar with a photograph of the dead person, flowers, and some favorite objects and foods of the deceased. After a day's vigil at their open home, the family transports the altar with its hanging objects and foods to the cemetery. Family and friends light tall candles and sit around the grave chanting and swaying. Close family members, particularly women and children, often sleep next to the grave, until the following morning, to "keep company to our poor dead ones" (*a nuestros pobrecitos muertos*). This ritual offers emotional release and continuing spiritual connection to the departed. Some household variant could be used as a therapeutic resource if the ritual was ever or remains meaningful to the particular family, as it would be hard to fathom an American cemetery as a place to spend the night with deceased relatives.

Less lavishly, Puerto Ricans and Cubans also celebrate the Day of the Dead. Their funerals, processions, or street caravans to accompany the dead are very expressive, especially for a child's funeral (Santiago, 1994). Gasping for breath, heart palpitations, or chest pains (*piquetes*) in the deeply bereaved are accepted as natural expressions of grief; emotional states are not conceived as being separate from bodily reactions in most Latino cultures. Although these practices appear to be more conspicuous among the poorer socioeconomic classes, elements of these beliefs exist among subgroups of middle- and upper-class Latinos.

Hallucinations of the deceased, including "visitations" of spirits and ghosts, may occur for several years following a loved one's death, especially among Puerto Ricans who practice *santería* and Cubans who engage in *macombe* (an Afro-Caribbean religion). Therapy may blend elements of religion and spirituality suggested by the client into mainstream modalities to fashion more meaningful and culturally congruent treatment.

### Locus of Control and Styles of Coping with Adversity

Many Latinos come from traditional cultures and social classes that share a core belief that is critical for therapists to understand: When illness or troubles strike, the cause is often attributed to sources outside or beyond the victim's influence or control. It is not unusual to attribute physical or emotional problems to external forces. Many Latinos automatically add "*si Dios quiere*" (God willing) or "*Dios mediante*" when speaking of their plans for the near or distant future. These statements transmit a recognition that their lives are not under their control and that they are governed by a higher power (Muslims similarly use the phrase "Allah willing"). The Chicana writer Sandra Cisneros (1997) sees the relatively infrequent use of this linguistic expression among Anglo-Americans as evidence that they must feel a great deal of control over their own destiny. For many Latinos, fate, destiny, or God is in charge.

## Fatalism

The notion that little in life is under one's direct control is a worldview that has sometimes been referred to as "fatalism" (Comas-Díaz, 1989) or external locus of control, and has been ascribed more frequently to underprivileged and underserved groups. Fatalism is more prevalent among poor people, because they learn through recurrent experiences that powerful others and unpredictable forces control their lives. Limited opportunities to get ahead and change life circumstances fuel feelings of helplessness, a sense of failure, and futility about pursuing an active orientation. This fatalistic outlook may increase psychological distress, but it is important for therapists to distinguish between this "deficit-oriented" theory of *fatalism* and a more "resource-oriented" perspective.

The ecology of lower socioeconomic status can indeed disempower individuals and limit their hopeful outlook, as would a marginalized position in the new culture. Such situations require the use of empowering therapeutic approaches to cope with the frequent external stresses. At the same time, accepting conditions and losses that are beyond one's control (e.g., an incurable disease, a job layoff, or an unexpected death) may be a strong resource based in a spiritual orientation. Holding a both/and frame in conversation with clients about how they view their control over problems and options is the most helpful approach. Resilience research supports this stance for positive adaptation: mastering the possible and accepting that which is beyond control (Walsh, 2003).

At first glance, it appears that belief in an external locus of control would "fit" with externalizations used by narrative therapists (White, 1989), who purposely separate a client's symptom from the client as an avenue to stimulate personal agency or choice. In fact, Wright et al. (1996) suggest that externalization techniques in which the illness, rather than the victim, is accused are similar to those employed by witch doctors. On closer examination, however, externalizing conversations are often based on talking about a problem as if it might eventually be defeated or escaped, so conversations about struggle and control prevail. This type of aggressive language use is very different from a worldview that encourages acceptance, resignation, and coexistence by making peace with an externally induced problem and belief in a higher spiritual power. Cultural inclinations to see problems as the result of fate, or of God's will, reveal several internal coping mechanisms that are more syntonic with the Latino worldview. These are discussed in the following section.

## Self-Control (Controlarse)

Various degrees of self-control are possible when dealing with life problems. *Controlarse*, or control of the self, is a dynamic theme of Latinos, a central cognitive and behavioral mechanism for mastering the challenges of life by controlling one's moods and negative emotions, particularly anger, anxiety, and depression (Cohen, 1980). The concept of *controlarse* includes the following ideas: *aguantarse* (endurance), or the ability to withstand stress in times of adversity; *no pensar* (don't think of the problem), or avoidance of focusing on disturbing thoughts and feelings; *resignarse* (resignation), or the passive acceptance of one's fate; and *sobreponerse* (to overcome), a more active coping that facilitates working through or overcoming adversity.

Mental illness may be seen as the result of poor luck, fate, or powers beyond the control of the individual, or as the fault of the parents. Sometimes it is God's test; other times, it is simply God's will. Quiet acceptance and resignation in the face of a chronic illness may represent a form of sensible, humble realism that contrasts sharply with the Western mastery orientation and optimism about endless possibilities for change.

## Somatization: The Mind–Body–Spirit Connection

Another form of coping related to locus of control is "somatization," those medically unexplained physical symptoms that commonly denote emotional distress. To explain the tendency to somatize rather than "psychologize," Canino, Rubio-Stipec, Canino, and Escobar (1992) argue that Anglo-Americans may be more likely to postulate a mind–body Cartesian dichotomy than other cultural groups, which are more likely to integrate mind–body experiences and express them somatically. Stigma toward mental illness may make it more socially acceptable to express psychological distress through physical complaints. Also, among the poor, health care is more readily available for medical than for psychological complaints. Herbal treatments are more affordable than drugs. Physical and emotional trauma and losses with migration may produce spiritual distress and bodily symptoms; research is now documenting the recursive influences of mind–body–spirit interactions in suffering and well-being. These many reasons may explain why somatization has been frequently found in immigrants and refugees (Castillo, Waitzin, Ramírez, & Escobar, 1995).

As therapists we need to be aware that physical complaints for which medical causes cannot be found may have a number of symbolic meanings, or emotional or spiritual explanations. These meanings may be accessed by asking Latino clients what they believe are possible sources of their physical symptoms, and what approaches to treatment they think would be helpful.

## CONCLUSION

Belief systems are enduring aspects of people's collective and personal cultures. Understanding and respecting immigrant clients' beliefs and traditional practices connected to family health, illness, and healing enhance the successful engagement and unfolding of psychotherapy. Therapists need to approach exploration of clients' belief systems as a way of tapping the ancient healing mechanisms that their cultural and spiritual resources can provide rather than viewing traditional beliefs and practices as useless magic and superstition. Mainstream religious practices, such as regular church attendance, praying, and confession, are important sources of comfort, solace, and moral guidance for many immigrants, and may coexist with other practices based on indigenous beliefs.

It is helpful in working with immigrants from different cultural traditions to envision a holistic mind–body–spirit connection that allows for emotions to manifest in bodily expressions, and for problems to reside in the mysteries of the spiritual domain or relational sin and revenge, thus entering the poetic realm of human drama. Solutions lie somewhere in the alchemy of religion, magic, and tradition, and their integration with both modern cultural practices and the therapist's openness to new perspectives for immigrant clients.

## REFERENCES

American Psychiatric Association. (1994). *Diagnostic and statistical manual of mental disorders* (4th ed.). Washington, DC: Author.

Aponte, H. J. (1994). *Bread and spirit: Therapy with the new poor.* New York: Norton.

Applewhite, S. L. (1995). *Curanderismo:* Demystifying the health beliefs and practices of elderly Mexican Americans. *Health and Social Work, 20*(4), 247–253.

Becerra, R. M., & Inglehart, A. P. (1995). Folk medicine use: Diverse populations in a metropolitan area. *Social Work in Health Care, 17*(2), 127–146.

Bergin, A. E. (1991). Values and religious issues in psychotherapy and mental health. *American Psychologist, 46,* 394–403.

Brandon, G. (1991). The uses of plants in healing in an Afro-Cuban religion: Santería. *Journal of Black Studies, 22*(1), 55–76.

Canino, I. A., Rubio-Stipec, M., Canino, G., & Escobar, J. I. (1992). Functional somatic symptoms: A cross-ethnic comparison. *American Journal of Orthopsychiatry, 62*(4), 605–612.

Castillo, R., Waitzkin, H., Ramírez, Y., & Escobar, J. I. (1995). Somatization in primary care, with a focus on immigrants and refugees. *Archives of Family Medicine, 4*, 637–646.

Cisneros, S. (1997). In two humors. *Sí Magazine, 1*, 68–70.

Cohen, L. M. (1980). Stress and coping among Latin American women immigrants. In G. V. Coelho & P. I. Ahmed (Eds.), *Uprooting and development: Dilemmas of coping with modernization* (pp. 345–372). New York: Plenum Press.

Comas-Díaz, L. (1995). Puerto Ricans and sexual child abuse. In L. Aronson Fontas (Ed.), *Sexual abuse in nine North American cultures: Treatment and prevention.* Thousand Oaks, CA: Sage.

Comas-Díaz, L. (2007). Ethnopolitical psychology: Healing and transformation. In E. Aldarondo (Ed.), *Advancing social justice through clinical practice* (pp. 91–118). Mahwah, NJ: Erlbaum.

Dossey, L. (1993). *Healing words: The power of prayer and the practice of medicine.* San Francisco: Harper.

Falicov, C. J. (1995). Training to think culturally: A multidimensional comparative framework. *Family Process, 34*, 373–388.

Falicov, C. J. (1998). *Latino families in therapy: A guide to multicultural practice.* New York: Guilford Press.

Falicov, C. J. (2002). Ambiguous loss: Risk and resilience in Latino immigrant families. In M. Suarez-Orozco & M. Paez (Eds.), *Latinos: Remaking America* (pp. 274–288). Berkeley: University of California Press.

Falicov, C. J. (2003). Immigrant family processes. In F. Walsh (Ed.), *Normal family processes* (3rd ed., pp. 280–300). New York: Guilford Press.

Falicov, C. J. (2005a). Mexican Americans. In M. McGoldrick, J. Giordano, & N. Garcia-Preto (Eds.), *Ethnicity and family therapy* (3rd ed., pp. 229–241). New York: Guilford Press.

Falicov, C. J. (2005b). The Latino family life cycle. In B. Carter & M. McGoldrick (Eds.), *Expanded family life cycle: Individual, family and social perspectives* (3rd ed., pp. 141–150). Boston: Allyn & Bacon.

Falicov, C. J. (2007). Working with transnational immigrants: Expanding meanings of family, community and culture. *Family Process, 46*(2), 157–172.

Fanon, F. (1967). *Black skin, White masks.* New York: Grove Press.

Gafner, G., & Duckett, S. (1992). Treating the sequelae of a curse in elderly Mexican Americans. *Clinical Gerontologist, 11*(3/4), 145–153.

Garcia-Preto, N. (2005). Puerto Rican families. In M. McGoldrick, J. Giordano, & N. Garcia-Preto (Eds.), *Ethnicity and family therapy* (2nd ed., pp. 242–255). New York: Guilford Press.

González-Wippler, M. (1996). *Santería: The religion.* St. Paul, MN: Llewellyn.

Guarnaccia, P. J., DeLaCancela, V., & Carrillo, E. (1989). The multiple meanings of the *ataques de nervios* in the Latino community. *Medical Anthropology, 11,* 47–62.

Harwood, A. (1981). *Ethnicity and medical care.* Cambridge, MA: Harvard University Press.

Lechner, N. (1992). Some people die of fear: Fear as a political problem. In J. E. Corradi, P. W. Fagen, & M. Garretón (Eds.), *Fear at the edge: State terror and resistance in Latin America.* Berkeley: University of California Press.

Levitt, P. (2002). The ties that change: Relations to the ancestral home over the life cycle. In P. Levitt & M. Waters (Eds.), *The changing face of home: The transnational lives of the second generation.* (pp. 123–145). New York: Russell Sage Foundation.

Martínez, R. (1996). The undocumented virgin. In A. Castillo (Ed.), *Goddess of the Americas–La diosa de las Américas: Writings on the Virgin of Guadalupe* (pp. 98–110). New York: Riverhead Books.

Minuchin, S., Montalvo, B., Guerney, B., Rosman, B., & Schumer, F. (1967). *Families of the slums: An exploration of their structure and treatment.* New York: Basic Books.

Organista, K. (2007). *Solving Latino psychosocial and health problems: Theory, practice and populations.* New York: Wiley.

Rumbaut, R. (2002). Severed or sustained attachments?: Language, identity and imagined communities in the post-immigrant generation. In P. Levitt & M. Waters (Eds.), *The changing face of home: The transnational lives of the second generation* (pp. 43–95). New York: Russell Sage Foundation.

Santiago, M. (1994). *A Puerto Rican view of death and dying.* Presentation at the quadrennial meeting of the *Family Process* Journal, San Juan, PR.

Scheffler, L. (1983). *Magia y brujería en México.* Mexico City: Panorama Editorial.

Shapiro, E. R. (1994). *Grief as a family process: A developmental approach to clinical practice.* New York: Guilford Press.

Smith, R. C. (2002). Life course, generation and social location as factors shaping second generation transnational life. In P. Levitt & M. Waters (Eds.), *The changing face of home: The transnational lives of the second generation* (pp. 145–168). New York: Russell Sage Foundation.

Tseng, W. S., & McDermott, J. F., Jr. (1981). *Culture, mind and therapy: An introduction to cultural psychiatry.* New York: Brunner/Mazel.

Walsh, F. (2003). Family resilience: A framework for clinical practice. *Family Process, 42*(1), 1–18.

White, M. (1989, Summer). Externalizing of the problem and re-authoring of lives and relationships. *Dulwich Centre Newsletter,* pp. 3–21.

Wright, L. M., Watson, W. L., & Bell, J. M. (1996). *Beliefs: The heart of healing in families and illness.* New York: Basic Books.

# "Honor Your Father and Your Mother"

## Intergenerational Values and Jewish Tradition

### MONA DEKOVEN FISHBANE

At the heart of the Jewish tradition, and at the center of the Ten Commandments, is the fifth commandment: "Honor your father and your mother, that your days may be long upon the land which the Lord your God gives you" (Exodus 20:12). According to rabbinic sources, this commandment belongs both to the first four commandments, which refer to acceptance of and obedience to God, and to the last five commandments, which deal with human relations. The fifth commandment is considered the link between divine and human realms.

This chapter considers the command to honor parents within the context of the Jewish tradition. It examines the nexus of values within which honoring parents is embedded, especially the values of multigenerational continuity and of parents' obligations to pass on the tradition to their children. Some of the laws and stories that exemplify the often difficult challenge of honoring mother and father are explored. These traditions of filial piety are considered as they affect and are affected by the modern American context. Finally, broader implications for families and family therapy are discussed, especially around intergenerational conflicts and reconciliation.[1]

## CLASSICAL TEXTS, MODERN CONCERNS

We confront classical Jewish texts, revered within the tradition, with modern sensibilities and concerns. Classical Judaism, like other world religions, traditionally has been patriarchal; the major voices and authors until recently have been male, as has the imagery and language describing God. There are significant exceptions, especially in the mystical tradition; for example, the Shekhina is the feminine dimension of God, and refers to the divine aspects of care. Likewise, there have been some notable examples of women heroines and scholars in the classical texts. Modern feminists and liberal Jews have worked to reclaim the tradition for themselves, seeking and developing narratives about women in the Bible and postbiblical texts, and altering prayer language to a gender-neutral form. Many women in recent years have taken on the central Jewish spiritual task of studying sacred texts—an opportunity not generally available to women historically. Within contemporary feminist Orthodox and liberal circles, women are attaining high levels of learning and scholarly and spiritual leadership.

Many of the classical texts cited in this chapter refer to fathers and sons as the prototypical intergenerational relationship (reflecting the patriarchal bias of the authors of these texts), even though both daughters and sons are commanded to honor their mother and father. I have chosen to cite these examples despite my discomfort with the male bias, because I believe there is much spiritual value in these ancient voices. In my own language in this chapter, where possible I use gender-neutral or inclusive terms, referring, for example, to "parents" rather than "fathers" and to "children" rather than "sons."

I find the narratives of the Jewish tradition around intergenerational connection to be resources of wisdom, especially in the open culture in which we live, with values in flux. Although the contemporary context is very different from that in which the laws and expectations around honoring parents evolved, many of the principles and difficulties involved in the fifth commandment remain relevant today. As we wrestle with intergenerational tensions and loyalty conflicts, it is helpful to consider how prior generations and traditions have dealt with these issues. Engaging in a cultural dialogue with the past can, I believe, inform our present and future.

## TRADITION AND NARRATIVE

Judaism is a religion of memory and narrative. The earliest and most central text, the Torah (the five books of Moses), tells of the formation of the ancient

Israelite nation and its complex relationship with God. The high points of this narrative are the Exodus from Egypt and the Revelation at Mount Sinai, in which the Ten Commandments and, according to tradition, the entire Torah was given by God to Moses on behalf of the people. The Torah is the foundation text, the core of a rich and varied tradition that extends from the ancient period to the present. Interpretation and study are key spiritual activities in Judaism; almost nothing is more highly valued than sacred learning (which includes study of the Torah as well as the commentaries on it, such as the Talmud and Midrash).[2] The study of older narratives, as well as the reworking of older texts into newer ones, allows the religion to evolve while staying attached to its roots. Through learning, prayer, and ritual, the emphasis on memory and making present the past is reinforced constantly. The Torah is read in synagogue throughout the year, and each year at specific holidays the nodal historical events are celebrated.

In passing on the tradition, there is a double vision about one's relationship to past generations. The sages are constantly interpreting and adjudicating legal and moral issues; the religion evolves and responds to the demands of the present historical period. At the same time, there is a reverence for the past and for the greatness of past scholars. This connection with the rabbis of earlier generations encourages a spiritual humility; one looks back as one moves forward.

## MULTIGENERATIONAL CONTINUITY

The Jewish God is referred to in many ways. One of the most common epithets in the Bible is "the God of Abraham, Isaac, and Jacob."[3] The original covenant was made between God and Abraham, in which Abraham, in return for embracing this God, was promised descendents who would become the nation Israel, later known as the Jewish people. The covenant with the biblical patriarchs includes the promise of multigenerational continuity. Subsequently, the complicated relationship between God and the Israelites revolves around the inconstancy and infidelity of the people, and divine threats to destroy or cut off the people in response. By contrast, the Israelites are promised divine blessing—in the form of the flourishing of generations of descendents and abundance in the land—if they are faithful to God.

The survival of the nation and of one's family through descendents is a theme that echoes throughout the biblical narratives. There is a deep anxiety that surfaces around childlessness, with the prospect of one's name not being continued through progeny. Filial succession is another central motif, especially in the Genesis narratives. Sibling rivalry abounds, as brothers vie for parental blessings (e.g., Isaac and Ishmael, Jacob and Esau, Joseph and his brothers).

The identification of oneself multigenerationally continues in the rabbinic period. In the Talmud and other classical texts, rabbis are identified by their familial line, for example, "Rabbi Joshua the son of Levi." Likewise, a rabbi frequently locates himself in his spiritual lineage by referring to his teacher: for example, "Rabbi Safra said on the authority of Rabbi Joshua the son of Hanania." In a world in which respect for parents and teachers is central, an individual's contribution to the rabbinic discussion is framed by his or her multigenerational context, both biological and spiritual. Credit, respect, and even reverence for parents and teachers characterize the rabbinic discourse.

## "AND YOU SHALL TEACH YOUR CHILDREN DILIGENTLY"

Multigenerational continuity is ensured in Judaism by the parent teaching the child. In the Bible, the parent is admonished: "And you shall teach [the laws] diligently to your children, and shall talk of them when you sit in your house, and when you walk on the way, and when you lie down, and when you rise up" (Deuteronomy 6:7). The teaching of Torah and its values to children is an ongoing, constant process, whether through instruction or through the modeling of one's daily behavior.

The same chapter in Deuteronomy further instructs the parent that when the child asks, "What are these commandments?," the parent should respond, "We were slaves in Egypt . . . and God brought us out of Egypt . . . and God commanded us to do these laws, to revere God" (6:20–24). This parent–child dialogue is woven into the Passover Haggadah,[4] which is recited at the Seder. The Haggadah is a supreme moment of ritual retelling, of multigenerational questions and answers. The Haggadah poses the drama of four sons, each of whom is facing the tradition in a different way. The parent is told to answer the child in a manner appropriate to each child's nature and capacity. The yearly drama of the Passover Seder is an invitation to ask, discuss, and wrestle with the tradition. The curiosity of the child is to be welcomed; the dynamics of questioning and teaching are cherished.

The value of passing on the tradition and of intergenerational dialogue is reiterated in the Babylonian Talmud (BT): "Whoever teaches his son Torah, Scripture ascribes merit to him as if he had taught him, his son, and his son's son until the end of the all the generations!" (BT, *Kiddushin*, 30a).[5]

Embedded in this statement is the understanding that although passing on the tradition happens one generation at a time, it affects all subsequent generations. Rabbi Joshua the son of Levi continues, "Whoever teaches his grandson Torah, Scripture attributes merit to him as if he had received the Torah [directly] from Mt. Sinai." The reward for passing on the tradition to the next generations is that one is in direct contact with prior generations, all the way back to the revelation at Sinai.

## THE DIVINE PRESENCE WITHIN THE FAMILY

The parent's obligation to teach the child is mirrored by the child's obligation to honor the parent. The tradition connects honoring one's parent with honoring God. A remarkable passage in the Talmud describes God as a partner with the parents in the creation of a person, and links honoring parents with divine presence in the family: "There are three partners in a person: The Holy One, blessed be He, the father, and the mother. When a person honors father and mother, the Holy One, blessed be He, says, 'I ascribe [merit] to them as though I had dwelt among them and they had honored Me'" (BT, *Kiddushin*, 30b). Reciprocally, when a person dishonors parents, we are told that the divine presence shrinks from dwelling among them. The Talmud comments: "When a person causes pain to mother or father, the Holy One, Blessed be He, says, 'It is good that I am not dwelling among them; for if I had dwelled among them, I would be pained'" (BT, *Kiddushin*, 31a).

## "HONOR YOUR FATHER AND YOUR MOTHER"

The Jewish tradition expands on the fifth commandment through a web of norms and instructive narratives. Honoring parents is defined in concrete terms in the Talmud; it entails giving parents "food and drink, clothing and covering, leading them in and out" (BT, *Kiddushin*, 31b). In this description, honor is behavioral and service-oriented; it is related to the need of the parent. In addition to honor, reverence is also commanded in the Bible (Leviticus 19:3). The Talmud defines reverence of parents in somewhat more psychological terms. Thus, reverence entails not standing or sitting in the parents' place, not contradicting their words, and not shaming them (BT, *Kiddushin*, 31b).

Beyond these pithy definitions, the challenges involved in honoring parents are fleshed out in the Talmud through exemplary narratives, anecdotes of adult children acting respectfully toward their elderly parents. In these narratives, "the son or daughter does not, ideally, respond to demands made of him or her but is responsible for a pattern and process of *kibbud* [honoring parents]. The temper is active, not submissive" (Blidstein, 1975, p. xii). The narratives exemplify the spiritual centeredness of the son or daughter in attempting to relate respectfully to the parent, even under difficult circumstances.

One of the most celebrated stories of honoring parents concerns a pagan, Dama from Ashkelon:

> They asked Rabbi Eliezer: "How far must one go in honoring father and mother?" He told them: "Go and look what a certain gentile did for his father in Ashkelon, and Dama the son of Netina is his name. The sages sought from him precious stones for the priestly breastplate, at a price of sixty thousand . . . and the key [to the jewelbox] was under his father's pillow, and he did not disturb him. The next year the Holy One Blessed be He gave him his reward; a red heifer was born in his flock.[6] The sages of Israel came to him [to buy the heifer] and he said to them: 'I know that if I ask of you all the wealth in the world you would give it to me; but I don't want from you anything more than the money that I lost in honoring my father.'" (BT, *Kiddushin*, 31a)

The rabbis considered Dama's behavior exemplary of the *mitzvah* (commandment; good deed) to honor parents. Dama's comportment is all the more laudatory because he did not seek personal gain as a reward. It is instructive to contrast this story with a very different, modern narrative, from Robert Bly's *Iron John* (1990): A boy in the process of attaining manhood has to steal a key from under his mother's pillow! The core values underlying these two very different anecdotes result in different "morals of the stories." In the Talmudic narrative, it is a virtue to restrain one's own desire for gain for the sake of honoring the father. In Bly's tale, the boy's freedom and masculinity depend on his stealing something valuable from his mother. It presumes a rejection of the mother as part of the individual's journey. Such a developmental trajectory could not be further from the traditional Jewish view.

The rabbis understood the complex dynamics involved in caring for parents. Rabbi Avimi offers the following somewhat puzzling observation: "A person can feed his father pheasant, and still be driven from the world [in punishment]; whereas another can make [his father] grind at a mill, and this brings him to the life of the world to come [the ultimate reward]." This pithy saying is unpacked by other commentators, who imagine the following scenario. In the first situation, the father eating the pheasant asks his son where he obtained such a delicacy; the son answers nastily, "Old man, what's it to you? Just chew and eat, like dogs chew and eat." In the second case, imagine the commentators, the son puts his father to work grinding at the mill because the father has been called to serve the king. The son, sensing that this royal service will entail difficult and long labor, offers to go in his father's stead, and asks his father to mind his mill in his place. The son thus protects his father from greater hardship (BT, *Kiddushin*, 31a). The value expressed in these stories is that honoring parents is not simply a matter of proper behavior—the manner in which the honoring is done is just as important. Caring for parents in a derogatory, resentful manner does not, in this view, fulfill the fifth commandment.

The principle of not shaming a parent is central to filial piety. The Talmud relates: "If a person's father [inadvertently] transgresses a law of the Torah, [the son] should not say to him, 'Father, you have transgressed a law of the Torah.' Rather, he should say to him, 'Father, thus it is written in the Torah'" (BT, *Kiddushin*, 32a). His correction of his father is to be indirect and gentle.

At times the challenge not to shame parents is sorely tested. Several episodes are related in which parents act irrationally and even physically attack their adult child. The child, while setting appropriate limits, is not to respond in kind, and is not to shame the parent in turn. "They asked Rabbi Eliezer, 'How far does honoring father and mother go?' He said to them, 'That [the father] would throw his wallet into the sea, and [the son] does not shame him'" (BT, *Kiddushin*, 32a). A more extreme case is told of Dama from Ashkelon: "One time he was wearing a golden robe and was sitting with the nobles of Rome; and his mother came and tore it off him, and hit him on the head, and spat in his face. Yet he did not shame her" (BT, *Kiddushin*, 31a). One wonders at Dama's self-control and calm in the face of his mother's emotional storm. Since Dama, a pagan, was not bound by the fifth commandment, his maturity seems to flow from an inner strength, a natural restraint. It is interesting that the rabbis chose Dama as their paragon of intergenerational virtue. We can see the command to honor parents— an external restraint—as pointing to the inner transformation that aims at Dama's intuitive piety and respect.

According to the Talmud, even when a child sets limits on disturbed parental behavior, this is to be done gently and without rage or humiliation of the parent. These vignettes convey the complex and at times painful choices adult children may face in dealing with parents. Balancing self-regard and self-protection with care and respect for parents is especially difficult when parents are unstable or abusive.

The tradition makes clear that honoring parents is not equivalent to blindly obeying arbitrary or outrageous parental requests. If the parent is frivolous and demands obedience in matters not based on the parent's genuine need, or if the parent is mentally disturbed and inappropriate in a request, the child is not required to obey the parent. Indeed, Moses Maimonides, the influential medieval philosopher and codifier of Jewish law, wrote in *Hilkhot Mamrim*, 6:10:

> A person whose father or mother is mentally disturbed should try to behave with them as their mental state requires, until God takes pity on them. And if it is impossible for him to tolerate because they are so extremely mentally disturbed, he should be allowed to leave and to have other people take care of [his parents] as they require.

Here Maimonides excuses the adult child from the obligation to provide direct service to parents; the concern for the child's welfare in this case takes precedence. The child is not free to leave the parents unattended, however; he or she must find substitute caregivers for the parents.

The spiritual and psychological self-control evidenced in the Talmudic anecdotes around honoring parents is remarkable. Indeed, these examples of filial self-restraint go much further than we would expect of an adult child in our culture. But honoring parents in classical Judaism is not limitless either. There are limiting conditions or competing circumstances that mitigate the obligation to honor parents even within that culture so devoted to filial piety. The limit cases reveal conflicting values, some of which override filial service and care.

One of these values is honoring the Torah. If a parent demands that the adult child act in a manner that violates religious law or encourages wicked behavior, the child is to disobey the parent. Even here, however, the parent is not to be shamed or unnecessarily rejected; disobedience should not result in discarding the misguided parent.

The adult child's spiritual and scholarly pursuits may take precedence over a parent's desire. Study of Torah, choosing a teacher, finding one's own place of worship, or going to Israel all may override the parent's plan for the child. Religious study is so central a value that honoring one's teacher or spiritual master can take precedence over honoring one's parents. The tradition is careful to point out, however, that honoring teacher over parent does not absolve the adult child from filial piety altogether; he or she is still obliged to care for the parent. But care for the teacher comes first if there is a conflict.

The manner in which the Talmud addresses honoring parents conveys the complexity involved in intergenerational relationships. Rather than simply preaching the value of fulfilling the fifth commandment, the rabbis discuss difficult questions and cases that exemplify the daily dilemmas and tensions inherent in parent–child interactions. Loyalty conflicts between the child's personal commitments and needs on the one hand, and obligations to care for parents on the other, are conveyed in these anecdotes. Fulfilling the fifth commandment is no simple task in the rabbinic view; it is composed of many moments of confusion and choice.

With all the difficulties involved, in the traditional Jewish perspective one is obligated to honor and respect parents whether or not they have been "good parents." This obligation is not based on their merit or on the spontaneous love of the adult child for the parent. Filial piety is considered a duty of the adult child, not an optional choice. This classical Jewish view is remarkably close to the contextual theory of Ivan Boszormenyi-Nagy and his colleagues (Boszormenyi-Nagy, Grunebaum, & Ulrich, 1991). In the contextual view, filial loyalty and filial debt are facts of life; if one does not find a way to care for and express positive loyalty to parents, one may become mired in invisible loyalty—negative and self-destructive ties to parents (Boszormenyi-Nagy & Spark, 1973). This calls to mind the reward stated in the fifth commandment for honoring parents: "that your days may be long upon the land" and, in the version given in Deuteronomy (5:16), "that it may go well for you." In both the Jewish and the contextual belief systems, honoring parents is inextricably linked with consequences for one's own life.

## MODERN DILEMMAS: A CLASH OF BELIEF SYSTEMS

The values and beliefs discussed earlier reflect the highly regulated worldview of traditional Judaism. They rest on a complex set of assumptions that is no longer widely shared among non-Orthodox Jews. Orthodox Jews adhere to the world of rabbinic law, which serves as a guide to daily life. Non-Orthodox Jews approach the tradition more optionally, as a focus of study or inspiration. In liberal Jewish American circles, personal autonomy and creativity tend to be more highly valued than strict adherence to religious law.

Furthermore, the notion of the person in traditional Judaism is very different from the notion of the person in mainstream modern American culture. Whereas Jewish law addresses the obligations and responsibilities of the individual, U.S. law is based on the notion of individual rights and freedoms. The trajectory of development in the dominant American culture is to become an independent self; within traditional Judaism, development is seen interpersonally in terms of ties to family and community. Obligation and duty are highly prized. Personal happiness is a by-product of an ethical life, not a goal in itself. Intergenerational loyalty and respect for parents are, as we have seen, core values. By contrast, popular psychology in the United States has made relationships with parents optional; growing away from or beyond parents is an acceptable normative development in this culture. In this view, the good of the individual is paramount, and the person is accountable primarily to self.

Many modern North American Jews, raised with the dominant cultural narrative, are caught between two worlds. Although they have imbibed the ethic of the individual, they may also be recipients of familial messages of obligation, guilt, and multigenerational accountability. These messages, characterized—and caricatured—by the guilt-inducing Jewish mother, can be seen as echoes of the Jewish belief system, attenuated and decontextualized from the larger Jewish tradition. Jewish parents who implore their adult children to marry Jews or to produce grandchildren to bring *nachas* (Yiddish: "joy") to the parents seem strangely out of place and are pathologized in the American context. Yet such parental claims are natural within a more traditional Jewish world. The American Jewish children receiving such messages may view their parents as overly controlling, and may distance themselves from what feels like intrusive parental behavior.

The tension between individual choice and intergenerational loyalty is by no means simply a Jewish dilemma; it is a common phenomenon within families of many backgrounds. Indeed, the fifth commandment is a shared foundation text for Christianity and Islam, as well as Judaism. Finding a balance between filial piety and personal autonomy is a challenge in many different cultures. This balance may be particularly difficult for families who immigrate to America from traditional cultures that value family priorities over individual preferences. Conflict often ensues between elders and their children raised in America, with its emphasis on individualism.

## CLINICAL IMPLICATIONS: INTERGENERATIONAL CONFLICT, LOYALTY, AND RECONCILIATION

Honoring one's mother and father is often a confusing prospect in contemporary life. For many in the dominant culture in the United States, filial piety is no longer integrated into a coherent worldview in which the self is defined in its intergenerational context (Walsh, 1999). The values of loyalty, obligation, and embeddedness in family and community that characterize many traditional cultures do not easily hold in modern American life. These

intergenerational values are often at odds with the more self-focused orientation that is prevalent in our culture and, increasingly, in many parts of the
world. They are also at odds with some therapeutic approaches that encourage personal liberation from the claims of the family of origin.

The values of honoring parents and maintaining a calm, nonreactive
position with one's family of origin are, however, quite consonant with intergenerational family therapy theory. Working toward intergenerational connection and reconciliation is central to multigenerational family therapy
(Boszormenyi-Nagy et al., 1991; Bowen, 1978; Carter & McGoldrick, 1999;
Fishbane, 2005; Framo, 1976; Grunebaum, 1987; Hargrave, 1994; Lerner,
1985; McGoldrick, 1995; Roberto, 1992; Rolland, 1994; Walsh, 2006).
The contextual approach of Boszormenyi-Nagy and colleagues (1991) most
explicitly deals with filial obligation and family loyalty, emphasizing honoring parents as a central task of adult development. The language of obligation and debt that characterizes contextual theory comes closest to the
traditional Jewish values discussed in this chapter. Although other intergenerational approaches do not use the language of obligation, they still carry
the implicit assumption that the individual is not free to cast away or cut off
from the family of origin without paying an enormous personal price. The
self is seen in its relational, multigenerational context.

The relational view of the self, implicit in intergenerational family theory, is emerging in other theories as well (Fishbane, 2001). In the fields of
human development, gender studies, neuroscience, and therapy, a relational
view of the person is replacing the individualistic view that has dominated
psychology, as well as North American culture in general. These relational
theories highlight interpersonal interdependence throughout the life cycle.
This shift to the relational dovetails with many of the classical Jewish values
discussed earlier.

A relational/intergenerational view informs my own clinical perspective. In working with couples or individual adults and their families of origin, I see the negative impact of individualistic, competitive stories on their
lives. Inviting clients to consider their dilemmas from a relational perspective, and helping them to create a dialogue with their parents and significant
others, is at the heart of my work (Fishbane, 1998, 2001, 2005, 2007, 2008;
Scheinkman & Fishbane, 2004). In particular, informed by intergenerational
theory, I try to help clients balance filial loyalty with personal authenticity,
boundaries, and self-respect—to honor their parents while still respecting
themselves. In this view, honoring parents does not imply giving up self;
rather, it entails appreciating personal autonomy within its relational context. This may include helping a client find ways to invite parents respect-

fully to a more mutually caring relationship (Fishbane, 2005). When this is done without blame or criticism, parents often responded enthusiastically, feeling respected by and connected with their adult child. In this context, it is much easier for the adult child to set limits, make requests, and be authentic in the relationship.

The challenge for the client is to have a voice and maintain his or her own position while staying connected with parents. Holding one's own intergenerationally—balancing autonomy with loyalty and respect for parents—is a complex relational skill. It includes learning to "make a relational claim" (Fishbane, 2001) in a way that honors both self and other. Parents are often able to respond with a reciprocal respect when approached in this manner. As this process unfolds, respect tends to beget respect, generating a "virtuous" rather than a vicious cycle between the generations. If the parent is unable to respond positively, the adult child has at least acted with integrity and generosity and, as in the previous examples from the Talmud, has not responded to the parent with rage or humiliation. I find, with Boszormenyi-Nagy and Spark (1973), that when an individual has found a constructive way to be loyal to his or her parents and is not stuck in blame or resentment with them, that person may be freer to live his or her own life without carrying burdens of resentment into other relationships.

The following clinical example illustrates this approach.[7]

Diana, a single woman in her 30s, comes to therapy because she is perennially disappointed in her relationships. She overaccomodates to others and becomes resentful, expressing her needs only when she is at the boiling point. Diana is chronically angry at her widowed mother Sarah, feeling controlled and guilt-tripped by her. Before her husband died in Diana's early adolescence, Sarah was disappointed in her relationship with him and looked to Diana, her only child, to meet her needs. After her father's death Diana felt even more burdened by her mother's sadness.

As a child, Diana complied and tried to please her mother; as an adult, she is so resentful that she has contemplated a cutoff from Sarah. Diana holds back a great deal from her mother, fearing that she will be engulfed if she doesn't protect herself with massive walls against maternal expectations. She tells me, "I can't be a daughter the way my mother wants me to be; therefore, I can't be my mother's daughter at all." As Diana sees it, she can either honor her mother by doing exactly what her mother wants, thus giving up self, or she can honor herself by distancing from and dismissing her mother. I suggest to Diana that she might find a way to honor her mother while honoring herself. I ask her,

"How do *you* want to be your mother's daughter?" Diana considers how she might connect with Sarah while staying authentic in the relationship and sensitive to her own needs. We discuss ways she can approach her mother that would facilitate dialogue and mutual respect.

Diana works on the boundary between herself and her mother through the "fence exercise" (Fishbane, 2005). She imagines her mother as her neighbor, with a fence between their yards. She considers the possibility that she can enjoy her own garden even if her neighbor's planting behavior isn't ideal. Diana finds it useful to conjure up the fence when she feels upset by her mother. She reports in a session, "I put my mother on her side of the fence this week, and it helped me not get reactive." Diana begins to hold her own reality side by side with her mother's. She no longer loses herself so easily in her mother's moods or needs.

As she feels stronger in relationship with her mother, Diana considers speaking more honestly with Sarah. Because she was so overaccommodating as a child and so withholding and angry as an adult, Diana hasn't found a way to share her pain and concerns with her mother. Diana has not given Sarah the opportunity to understand her experience, nor has she given her mother the chance to work on improving their relationship. Diana decides to invite her mother to a joint session to explore these issues and, she hopes, open up more dialogue.

Diana's mother joins us for a session. Diana states her hope that they can improve their relationship, and acknowledges that in recent years she has been distancing from her mother. She gently lets Sarah in on some of her experiences of burden with her childhood role of making her mother happy. She expresses a desire for a healthier relationship now, in which she can be more honest about her own needs with Sarah. Sarah is relieved by Diana's invitation to a better relationship, and takes in Diana's painful recollections of her childhood. She is able to acknowledge how she inadvertently hurt Diana through overinvestment in her daughter, and she apologizes to Diana. Sarah then explains—without justifying—the origins of her clingy behavior with her young daughter. For the first time, Sarah shares with Diana stories of her own father's alcoholic rages, and of her mother's depression and unavailability. Sarah had determined that when she became a mother, she would never replicate the abuse and abandonment she experienced as a child. She would devote herself totally to her daughter. Furthermore, she had decided not to tell her young daughter about her own childhood to protect Diana from experiencing Sarah's pain. While raising her daughter, Sarah had felt isolated; her husband was nonabusive but also noninvolved. Following the societal dictates of the times, she stayed home and gave herself full-time to Diana, living through Diana's successes and seeking the closeness she craved with her daughter.

As Diana hears her mother's story, she softens. Whereas before she has seen only her mother's pathology and demands, now she sees her mother's pain and her attempts to protect and care for her daughter. Diana develops a more sympathetic and systemic view, seeing her mother's behavior in the context of Sarah's own family of origin, as well as her loneliness in marriage. Diana feels grateful for her mother's courage in breaking the intergenerational cycle of abuse, as well as her sincere apology for the pain she caused Diana. In therapy, Diana works on a "loving update" (Fishbane, 2005) with her mother. She invites her mother to help create a more satisfying relationship for them both, based on appreciation and respect for differences—a kind of "mutual honoring"—rather than resentment and criticism. Diana learns to articulate her own experience, and sets limits and healthier boundaries with her mother in a nonaccusatory, connected manner. Reciprocally, Sarah is less defensive as she senses Diana's rejection shift to acceptance. When Diana tells her mother she needs space or feels guilt-tripped, Sarah no longer feels like the enemy; she is part of their joint project to have a better relationship. They even develop some humor around their old patterns when they emerge. Sarah, concerned with her own worth and the meaning of her life as she ages, is deeply moved by Diana's acknowledgment of her strengths as a mother. It is important to note that Diana is not simply reverting to her childhood role of serving her mother's needs. Rather, she is able to be aware of her mother as a whole person, with strengths as well as flaws. In this process, Diana is developing "filial maturity" (Fingerman, 2003), the ability to see her mother as a real human being.

The repair process between Sarah and Diana, in which Sarah, acknowledging the harm she has inadvertently caused, offers a heartfelt apology and seeks to make amends, is consistent with Jewish views on forgiveness. The Jewish tradition holds that forgiveness is a dyadic, relational process: When a person has been harmed by another, forgiveness is called for after the offender has recognized the wrong, apologized, and engaged in a process of inner transformation (*teshuva*, or "turning") that lessens the chance of that person committing the same wrong in the future (Schimmel, 2002). The rabbis also attended to the human tendency to bear grudges and to hold on to resentment. Maimonides recommended that, if necessary, the one who harmed another, having done *teshuva* and shown remorse, should ask for forgiveness from the offended person up to three times—even bringing along some of the victim's neighbors for support. If, after all this, the victim still refuses to forgive, the sin, according to Maimonides, now belongs to the unforgiving victim. In the face of genuine *teshuva*, remorse, and apology, the wronged party is obliged to forgive. The rabbis understood that ongoing resentment is corrosive and damaging, and that interactive repair can be a healthy process (see also Hargrave, Froeschle, & Castillo, Chapter 16, this volume).

Sometimes in parent–child relationships, there is a clear offender and a clear victim. But more often the harm a child experiences stems from complex family dynamics or from parental good intentions gone awry, as in the case of Sarah and Diana. Sarah was well-intentioned in her clingy maternal behavior, but Diana was hurt nevertheless. So it was healthy and appropriate for Sarah to apologize once she realized the impact her behavior had had on Diana. For her part, Diana's forgiveness was bolstered by growing compassion for her mother, and by appreciation for her mother's courage and love. Sarah's apology had a profound impact on Diana, as Diana felt fully seen and understood by her mother.

> In addition to forgiveness, Diana considers ways she can care for her mother as she ages without feeling overburdened, and she examines her old reactivity around Sarah's needs. Diana struggles with the balance of caring for her mother and respecting her own needs and boundaries. Perhaps most importantly, as Diana confronts these moments of choice with her mother, she no longer feels resentful and victimized in the process. Diana begins to see honoring as a positive opportunity, not just a burden.
>
> In this work, Diana has achieved a spiritual centeredness; she is no longer dominated by resentment and suspicion of her mother. Diana's spiritual focus and her ability to honor and to forgive her mother have ramifications beyond their relationship. Diana finds that she has more flexibility and choice in her other relationships as well; she feels less caught in her old pattern of either overaccommodating or asserting her needs angrily. She finds that "mutual honoring" works more generally in her relational life.
>
> Diana reexamines her feelings about her father as well. Because he died when she was 13, she never had a chance to get to know him from an adult perspective. In therapy she explores him as a real person, with his own strengths and limitations. She speaks to relatives and friends who knew him in different phases of his life. Honoring her father includes developing a more complex, nuanced view of him and of his relationship with her mother. The two women visit his grave, sharing memories and enlarging their stories about him.

There are clinical situations in which the parent is not as responsive as Diana's mother, in which the difficult or even abusive behavior of the parent is not affected by the adult child's attempt at "mutual honoring." If the parent is unavailable to do the dyadic relational work of forgiveness, the adult child is in a dilemma. Interpersonally based forgiveness may be impossible, yet chronic resentment is unhealthy. Janis Abrahms Spring (2004) offers an alternative when the person who caused harm cannot participate in the relational work of forgiveness: Acceptance. When the parent is unable or unwilling to enter into a dialogue, to repair or make amends, the adult child can choose to accept the parent's limitations, protecting the self from future violations, and still relinquish the burden of chronic anger and resentment. Indeed, in such cases, it is still in the interest of the child to maintain a nonreactive, respectful stance with the parent, while setting firm limits and protecting the self from abusive or unsafe interactions. Even if problematic parental behavior requires limited contact, this need not result in a cutoff or in chronically angry reactivity in the adult child. As contextual theorists have suggested, when the adult child carries a burden of resentment and victimization, that individual is likely to victimize others through the "revolving slate of vindictive behavior" (Boszormenyi-Nagy & Ulrich, 1981, p. 167), or to assume a lifelong role as victim. Maintaining a nonreactive position with the parent, and not becoming abusive in kind, contributes to the adult child's own well-being, and to the well-being of subsequent generations.

Respecting parents in the contextual view—as in the rabbinic tradition—is not contingent on whether the parent is a "good parent"; rather, it is a position that the adult child adopts through personal spiritual centeredness. Such a filial position is characterized by differentiation of self (Bowen, 1978); the child is not a victim of the parent, but rather is the author of his or her own behavior. Clients experience such a position as empowering and report a sense of freedom when they are able to resist getting hooked in reactivity with their parents. The adult child shifts from "power over" thinking with parents, in which either the parent or the child prevails, to a "power to" or "power with" position (Goodrich, 1991; Surrey, 1991), maintaining a focus and a clarity of purpose in the context of generosity and respect for the parent. In the "power over" mode, the adult child is stuck in a *hierarchical* relationship with the parent. Shifting to a "power with" mode allows for the development of a *generational* view of the parent–child relationship (Fishbane, 1998). Whereas in the hierarchical view the parent has power over the child, which the child is likely to resist, in a generational view the parent is seen in terms of his or her own life journey. The parent who thus emerges is a three-dimensional person, and is not perceived only as a good or bad parent. The adult child is then in a better position to honor parents as they are, flaws and all.

The shift to a generational view of parents may entail some grieving as the child lets go of the project of shaping parents up and lets go of some of the disappointments and hopes of the past (Framo, 1976). On the other side of this sadness, clients often report a sense of peace. In acknowledging and accepting parents as they are today, the adult child can "wake from the spell of childhood" (Fishbane, 1998) and become an equal partner in the process of intergenerational healing. This is facilitated when the adult child focuses on changing his or her own position in the relationship rather than on changing the parent (Bowen, 1978; Lerner, 1985). A clinical paradox often emerges in this process. As the child stops trying to change the parent, the parent often does change. With the shift in the parent–child relationship away from an adversarial, mutually mistrustful, "power over" tone, interactions assume a more collaborative, relaxed, "power with" tone. When the adult child genuinely gives up the project of changing the parent and becomes more accepting and respectful, that parent often feels freer to respond generously as well.

In the "power to" mode, one acts thoughtfully and in accordance with one's higher goals. This is a kind of self-mastery, in keeping with the Roman philosopher Seneca's maxim, "Most powerful is he who has himself in his own power." The classical Jewish version is "Who is mighty?—The one who conquers his own instincts" (*Ethics of the Fathers*, 4.1). It is interesting to note that these ancient depictions of personal empowerment are very close to the emerging visions of resilience and mental health in current research on neurobiology. Integration of thought and feeling, and the ability of higher brain processes to calm the emotional brain, are central in this literature (Fishbane, 2007, 2008; Siegel & Hartzell, 2003). I use imagery techniques in therapy to facilitate this process. Adapting Internal Family Systems parts work (Schwartz, 1995), I help clients learn to self-soothe when they are upset, as a good parent would with a child. As clients learn to calm and parent themselves when agitated, they have less need for their (actual) parents to do this for them, so they are less reactive if their parents disappoint them. This greater intrapersonal empowerment benefits clients in their relational lives, including with parents. With this self-transformation, clients are able to honor parents "from the inside out" (Siegel & Hartzell, 2003), a generosity that flows from an inner peace.

I have witnessed the profound shifts that clients experience when they develop this self-mastery and relational empowerment, find a way to balance honoring parents with respecting self, and are relieved of burdens of resentment and victimization. As I see it, the consequence of the fifth commandment, "that it may go well with you," is not just a moral reward, but flows from the very nature of being one-who-honors, rather than one-who-does-not-honor. In the intergenerational view, and in the traditional Jewish view, honoring parents benefits the adult child as much as it benefits the parents.

## NOTES

1. My husband, Michael Fishbane, has been my study partner in the classical Jewish texts for this chapter. I am grateful for our dialogue and for his wisdom.
2. The Talmud, a central text in Judaism, is a collection of legal and ethical discussions of the rabbis during the first five centuries of the common era. Classical Midrash consists of ancient and early medieval rabbinic Bible interpretation, found in various collections and volumes. Midrash continues as an ongoing process of textual interpretation and creative narrativization into the present.
3. Some contemporary worshipers add "the God of Sarah, Rebekah, Rachel, and Leah," the four matriarchs.
4. The Haggadah is a rabbinic text from the early medieval period.
5. The citations from the Talmud are from a traditional edition of the Babylonian Talmud (BT) redacted in the fifth century (C.E.) All translations are my own.
6. A pure red heifer was especially valuable in ancient Israel, as its ashes were used in ritual practices in the Temple.
7. The case is a composite, reflecting a relational/intergenerational approach to clinical dilemmas in honoring parents.

## REFERENCES

Babylonian Talmud (BT). Tractate *Kiddushin*, traditional ed. (First redacted 5th century C.E.)

Blidstein, G. (1975). *Honor thy father and mother: Filial responsibility in Jewish law and ethics.* New York: Ktav.

Bly, R. (1990). *Iron John.* Reading, MA: Addison-Wesley.

Boszormenyi-Nagy, I., Grunebaum, J., & Ulrich, D. (1991). Contextual family therapy. In A. S. Gurman & D. P. Kniskern (Eds.), *Handbook of family therapy* (Vol. 2). New York: Brunner/Mazel.

Boszormenyi-Nagy, I., & Spark, G. (1973). *Invisible loyalties: Reciprocity in intergenerational family therapy.* New York: Harper & Row.

Boszormenyi-Nagy, I., & Ulrich, D. (1981). Contextual family therapy. In A. S. Gurman & D. P. Kniskern (Eds.), *Handbook of family therapy.* New York: Brunner/Mazel.

Bowen, M. (1978). *Family therapy in clinical practice.* New York: Aronson.

Carter, B., & McGoldrick, M. (Eds.). (1999). *The expanding family life cycle: Individual, family, and social dimensions* (3rd ed.). Boston: Allyn & Bacon.

*Ethics of the Fathers. Mishnah,* Order of *Nezikin,* traditional ed. (Redacted beginning of 3rd century C.E.)

Fingerman, K. (2003). *Mothers and their adult daughters: Mixed emotions, enduring bonds.* Amherst, NY: Prometheus Books.

Fishbane, M. D. (1998). I, thou and we: A dialogical approach to couples therapy. *Journal of Marital and Family Therapy, 24,* 41–58.

Fishbane, M. D. (2001). Relational narratives of the self. *Family Process, 40,* 273–291.

Fishbane, M. D. (2005). Differentiation and dialogue in intergenerational relationships. In J. Lebow (Ed.), *Handbook of clinical family therapy.* Hoboken, NJ: Wiley.

Fishbane, M. D. (2007). Wired to connect: Neuroscience, relationships and therapy. *Family Process, 46,* 395–412.

Fishbane, M.D. (2008). "News from neuroscience": Applications to couple therapy. In M. E. Edwards (Ed.), *Neuroscience and family therapy: Integrations and applications.* Washington, DC: American Family Therapy Academy Monograph Series.

Framo, J. (1976). Family of origin as a therapeutic resource for adults in marital and family therapy: You can and should go home again. *Family Process, 15,* 193–210.

Goodrich, T. J. (1991). Women, power, and family therapy: What's wrong with this picture? In T. J. Goodrich (Ed.), *Women and power: Perspectives for family therapy.* New York: Norton.

Grunebaum, J. (1987). Multidirected partiality and the "parental imperative." *Psychotherapy, 24,* 646–655.

Hargrave, T. (1994). *Families and forgiveness: Healing wounds in the intergenerational family.* New York: Brunner/Mazel.

Lerner, H. G. (1985). *The dance of anger.* New York: Harper & Row.

Maimonides, M. *Hilkhot Mamrim, Shoftim, Mishna Torah,* traditional ed. (12th century C.E.).

McGoldrick, M. (1995). *You can go home again: Reconnecting with your family.* New York: Norton.

Roberto, L. G. (1992). *Transgenerational family theories.* New York: Guilford Press.

Rolland, J. (1994). *Families, illness and disability: An integrative treatment model.* New York: Basic Books.

Scheinkman, M., & Fishbane, M. (2004). The vulnerability cycle: Working with impasses in couple therapy. *Family Process, 43,* 279–299.

Schimmel, S. (2002). *Wounds not healed by time: The process of repentance and forgiveness.* New York: Oxford University Press.

Schwartz, R. C. (1995). *Internal family systems.* New York: Guilford Press.

Siegel, D. J., & Hartzell, M. (2003). *Parenting from the inside out.* New York: Penguin.

Spring, J. A. (2004). *How can I forgive you?: The courage to forgive, the freedom not to.* New York: HarperCollins.

Surrey, J. L. (1991). Relationship and empowerment. In J. V. Jordan, A. G. Kaplan, J. B. Miller, I. P. Stiver, & J. L. Surrey (Eds.), *Women's growth in connection: Writings from the Stone Center.* New York: Guilford Press.

Walsh, F. (1999). Families in later life. In B. Carter & M. McGoldrick (Eds.), *The expanding family life cycle: Individual, family, and social dimensions* (3rd ed.). Boston: Allyn & Bacon.

Walsh, F. (2006). *Strengthening family resilience* (2nd ed.). New York: Guilford Press.

# A Spirituality for Family Living

## HERBERT ANDERSON

Spirituality is both a way of seeing and a pattern for living. It is the commonplace attitude that influences how individuals and communities act and react habitually throughout life. Because spirituality is about meaning making as well as authenticity, it is a highly personal reality. Tibetan monks and Christian mystics and Sufi mullahs each have their own spiritualities. So do joggers and potters, birdwatchers and bread bakers, and elementary school teachers and family therapists. When there is openness to transcendence in human life, spirituality is fashioned by the urgings of spirit, both human and divine, that move us toward wholeness and community.

Spirituality is communal as well as individual. Human systems like families are meaning-making communities with directionality and a life of their own. From a spiritual perspective, to say that a family is an organism with a life of its own makes it possible to say that it is a communal soul. For that reason, each family has its own spirituality. Despite this diversity of communal or individual perspectives, the general aim of spirituality remains constant: to be open to the transcendent dimension of life present in ordinary, everyday activity. Spirituality is about accepting the complicated and muddled bundle of human experience as the theater for God's creative and transforming work. In that sense, ordinary human experience as individuals and as families becomes a window to the divine.

Seeing life through spiritual eyes enables one to link the fullness of being human to a relationship with the divine, with others, and with the world of creation. Spirit is often identified as the fundamental dynamic or energy in life that penetrates feeling or action and adds vitality to thought. The ancient Hebrews were clear, however, that spirituality is always an earthy matter. Souls yearn and the flesh cries out. In support of embodied spirituality, Thomas Moore (1992) has suggested that "a piece of sky and a chunk of the earth lie lodged in the heart of every human being" (p. 20). Spirituality that is not embodied is in danger of drifting toward disembodied vagueness or unrestrained individualism.

The renewal of embodied spirituality in ordinary life leads to a reexamination of the metaphors used to describe the human person. Images linked with *self, spirit, ego,* or *psyche,* useful as they may be, do not adequately express the biopsychosocial–spiritual unity of the human person. The recovery of *soul* is therefore simultaneously a retrieval of the earthy *and* the transcendent in human life. We have life from the earth and from God. The spiritual quest happens in the ordinary, everyday activities of families, as well as individuals, as we seek to hold together "a piece of sky and a chunk of the earth" in the human soul. *Soul* is also both communal and individual, and may be described with the paradoxical phrase *communal autonomy.*

## FAMILIES AS COMMUNAL SOULS

A spiritual perspective deepens what we have come to know about human systems. The family is a communal soul constituted by relationships that fashion an organism with a life of its own. *Soul is what gives a living organism, such as a family, unity and direction, making the parts into a composite whole, uniting with others and with the divine.* This is the first and most obvious consequence of introducing the perspective of spirituality into family therapy. Mona D. Fishbane (1998), among others, has described this perspective as a dialogical or relational approach to couple therapy. Autonomy and relational accountability are inextricably linked. Egocentric perspectives cannot be separated from sociocentric or communal realities. *The family is a communal soul.*

Whereas human communities, like families, are fiercely committed to promoting the unique gifts and autonomous intentionality of each member, their vitality depends on seeing how deeply they belong to each other. William Doherty has observed that people who seek therapy today have often lost the capacity to belong deeply to each other (1995). They are lonely and disconnected souls, "weakly moored in family and community who find less and less personal meaning in their roles as consumers and citizens—the two major roles offered by the market and the state" (p. 96). The self is relational, and personal identity is derivative from community. The African dictum

"Because we are, I am" is a challenge to the individualism that is largely unchecked in Western cultures. The *soul* is in peril when we lose sight of this fundamental human connectedness.

The great enemy of soul, whether individual or communal, is pretense and deception. We also endanger the soul when we obscure human vulnerability. By vulnerability I mean simply our susceptibility to being wounded. Being a soul, whether individual or communal, is like being a trapeze artist swinging above the earth, with feet planted firmly in midair. What is certain in being *soul* is ambiguity and uncertainty. We are always in danger of losing soul when we seek to sink our feet into concrete or eliminate ambiguity with rationality, or cover vulnerability with pretense or power. We are free to live without pretense when we believe that the soul is ultimately hidden in God, whose graciousness transforms everything we have hated or feared in ourselves. The family *soul* is constituted by its relationships. In turn, *soul is what gives a living organism, such as a family, unity and direction, fashioning the parts into a whole and uniting the whole with others and with the divine.*

To be a lover of souls, both individual and communal, including one's own, one needs to have some appreciation for human complexity. Troubled souls often long for simplicity. They seek prescriptions that will eliminate emotional pain or erase ambiguity. The care of soul begins, as Moore observes, with "an appreciation of the paradoxical mysteries that blend light and darkness into the grandeur of what human life and culture can be" (Moore, 1992, p. xix). When spirituality informs our therapy with individuals and families, the aim of care includes empowering people to *embrace paradox, seek justice, acknowledge finitude, and practice hospitality in the face of fear and contingency.*

## EMBRACING PARADOX: LIVING CONTRADICTIONS

The philosopher Jacob Needleman once observed that the deepest and most fundamental contradictions of existence "have been placed there not to be resolved but to be lived in full consciousness of their contradictoriness" (1982, p. 7). These contradictions are not accidental. Nor are they new. They are inherent in human nature, in human community, and most particularly in family living. I understand paradox as a seeming contradiction that may in fact *be* a contradiction: Two things are true that do not seem to be true in relation to each other. Living contradictions or embracing paradox is seldom easy, because paradox is messy and chaotic, and fraught with uncertainty and ambiguity. Embracing paradox is too much like walking a tightrope or speaking with a forked tongue, or straddling two paths. We would rather believe that things are this way or that way.

If, however, the deepest spiritual truths are most likely expressed in paradox, then living with ambiguity and incomprehensibility is a mark of spiritual maturity. The ideal in human life is to be capable of being engaged in mysteries, uncertainties, and doubts without insisting on fact or reason. By contrast, the inability to live with ambiguity leads to arbitrary and rigid absolutes. As Alfred Margulies has described it, "The holding of a searching attitude of simultaneously knowing and not-knowing, of finding pattern and breaking apart, goes against the grain of our organizing mind, but is intrinsic to the creativity of introspection, art, and empathy" (1989, p. xii). Our aim as therapists is to help individuals and families deepen their spirituality by living paradox.

Ordinary categories that measure health and well-being are insufficiently ambiguous to capture the deeper truths that are almost always carried by paradox. The language of ambiguity is more narrative and ritual than carefully delineated, statistically verified diagnostic categories. As I use it here, *ambiguity* refers to the multiple meanings, contradictions, and mystery in human life at its depth. Paradox is also a window to the holy. Max Jacob, the 20th-century French, Jewish–Christian mystic, once said that we must live things, not define them. Theology and psychology depend on definitions; spirituality does not.

Embracing paradox or living paradox is a psychological necessity and a mark of spiritual maturity for families as well as individuals. The modern malaise of the soul stems in part from the desire to handle unmanageable ambiguity and contradiction by means of pretense and subterfuge, or the insistence on certainty when there is no certainty. A spirituality that embraces paradox includes epistemological humility that eschews absolutizing of any kind and is willing to wait in ambiguity to be part of larger movements of spirit. Living contradictions and embracing paradox require humility about what is right and a willingness to entertain the possibility that two opposing things might be true. Because there is another side to everything, we need to practice listening to one another in families, so that no one's idea or perspective is disregarded or left out. We are more likely to embrace paradox if we believe that there is more than one truth.

### Paradoxical Spirituality: Being Separate Together in Marriage and Family

Family vitality depends on embracing paradoxical living. *To be totally committed to the well-being of the family as community and totally committed to the development of each person in the family is as impossible as it is necessary.* In *The Family Crucible*, Augustus Napier and Carl Whitaker described this paradox in a very useful way: "We feel that the family's capacity to be intimate and caring and their capacity to be separate and divergent increase in careful synchrony. . . . The more closeness, the easier it is to risk independence" (1978, p. 93). The aim of a paradoxical spirituality for family living is to achieve differentiation within the context of intimate relationships. The primary psychosocial challenge for both individual and family living is to maintain this tension between differentiation and intimacy.

Marriage is sustained by holding in vital, paradoxical tension this fundamental human need for intimacy and the fundamental human need for autonomy. One manifestation of this paradox is suggested by Rainer Maria Rilke's observation that "a wonderful living side by side can grow up, if they [the couple] succeed in loving the distance between them which makes it possible for each to see the other whole and against a wide sky" (1975, p. 28). Distance makes intimacy possible, although it does not guarantee that it will happen. Nor does living side by side ensure clear seeing of the other. Couples who are able to love the distance that exists between them are more likely to see clearly the uniqueness of the partner and form a marital relationship grounded in respect. *A spirituality that embraces paradox is particularly necessary for modern family living.*

### The Paradox of Mutual Recognition

Each person in a marriage may be a fully defined self, but the recognition of that uniqueness by the other is necessary for a marriage to work. The freedom to develop one's gifts within the bonds of marriage is enhanced by the willingness of each partner to recognize that growth and those gifts in the other. In *The Bonds of Love*, Jessica Benjamin makes the following observation about paradox:

> The vision of recognition between equal subjects gives rise to a new logic—the logic of paradox, of sustaining the tension between contradictory forces. Perhaps the most fateful paradox is the one posed by our simultaneous need for recognition and independence—that the other subject is outside our control and yet we need him or her. (1988, p. 221)

There is no theme more necessary or more complex for a vital marriage or family than the paradox of mutual recognition of equal subjects.

The experience of being recognized is not only a prerequisite for community but it is also fundamental for human growth and identity. Recognition precedes empathy and is a prelude to mutual respect. What begins in infancy in the interaction between a newborn child and its mother is a lifelong need for humankind. Marriage becomes a context for growth if two people are able to see one another "whole and against a wide sky," as Rilke (1975) put it. When each partner is able to see the particular gifts of his or her spouse, domination is diminished and the possibility of equality is increased. That kind of seeing is necessary so that the distinctive gifts and abilities of women can be recognized. Once recognized, they can be actualized and honored both at home and in the marketplace.

*Remembering Babylon*, a novel by David Malouf (1993), is about the unexpected visit of Gemmy, a shipwrecked British cabin boy raised by Aboriginal people, to a British settlement in northern Australia in the mid-19th century. To the people of the settlement, Gemmy was not a Black person, but he was not a White person either. Rather, he was an unsettling combination of "monstrous strangeness and unwelcome likeness." One of the people most affected by Gemmy was Jock McIver. Because of his encounter with Gemmy, the tall grass that Jock walked through all the time had "tips beaded with green" he had not seen before. He saw himself more honestly, his neighbors differently, and his wife more clearly than ever before:

> He had turned his full gaze upon her—that is what she felt. He wanted to know now what her life was beyond what he saw and had taken for granted, a shift washed and shaken to make it soft, food on the table; to inquire into her affections. It was amazing to him—that is what his tentativeness suggested— that he had known so little and had not looked. (pp. 108–109)

Because many men resemble Jock McIver, we know little about the women we live or work with, yet do not look or ask in order to understand more. Because men do not always see their wives "whole and against a wide sky," women easily become objects rather than subjects, people whose uniqueness is covered over by role definition and stereotypes. *Recognition is a prelude to equal regard between men and women, because it helps us see the gifts each brings to our common life and work together.* A *spirituality of mutual recognition* that embraces paradox enables marriages to endure and flourish "in the spirit" of mutual recognition.

### Implications for Couple and Family Therapy

1. Not all paradoxes in family living or individual life are life enhancing. Some are crazy making. Sometimes we set up contradictory expectations in children or spouses from which the only escape is to get sick. When that happens, however, paradox has been distorted. There is always the possibility that a series of contradictions will immobilize rather than energize a

family. *The paradoxical nature of life presses us to explore deeper metaphors of living in which oscillation between two sides does not immobilize, because we understand that both sides of a paradox are true.*

2. The use of *paradoxical intervention* as an intermediate therapeutic strategy needs to be reconsidered if paradox is an enduring reality in family living. Paradoxical directives, as Jay Haley (1976) and others have devised them, are useful in breaking open distorted paradoxes. If, however, paradox is not just a means but an end, or a normal state of family living, the therapeutic task includes helping people live with both sides of paradox. *In that sense, paradoxical intervention becomes paradoxical intention.*

3. If the ultimate mystery of family living is paradox, then "saying the other side" becomes a therapeutic strategy that heightens contradiction to expand the arena of truth. Because we are emotionally wedded to our deep metaphors and preferred absolutes, we are often reluctant to acknowledge that every story has at least two sides. The therapeutic task with conflicted families or with troubled couples is to make sure that the other side of the story is told. This paradoxical approach to therapy requires an ability to see the less obvious side of reality and appreciate the complexity of every story. It takes accurate empathy and moral courage on the part of the therapist to insist that there is another side. *"Saying the other side" is a liberating method only if everyone agrees that the deepest truths in life are paradoxical, and that learning to live with contradiction is one road to spiritual transformation, marital peace, and family vitality.*

## SEEKING JUSTICE:
## MUTUALITY BETWEEN WOMEN AND MEN

Families constantly face questions of justice, whether they realize it or not. Some issues of justice are raised by major decisions, such as whether to move the family so that the mother can accept a very attractive job offer; whether one of the parents should switch to a part-time position after the birth of a child—and if so, which parent; how to deal with vastly different needs of older and younger siblings; and how the responsibilities for the care of elderly parents can be distributed fairly. Often significant issues of justice arise from everyday contexts of choice: Who's going to change the diaper this time? How many out-of-town business trips are too many? Who will pick up a child from soccer practice? How should children be expected to treat one another? Considering a new job offer or dividing the long list of chores can all too easily devolve into conflicts over who is doing more work to sustain the family, or who should give way to whom.

These family matters are typically not treated as matters of justice by social and religious conservatives. Moreover, it is widely thought that treating them as matters of justice would undermine healthy, stable, and fulfilling family life by introducing an alien issue. From that perspective, the concern for justice in intimate relationships is thought to be in opposition to (or at least in tension with) the kinds of concerns that are characteristic of loving families. Those who have worried most about the decline of the family often view feminist campaigns for justice with a similar degree of suspicion and hostility. Love is enough, they would say. On the other hand, those who have fought hardest against gender-based inequality and injustice often regard public policies or cultural movements aimed at strengthening families as thinly veiled efforts to return women to subordinate roles.

In the radical democratization of intimacy that has occurred over the last few decades, it is increasingly clear that love is not enough. Fixed roles and obligations of headship for men and presumptions of submission and sacrifice for women in the family have been replaced by more fluid bonds of equality, mutual trust, and mutuality. To maintain this new vision of mutuality in relationships between women and men, we need to reconceive the ideal of marriage in terms of justice, as well as love. This is a major theme in a collection of essays entitled *Mutuality Matters: Family, Faith, and Just Love* (Anderson, Foley, Miller-McLemore, & Schreiter, 2004). Because spirituality is about connectedness, mutuality is an essential dimension of family living: Adding justice to love at the core of marriage makes mutuality possible.

## Seeking Justice at the Core of Marriage

Marriage is not simply a relationship of love but a shared commitment to justice. Pauline Kleingeld (1998), in an essay entitled "Just Love?: Marriage and the Question of Justice," has proposed that we reconceive of the ideal of marriage as essentially *"not only* a matter of love, *but also* of justice. On this view, married couples ideally would think of themselves as sharing at least two overarching aims: a loving marriage and a just marriage" (p. 271). What Kleingeld is proposing fundamentally changes the framework for negotiating mutuality and role equality in marriage. It is not simply that two people who love one another seek to work out some arrangement regarding role responsibilities that is acceptable, beneficial, and even fair for everyone involved, but that the commitment to work for justice in the relationship and for each other is part of the marital bond. Just love is a value necessary for the family's future.

Justice is an issue for men and women alike. Positive changes in gender roles in some aspects of society and in many marriages have not altogether eliminated injustice from marriage, nor have they eradicated injustice toward women at home or at work. More jobs are available to women, even though women are still paid less for the same or equivalent work. Men today do more housework and parenting than they used to, but it is still perceived as *helping women*. (Men also think they do more than they do.) Women feel guiltier than do men about work-related absence from the family. Moreover, as long as the responsibilities for a family's well-being remain with women, maintaining a marriage and parenting children will be a woman's work to do. We need just laws and social policies, but just laws do not guarantee just action in the privacy of family life. We need a new framework for thinking about gender in the family.

Couples who are determined to work toward an equal division of household and parenting responsibilities often find themselves torn by the limits of time. Even when the intent is to establish equality, there is simply too much to do and not enough time in which to do it. Moreover, a free market economic model continues to presume that workers are unencumbered by obligations to marriage or family. A combined 60-hour work week for couples with children (Browning, 2003) would not help couples who must work a combined total of four and five jobs to make ends meet. The application of a cost–benefit analysis is perhaps the most pernicious factor undermining our best intentions to realign the gender distinctions between the public and private spheres and to establish equality of responsibility between women and men at home, as well as at work. Even when we do not consciously ascribe economic value to attending a child's soccer game or piano recital, the fact that we schedule family time and work time alike makes it easy to confuse them, then measure them both according to cost-effective market standards.

Seeking justice is not antithetical to loving one another. It is the *shared goal of life together.* Joel Anderson has observed that seeking to return to traditional role patterns for women and men at home and at work is not really an option in modern industrial societies. "When a couple picks the traditional male-breadwinner–female-homemaker pattern today, the modern understanding of mutual and just respect requires that it be a *choice* made by *equals*" (1998, p. 371). If couples make a commitment to form a just marriage, they inevitably experience unexpected conflicts and unseen rocky shoals that require a wide array of skills, virtues, and practices that must be developed. These practices include recognizing the other, empathic listening, the ability to postpone gratification, clear expression of wishes, renegotiating previously agreed-to promises, and a short-term memory that does not keep score of mutual sacrifice.

This commitment to justice does not, however, eliminate the need for sacrifice. But the deeper meaning of sacrifice is not about giving up but about giving over our freedom or our preference to a larger reality. That larger reality is a marriage of *both* love *and* justice. If both partners in a marriage are committed to a just relationship, then neither person will do all the accommodating. If both the husband and the wife are committed to forming a just marriage, then one's willingness to set aside needs for the sake of others becomes a positive expression of a common bond. Sacrifice deepens a marital bond as long as each person in a relationship is committed to justice. When one partner does all the accommodating, or when the sacrifices are not evenly distributed over time, the commitment to justice is undermined and the marriage is not just. Husbands and wives work together toward a just division of responsibilities only if both partners *seek justice as an expression of spirituality for family living.*

People who are committed to justice as a family value need to develop a wide array of skills, virtues, and practices to make sure no one is inadvertently silenced and that even seemingly outrageous solutions are given due consideration. The capacities that are needed for maintaining justice within the family—such as capacities for listening and a willingness to take the wishes of the other seriously and see the other side of everything—are clearly conducive to maintaining genuinely loving family relationships. In this sense, a commitment to justice actually serves to make loving relationships more flexible, adaptive, and enduring. A family that is committed to justice becomes a crucible for learning how to practice justice in relationship to the wider public good. Bonnie Miller-McLemore (2006) has observed that parents are a bridge or a hinge standing between children and the wider world, helping children move from love of self to love of others in the wider community. "Precisely at the point where one's heart might turn away, might curve in on itself—on the doorstep, at the gate, from the center of one's most primal, passionate, intimate love of our children—we are called to realign our passions and help our children do likewise" (Miller-McLemore, p. 9). A family's commitment to justice also becomes a passion for a just society.

### Implications for Therapy with Couples and Families

1. The kind of changes that once marked shifting family living patterns over time now occur within the lifetime of a marriage. Because we can regularly anticipate changes in roles and disruptions in living that destabilize the family as a system, we need to develop an understanding of *promising*

*again and again* to keep the marriage covenant alive. I understand "promising again" as an act of fidelity beyond the initial promise. "Promising again is an act of *creative fidelity* because we see and understand implications and dimensions of the initial promise we could never have anticipated when we first made it" (Anderson, Hogue, & McCarthy, 1995, p. 8; emphasis in original). Effective marital therapy attends to the inevitable changes that occur over time even in traditional marriages, and the grief that follows from those changes.

2. Couples need to practice making promises that are time limited, situational, circumstantial, and frequently renegotiated to accommodate the inevitable and sometimes necessary changes that occur in postmodern marriage. Obviously, these promises build on the primary promises of love, respect, and mutual recognition that are foundational for marriage. One parent's situational promise to stay home with young children so the other can invest fully in a career opportunity need not last for the duration of a marriage. One partner's adjustment of his regular schedule while his mother-in-law recovers from surgery is a time-limited response to a particular circumstance. Afterwards, another negotiation is needed. If modern marriages are to move toward greater and greater equality and mutuality for both partners, couples need to develop the capacity to negotiate, modify, and renegotiate or give up circumstantial, time-limited promises.

3. Because conflict, disappointment, and grief are inevitable dimensions in the life of a couple that seeks to establish a just marriage, men and women need to learn how to practice reconciliation in advance. *Reconciliation*, as I mean it here, is more than restoring relationships broken by conflicts over contending views of what is just: It is about a way of living and thinking that seeks to promote a peaceable environment in which husbands and wives can sort out *very* complex and competing demands on their time from work and home. Peaceableness is important because it creates a safe environment in which bonds of trust are sustained or rebuilt. Such a vision requires that partners work together for the common good at home and at work. *This is most likely to occur when we live gently with the contradictions of our lives.*

## FAMILIES ARE FINITE AND CONTINGENT REALITIES

In their introduction to the second edition of *Living beyond Loss*, Froma Walsh and Monica McGoldrick suggested that "the systemic impact of loss had remained largely unexplored within the field" (2004, p. xxi). This denial of death in family living mirrors society's inability to deal honestly with finitude and loss as human realities. Walsh and McGoldrick have introduced important themes that need to be explored about legacies of loss, the impact of death on a family system, and the complexity of any family mourning process. The fear of death, they argue, is our deepest terror, and the loss of a family member, our most profound sorrow. In the first edition of this important work, therapists were challenged in this way: "We need to come to terms with our own fears of death and the limits of our control in order to detoxify issues of loss so that we do not continue to deny their significance or neglect them in our theory and practice" (Walsh & McGoldrick, 1991, p. 27; see Walsh, Chapter 4, this volume). I concur with both their observations and their challenge. Families and therapists alike need help in understanding how their own legacies of loss affect their lives together. Families and therapists also need to learn how to mourn the loss of loved ones when that occurs. But there is more. We need to understand that all of life is framed by birth and death. *And we are more likely to discover the deeper truth about human finitude through a spiritual pilgrimage than through a psychological exploration.*

Each human journey has a beginning and an end. This existential paradox for humankind, according to Ernest Becker (1973), is *individuality within finitude.* The human creature is literally split in two: aware of a splendid uniqueness that transcends creation and enables humankind to stick out of nature with a "towering majesty"; aware at the same time, as the Eastern sages (and William Shakespeare) knew, that we are worms and food for worms. The human creature is out of nature and hopelessly in it: up in the stars, yet housed in a heart-pumping, breath-gasping body that goes back into the ground to rot and disappear forever. The human creature is a union of opposites—of self-consciousness and of physical body. The fall into consciousness is the beginning of dread: We are creatures who know we will die.

Human beings get into trouble, according to Becker, because of their inability to live with finitude and death. Families face the same challenge. The elaborate artifacts we fashion, the grand illusions we spin, or the vital lies we live are all designed to repress the terror of finitude as individuals and as families. Living with a deeper awareness of the limitations of existence sharpens paradox, deepens ambiguity, and clarifies that "reality is remorseless because gods do not walk upon the earth" (Becker, 1973, p. 281). When this spiritual agenda is translated into family living, it is clear that loss and death are only part of the struggle. Families flourish and grow when they are able to factor finitude into their self-understanding and daily strategies. Spirituality that enhances the capacity for contingency becomes a necessary dimension of individual and family living.

## Instances of Family Finitude

One of the most disturbing observations about the tension between work time and family time has come from German sociologist Ulrich Beck in a book with the translated title *The Risk Society* (1992). He has observed that a free market economic model presupposes a society without families or marriages. "The market individual is ultimately a single individual unhindered by a relationship, marriage or family. . . . [In fact] a fully realized market society is also a society without children—unless the children grow up with mobile, single-parent mothers and fathers" (p. 116). According to Beck, and I am inclined to believe that he is right, the crisis of the family today is built into the organization of modern, industrial, market-driven societies. It is not surprising, therefore, that the family is a constant juggling act of disparate, multiple ambitions, requiring maximum mobility on the one side *with* the obligations of being married and raising children on the other side. A society that rewards people for selfishness should not be surprised that it faces a crisis in families. If both women and men are equally devoted to the marketplace and its demands, then children obviously suffer. But so does the marriage, even if there are no children.

The second illustration of how families struggle with finitude is equally common. It was Kahlil Gibran, the Lebanese philosopher and poet, who reminded us that our children do not belong to us. They come from us, but we do not own them. We may house their bodies but not their souls, because their souls "dwell in a place of tomorrow you [parents] cannot go, not even in your dreams" (Gibran, 1923, p. 18). There is nothing we human beings do that is more important than welcoming a child into our family and society. We love our children outrageously and protect them fiercely and discipline them carefully, but we never possess them. They are not ours. So, from the beginning of life, as we love our children, we must let them go. It is another instance of understanding finitude at the core of family spirituality. *The greatest gift that parents can give their children is to love them tenderly and fiercely and let them go respectfully and graciously.*

## Implications for Therapy with Couples and Families

1. Every individual and every family experiencing loss has a story to tell about how that loss changed their experience of the world. The primary therapeutic task in such circumstances is to attend carefully to the story of loss and the pains of grief. Our grieving is an intermediate stage between life as it was before a death occurred and life as it can be again in spite of

the death. When families mourn, the story is inevitably more complex than individual grief. Neither the loss nor the grief will be the same for everyone in a family, because the relationships with the deceased varied. Grief rituals in a family context need to be expansive enough to hold differing realities simultaneously, and express conflicting thoughts and emotions in response to the death of a loved person.

2. Apathy, as a way of coping with pain and suffering by not feeling, is a common malady of our time. When we become apathetic, nothing matters. When we become apathetic, we die before we are dead. To live without apathy in the midst of suffering and injustice, we need to learn to lament. Sometimes it is the only alternative because change or restoration is not always possible. *If, however, we have incorporated finitude and contingency into a spirituality for family living, it will be easier to practice lament and teach it to others. Therapies of the future that are attentive to human contingency and finitude will also be willing to practice and teach lament.*

3. If we allow death to be a teacher of wisdom as well as the liberator of soul, ordinary moments become signs of the holy. When we learn to live with finitude and contingency, there is a new urgency to living. It is no longer sufficient to promote individual health or even family well-being disconnected from larger frameworks of meaning and commitment to the common good. From a spiritual perspective, the aim of health is greater service. We find ourselves to give ourselves away. We establish a life in order to lay it down. William Doherty's challenge to psychotherapy to promote moral responsibility is germane just here: "There is no fundamental contradiction between pursuing personal needs and promoting the welfare of the community. . . . Like responsible parenting, responsible participation in activities to preserve and promote that environment is at once generous and self-serving" (1995, p. 100). *When we view life through the lens of a spirituality that is aware of contingency and death, the aims of our therapy will be modified.*

## FAMILY HOSPITALITY

When I wrote the earlier version of this chapter for the first edition of this volume, the specter of terror and the consequent fear of the stranger did not yet dominate the cultural landscape in which we live. In March 2002, 28 people gathered in our home to talk about this question: *Is hospitality possible in a dangerous time?* The conversation was both sobering and hopeful. It was sobering because of the ways in which fear diminished our willingness to practice hospitality in our homes. It was hopeful because we recognized how critical hospitality is for the future of the human family. The only way to stop genocide in our world, a participant said, is by extending hospitality to the stranger.

Hospitality is central to family functioning in the midst of diversity, and it is the spiritual heart of family living. The purpose of family is to make a home in which the husband and wife thrive and into which children are welcome and in which they may grow. Showing hospitality to the children in our midst is the prelude to honoring them in all their vulnerability and uniqueness. Hospitality is an essential family value if we are to create a space in which children are free to grow and to be all they can be. The characteristics of hospitality that are essential for welcoming a child continue throughout a family's history. When families are unable to welcome new people and ideas, adolescent children may need to run away to grow up; college-age children may not bring home new friends or ideas; and adult children may find endless excuses not to go home if their families disapprove of whom they love or how they live.

Experiencing the practice of hospitality is also critical for our time, because it invites us to explore different ways of thinking about what is public and what is private. To maintain the distinction between the public and private, we have kept separate the public sphere of work and the private, domestic sphere, public laws and policies from the personal and private spheres. Justice, as noted earlier, belonged to public realm, and love was enough for the private realm of marriage and family. The practice of hospitality makes it possible to bridge this division between what is private and what is public and to create, if only for a brief time, common space in which no one is a stranger. Love and justice meet in the practice of family hospitality.

Hospitality refers to how we think, as well as what we do. Hospitality is the central family value, because it transforms our attitude toward those who are "other" from one of fear or indifference to respect. When a family welcomes a child or shows hospitality to a daughter's boyfriend from Turkey, or even entertains new ideas that children bring home from school, it is possible that the family may be transformed from a company of strangers to a community of shared meanings. *Home* is no longer just a private sphere, because hospitality has made it something common. Hospitality gives a new meaning to *home* that is grounded in common responsibility and commitment to the common good. When the values of justice and reconciliation and hospitality are dimensions of a family spirituality, the homes where we live are transformed into places where people of all ages grow and flourish, and in which the bonds of just love build sustaining communities of care.

## Implications for Therapy with Couples and Families

1. If hospitality is understood to be the spiritual heart of family living and the principle by which homes function, then we have an alternative for people who struggle with privacy issues. Unavoidably, the home is more than a private sphere, because hospitality makes it something common. Whenever another person is invited into the space I call my own *home*, I give up, at least temporarily, a measure of my own privacy. It is not enough to make our homes safe shelters from a heartless world.

2. Modern communication technology has created a real contradiction about the privacy of home. It is increasingly possible to cocoon, to construct a home that is a private haven from the world. And yet our private world is increasingly porous and susceptible to invasion from the outside. Learning to practice hospitality makes it possible to fashion common ground. It also fosters the emotional and moral capacities to live between the private and the public, which is both a spiritual and therapeutic necessity for family living.

3. Attending to *soul* also adds new dimensions to the therapeutic task. Understanding therapy from a spiritual perspective means that one aim is to enable individuals and families to fashion narratives that weave together human and divine realities in a single fabric. Divine stories may originate in the memory of a religious tradition or they may be a particular experience of transcendence that confirms the belief that there is *something more* in human living. When human stories are retold with transcendence in view, lives are transformed in the telling. And when lives are transformed, it is possible that both individuals and families are liberated from confining worldviews, confirmed in their sense of belonging in the world, and strengthened to live responsibly for the common good.

## CONCLUSION

There is a new urgency about family spirituality since the first edition of this book was published. We are all one family—all peoples of the earth. The families we live in and the families of poverty in Appalachia or Cleveland or rural Pennsylvania are linked together with the Sunni or Shiite families in Iraq or those in refuge camps in West Africa. Hospitality is the spiritual heart of family living. Being formed in the practice of hospitality is critical for this time because the primary contexts of our lives are increasingly diverse. How will families foster respect for difference to prepare people for living in an increasingly pluralistic world? Will families of the future be havens of hospitality in a world that seems to be increasingly dangerous? How will families form future citizens with a commitment to the common good in a society that is preoccupied with individualism and privatism? Because we live simultaneously in very different social or cultural networks, we need to be prepared by our families to live in uncertainties, contradictions, ambiguities, and conflicting interests.

To develop a spirituality that embraces paradox, seeks justice, acknowledges contingency, and practices hospitality, we need families that will raise people of courage and compassion, with a willingness to embrace ambiguity. It is not enough to make homes that are safe shelters from a heartless world. Nor is the family an end in itself or the final aim of existence. Individuals come together in families to do something in the world separately and together. This vision of marriage and family living prevents us from being preoccupied with just our little group. We are all interdependent—linked together in a common human family. There is a saying from Zimbabwe that helps us understand the interdependence of families and the larger human family: *I am well if you are well.* The human future depends on such a vision.

## REFERENCES

Anderson, H., Foley, E., Miller-McLemore, B., & Schreiter, R. (Eds.). (2004). *Mutuality matters: Family, faith, and just love.* Lanham, MD: Rowman & Littlefield.

Beck, U. (1992). *The risk society: Towards a new modernity.* Newbury Park, CA: Sage.

Becker, E. (1973). *The denial of death.* New York: Free Press.

Benjamin, J. (1988). *The bonds of love: Psychoanalysis, feminism, and the problem of domination.* New York: Pantheon Books.

Browning, D. S. (2003) *Marriage and modernization: How globalization threatens marriage and what to do about it.* Grand Rapids, MI: Eerdmans.

Doherty, W. (1995). *Soul searching: Why psychotherapy must promote moral responsibility.* New York: Basic Books.

Fishbane, M. D. (1998). I, thou, and we: A dialogical approach to couples therapy. *Journal of Marital and Family Therapy, 24*(1), 41–58.

Gibran, K. (1923). *The prophet.* New York: Knopf.

Haley, J. (1976). *Problem solving therapy.* San Francisco: Jossey-Bass.

Kleingeld, P. (1998). Just love?: Marriage and the question of justice. *Social Theory and Practice, 24*, 261–281.

Malouf, D. (1993). *Remembering Babylon.* New York: Vintage Books.

Margulies, A. (1989). *The empathic imagination.* New York: Norton.

Miller-McLemore, B. (2006). *Midst of chaos: Care of children as spiritual practice.* San Francisco: Jossey-Bass.

Moore, T. (1992). *The care of soul.* New York: HarperCollins.

Napier, A., & Whitaker, C. (1978). *The family crucible.* New York: Harper & Row.

Needleman, J. (1982). *Consciousness and tradition.* New York: Crossroad.

Rilke, R. M. (1975). *Rilke on love and other difficulties* (J. Mood, Ed.). New York: Norton.

Walsh, F., & McGoldrick, M. (1991). *Living beyond loss: Death in the family.* New York: Norton.

Walsh, F., & McGoldrick, M. (2004). *Living beyond loss: Death in the family* (2nd ed.). New York: Norton.

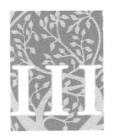

# SPIRITUALITY IN THERAPEUTIC PRACTICE

# Morality and Spirituality
# in Therapy

## WILLIAM J. DOHERTY

Now that there is a consensus that the spiritual and moral realms are inescapable in therapy, it's important that we figure out how to integrate them into everyone's clinical practice. Since therapy is basically a form of conversation, I focus on how we can interweave clinical, moral, and spiritual language in therapy in an integrated way. I offer specific clinical guidelines for how to use spiritual language in therapy in a way that respects clients' worldviews, uses the self of the therapist, and is sensitive to the boundaries that separate secular therapy in mental health settings from spiritual counseling within religious settings.

## MY PERSONAL RELIGIOUS CONTEXT

In reading the literature on spirituality and therapy, I have been struck by the silence of most authors about their own religious backgrounds and current context. Nowhere in comprehensive volumes such as *Religion in the Clinical Practice of Psychology* (Shafranske, 1996) and *The Psychology of Religion* (Spilka, Hood, Hunsberger, & Gorsuch, 2003) does an author declare his or her own religious or spiritual beliefs or affiliations. Journal articles on the topic rarely give the author's religious or spiritual context. Exceptions are noteworthy: Dorothy Becvar (1996) elaborates her own spiritual journey in her book *Soul Healing*. This omission of autobiographical information is unfortunate, because readers inevitably wonder how an author's religious background and current orientation affect the research or writing. No one can be fully neutral or objective about the values-saturated domain of religion and spirituality.

So here's my context in brief. I was raised Irish Catholic in the 1950s and early 1960s, spent 7 years in a Catholic Paulist Fathers' seminary, left the seminary in 1970 amid the turmoil of that era, remained a Catholic until 1975, was "unchurched" for a couple of years, then became a Unitarian-Universalist in 1977. Along this spiritual and religious path, I moved from being a traditional Christian to being a religious humanist and a naturalistic theist. I moved from a traditional Christian prayer life to no prayer life to Chinese *qigong* meditation. As a religious humanist, I appreciate the power and importance of religious and spiritual issues and questions. Religious beliefs and spiritual practices can be positive and life-enhancing for individuals, families, and communities, and also constricting and destructive. I see religion, spirituality, and morality as human creations in the context of a broader natural universe rather than revelations from a supernatural God. As a naturalistic theist, I view God as a force within the universe, the ultimate source of creativity that draws us toward lives of integrity and love. My theological perspective is most influenced by naturalist theologians Henry Nelson Wieman and Gordon Kaufman. Kaufman (2004) views God as "the creativity manifest throughout the cosmos." For Wieman (1946/1995), God is the name we give to the creative force that transforms us in ways we cannot transform ourselves. This transformative power shows itself most emphatically in history through individuals such as Jesus and Buddha, and through the human communities that sprang up around them. A connection of these beliefs to psychotherapy is Wieman's (1958) idea that the experience of the divine occurs most powerfully in creative interchange between people when we bring our whole selves and are open to the whole selves of others. In that sense, therapy at its best is a spiritual practice in which lives are transformed.

## PROBLEMS WITH THE LITERATURE ON SPIRITUALITY AND THERAPY

When asked to write for the first edition of this volume, I had never written on the topic of spirituality and therapy, although I had written about morality and therapy (Doherty, 1995). So I set about sampling the burgeoning professional literature on spirituality and therapy. Nearly every author, following the lead of pioneer psychologist Allen Bergin (1980), criticized (to some degree) the field of psychotherapy for its avoidance of dealing with spirituality and religion. Nearly every author distinguished between *religion*—a set of organizational beliefs, structures, and practices—and *spirituality*—a more personal set of sensibilities about the meaning of life and one's relationship to transcendent reality (Becvar, 1996; Stander, Piercy, MacKinnon, & Helmeke, 1994). And most authors stressed the importance of following the client's lead in the spiritual domain and not coercing the client into a spiritual or religious discussion (Tan, 1996). Recent literature appears to reflect the same consensus (e.g., Carlson & Erickson, 2002; Onedera, 2008). Although much of this literature is valuable and enlightening, I see five continuing problems with how spirituality is dealt with in contemporary professional literature.

First, sometimes the definition of spirituality becomes so large as to encompass most of the mental health domain as well, as in Elkins's (1990) definition of spirituality using terms such as *realism, idealism, ultimate satisfaction,* and *altruism.* A term that means too much soon means nothing—and risks become everything. (See Spilka et al.'s [2003] critique of the vagueness of the term *spirituality* and Walsh's more balanced and focused definition in Chapter 1, this volume.)

Second, the emphasis in the therapy literature is primarily individualistic. Religion, with its corporate, community nature, is frequently disparaged in contrast to spirituality as a fundamentally personal phenomenon. The image is that of the individual searcher for meaning, free to choose or to discard whatever beliefs make sense at the time, and not anchored in a faith tradition. Wendell (2003), trained in both therapy and theology, argues that spirituality cannot be separated from communal religious traditions, because it is inherently tied to them. No one is a spiritual island.

Third, there is too little attention to the family dimension of spiritual beliefs and practices. Despite a large literature on interfaith marriages, there is relatively little discussion of intrafamilial differences in spirituality. What happens to a couple when one partner becomes focused on New Age spirituality, while the other continues to be a traditional Presbyterian? Or when religious and spiritual paths of parents and children diverge? Similarly, there is insufficient attention to spirituality as a resource for couples and families, although this gap is now being addressed (e.g., Marks, 2004; Lambert & Dollahite, 2006).

Fourth, spirituality is often disconnected from the moral realm of interpersonal responsibilities and obligations. At its worst, the literature treats the individual as an unencumbered spiritual self, free to grow and explore meaning, with little attention to the contextual responsibilities to family, friends, and community. Some authors seem to imply that spiritual enlightenment automatically guarantees morally sensitive behavior, a position out of keeping with the historical fact that most spiritual leaders throughout history supported, or at least did not protest, the institution of slavery. Fortunately, authors such as Walsh (2008) now explicitly connect spirituality and morality in their new writing.

Fifth, there is still too little discussion of how to use spiritual language in clinical practice. In therapy, a conversational healing medium, how do we engage in spiritual discourse with clients? Although progress is being made (e.g., Griffith & Griffith, 2002), too much of the literature stays at a fairly high level of abstraction and lacks guidance about how to talk about these issues in a therapy session.

The rest of this chapter addresses some of these issues. It distinguishes between the language of the spiritual domain and those of the moral and the clinical domains. It addresses how to use the language of spiritual dialogue in therapy and touches on ways to incorporate a family systems perspective in working on spiritual issues.

## THREE DOMAINS OF LANGUAGE AND MEANING

My prior work on morality and psychotherapy led to the book *Soul Searching: Why Psychotherapy Must Promote Moral Responsibility* (Doherty, 1995). In that work, I deliberately focused only on the moral realm, not on the religious or spiritual realms. I believed that in therapy one could deal with issues of *morality* (defined as the domain in which one's actions have good or bad consequences for the welfare of others), without explicitly dealing with spiritual and religious issues. Note that the moral realm, as defined here, is also distinct from *professional ethics*, which refers to principles, values, and rules for professional conduct, often articulated in codes adopted by professional associations and licensing boards. This chapter focuses on morality and spirituality in clinical practice, but not professional ethics.

As an example of the distinction between morality and spirituality in therapy, consider a newly divorced father deciding whether to cut off from his children and start a new life away from his difficult ex-wife. This issue can be dealt with at the clinical level (his identification with the father role, his anxiety about coping with his ex-wife, his family-of-origin cutoffs) and the moral level (his sense of responsibility to his children vs. concern for his own well-being), without moving into the spiritual realm (e.g., a sense of being called by a higher power to do the right thing). The distinction between morality and ethics can be shown in the same illustration: The man's therapist might be seen as practicing ethically (respecting autonomy and boundaries, keeping confidentiality, etc.), while not explicitly addressing the moral dimension of the man's issue. Indeed, many therapists are perhaps even more skittish about dealing with moral issues in therapy than with spiritual issues.

Because therapy is a conversational healing modality, I will focus on language and meaning to illuminate the moral and spiritual domains of clinical practice. I outline in Figure 11.1 three domains of language and meaning in therapy: the clinical world of mental health, the moral realm of obligations, and the spiritual realm of transcendent meaning. I argue that

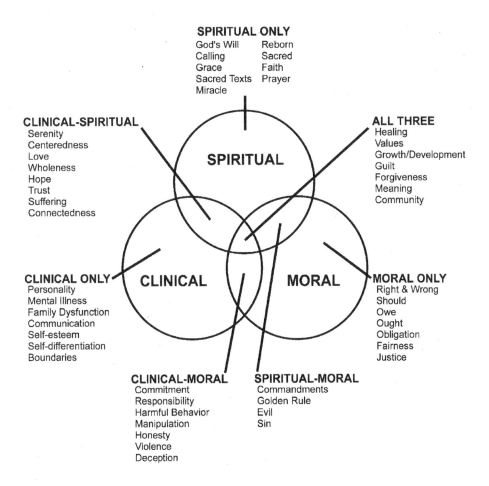

**FIGURE** 11.1. Three domains of language and meaning.

these domains should be kept distinct both for purposes of clarity and so that one domain does not "trump" the others. Trumping occurs when the distinctive meanings of one domain become appropriated by another, as with Freud's subsuming of religion into psychoanalytical theory or televangelist Jimmy Swaggart saying that he would treat his compulsive sexual problem with prayer only, because the devil caused his problem, rather than with mental health treatment. To repeat, the three domains have different modes of language and knowledge generation, different epistemologies and standards of evidence. They represent different traditions and cultures, and cannot be subsumed into one another without committing disciplinary imperialism.

Figure 11.1 gives examples of language specific to each domain. In examining the figure, look first at the circles that reflect language specific to the three main circles: the clinical domain, the moral domain, and the spiritual domain. Clinical-only terms include *personality, mental illness, self-differentiation*, and *boundaries*—terms that reflect the language and scholarly tradition of mental health professionals. Moral-only terms include *right and wrong, should*, and *obligation*—terms that most people use every day to describe human behavior but that have historically been outside the discourse of therapy. I am not suggesting that therapists never use these terms; rather, when they do so, they are clearly borrowing language from the moral domain rather than drawing on models of therapy (an exception being Ivan Boszormenyi-Nagy's [1987] contextual family therapy). Spiritual-only terms include *God's will, calling, faith*, and *prayer*—terms that have historically been used within religious traditions.

Before moving on to the overlap areas among the domains, I want to reemphasize that it is important to respect the conceptual and linguistic autonomy of terms that are specific to each domain. When the idea of a *calling* in the spiritual domain is reduced to a *need* in the psychological domain, conceptual imperialism is at work. Similarly, when ancient biblical texts are used to justify harsh parenting practices in contemporary society, imperialism is evident. And when the morality of sexual abuse is obfuscated in clinical language of *poor boundaries*, both the moral domain and the clinical domain are impoverished.

After developing this model, I came upon a similar exposition in the work of Don S. Browning (1987), a professor of religious ethics and the social sciences at the University of Chicago. Browning argues that the domains of ultimate metaphors (theology), obligation (ethics), and psychology are categorically distinct, although they have implications for one another. Beyond this basic set of distinctions, however, things get more complicated. Browning argues that all psychological theories have implicit metaphors that concern ultimate meaning in life, along with an implicit ethic about human obligations. For their own part, theologies and ethical models have implicit theories of psychological and family functioning. Thus, there is resonance across the categorically separate domains of spirituality, morality, and clinical care.

Figure 11.1 illustrates this resonance by showing overlap areas in which certain words and phrases carry meanings in two or even three domains. The clinical–spiritual overlap can be seen in terms such as *serenity, wholeness, hope*, and *trust*. The clinical–moral overlap can be seen in terms such as *commitment, honesty, responsibility*, and *violence*. Examples of the spiritual–moral overlap are the Ten Commandments, sin, and the Golden Rule. Finally, in the center of Figure 11.1 is the zone of overlap among all three domains, evident in terms such as *healing, values, guilt*, and *forgiveness*. These words resonate across spirituality, morality, and therapy. I do not defend the placement of every specific term in the model; rather, my aim is to illustrate the kinds of words that convey different kinds of spiritual, moral, and clinical meaning in contemporary English-speaking societies. I also note that historically clinical language has been the most recent entry into human discourse, the most rational and least emotive, and the most individualistic.

## CLINICAL USE OF THE THREE-DOMAINS MODEL

Because it deals with the language of spirituality, morality, and clinical care, the three-domains model has several implications for how therapists can approach spiritual issues in clinical practice. This discussion is intended for therapists working in secular settings in which they cannot assume or readily call upon a common religious affiliation and spiritual orientation.

First, without knowledge of the client's spiritual beliefs and preferred spiritual language, the therapist is advised to avoid introducing terms in the "spiritual-only" domain in exploring the client's experience. It would generally be a mistake for a therapist to ask the client whether he or she is praying about a problem unless the client had already opened up the spiritual domain by referring to prayer or at least a belief in a personal God. Similarly, the secular therapist ought not to refer to the Bible without a prior understanding that the client gives allegiance to the Bible. This first implication reflects a clear consensus in the spirituality and therapy literature about the therapist following the client's lead rather than taking the lead (Becvar, 1996; Tan, 1996).

Second, therapists should be wary about self-disclosing their own spiritual beliefs and practices without establishing that the client shares them in some way or wishes to hear about the therapist's orientation. Wulff (1996) makes the incisive point that every religious claim implicitly asks for the listener's assent. For me to tell a depressed client that I know God loves her is more than a statement of my faith. It is a statement that asks for agreement and appropriation by the client, and it could be a misuse of my position of power and responsibility in the therapeutic conversation unless I am confident that the client shares my belief in a loving God. Self-disclosure that follows the client's lead, on the other hand, can sometimes be quite therapeutic, if the timing is right.

Third, if the therapist is familiar with the client's spiritual language and faith tradition, and if the client is interested in using this language and calling on this faith tradition, then the therapist can serve as a spiritual consultant and co-explorer. For example, a man had worked hard in individual and marital therapy to deal with the aftermath of his extramarital affair. But in a marital therapy session he said he was planning to attend a Catholic retreat (he had just converted to Catholicism) and seek forgiveness in Confession. When his wife objected, saying that she thought they both had put the issue behind them, he said he couldn't explain it better than to say he needed to go beyond himself and their relationship. I then said the following: "It sounds like you believe your affair offended a higher moral order than just you and your wife, and that you want to seek forgiveness from God, now that you have been forgiven by your wife." He affirmed that I had got it right, and his wife understood for the first time that he was not trying to dig up an old, settled issue but was seeking spiritual and moral healing. This case is also an illustration of the power of relational therapy in dealing with spiritual issues and moral issues, because his wife at first could not support him on the last leg of his journey of reconciliation.

In another case, Martha had finally decided to divorce her emotionally abusive husband, who had shown no willingness to look at his own destructive behavior. Martha, who had been her husband's emotional caretaker for many years, was tormented by the thought of not being able to help him now that he was facing this rejection and was at risk for relapsing into alcoholism. She knew that she had to keep her boundaries with him, but it was hard. She said, "There is nothing I can do for him, is there?" I replied, "Not without making things worse; others will have to look out for him now." After a pause, and pondering her strong religious faith, I added, "But you can pray for him." She sat up straight for the first time in the session and said, "Thanks for saying that. I do pray for him every day, and I'll continue to. That is the one thing I can do without confusing him and me and the kids about this divorce." I introduced the spiritual term *pray* because I was confident she would relate to it and find it helpful.

Fourth, if the therapist does not know the client's spiritual beliefs, then spiritual issues can be broached implicitly through the language of the overlap areas. The famous serenity prayer can be used without the "God grant me" introduction. A woman struggling courageously against her breast cancer did not believe in God; she said that she would keep fighting, although she knew that the outcome was out of her control. I introduced *serenity* as a term that resonates across the clinical and spiritual domains: It goes deeper than the term *acceptance* and connotes for many people surrender to a broader reality than our own. Similarly, like many other therapists, with clients I make a distinction between *optimism*, which denotes a rational process of assessing likely outcomes, and *hope*, which runs deeper and is connected by some people with spirituality. Terms such as *suffering* instead of *pain* also resonate across the clinical and spiritual domains in a safe way that does not risk alienating the client but does deepen the therapeutic conversation.

Fifth, when the therapist senses that a religious client is using spiritual-only language in a rote or empty way, introducing clinical–spiritual or clinical–moral–spiritual overlap language can enhance the client's experience. For example, should the client use the term *reborn* with little emotional resonance or conviction, the therapist could inquire about the ways in which God's love has brought growth and healing to the client. Or partners who consider rejecting their son because he is gay, based on statements of Christian doctrine and biblical texts, might be offered the chance to pursue the other side of the Christian story about love and faithfulness. It is important not to pit the overlap language against the client's core spiritual beliefs, but to create the possibility of an expanded conversation and an altered spiritual narrative when the current one seems to be compromising personal or family health.

Sixth, when a family is in conflict over different spiritual beliefs or religious tradition, the therapist can use the overlap areas to search for core beliefs and values that are shared by family members. Both a fundamentalist Christian and an atheist can believe in the importance of moral responsibility and constructive guilt when they transgress in their responsibilities, but they might well agree to disagree about whether the moral order originates with God or humanity. In other words, family members can meet at the level of values that connect the clinical, moral, and spiritual domains rather than stay stuck with their theological differences. In one family therapy session, both the conservative Catholic father and the gay agnostic son were surprised that they held similar desires to make the world a better place through their lives.

In summary, an appreciation of the language differences and points of connection among the clinical, moral, and spiritual domains can guide therapists through these waters. Because therapy is basically a form of conversation, the appropriate role of spirituality in therapy has to be played out in terms of the language we learn to use with our clients and the language they use with us. In the next section, I apply to spiritual consultation a model I originally developed to map different degrees of intensity of moral language in therapy.

## DEGREES OF INTENSITY
## OF SPIRITUAL CONSULTATION IN THERAPY

When authors write about their use of spirituality in therapy, they often describe their most dramatic cases and outstanding interventions. This can suggest to readers who are tentative about this area that spiritual interventions are generally intense, and therefore risky. I have dealt with a related concern about moral consultation in therapy: Many therapists tend to view their role as (preferably) keeping quiet about moral issues or (if all else fails) telling the clients that their behavior is wrong—the *a* or *z* approach. I have developed a model of graduated levels of intensity for moral consultation, with the advice that therapists stay mostly in the low-intensity zone of affirming and asking questions (Doherty, 1995). The quintessential moral *intervention* is the simple question about how the client believes his or her behavior might affect the welfare of another person or group of persons, for example, "How do you think moving to another state after the divorce would affect your children?" Only occasionally is the therapist called upon to increase the intensity by direct moral challenge, as I did when I challenged a father who was about to leave town and not see his children again. Following is my adaptation of this model for the use of spiritual language in therapy. Therapist statements are arranged in order from less to more intense.

1. *Acknowledge the client's spontaneous statements of spiritual beliefs.* This may seem obvious, but many therapists historically have kept silent and seemed uncomfortable when clients uttered spiritual statements. When I asked a married woman where she got her courage to keep trying to salvage her marriage, she replied that although she knew that divorce was a possibility, "The heart of God would be sad if I ended this marriage right now." I told her I was moved by what she said, thereby acknowledging and validating her spiritual sensibility.

2. *Inquire about the client's spiritual beliefs and practices.* The therapist can ask clients both at the start of therapy and later whether religion and spirituality are important in their lives or in their thinking about their prob-

lems and how to get past them. For example, I asked a Turkish man if his religious beliefs were a resource for him during his years of intense back pain. He responded, "No, I am not a religious person." No harm was done, and I had directly checked out this potential resource in his life. But I do not routinely ask every new client this kind of question in the first session; mostly I let the topic unfold.

3. *Inquire about how the client connects the spiritual, clinical, and moral dimensions of his or her life or problems.* Here the therapist explores clients' beliefs about how their spiritual beliefs ought to shape the rest of their lives. A therapist might ask a woman who is a caregiver for her husband with dementia what role her faith plays in her decision to keep him at home as long as possible. The goal would be to help her connect the strands of her moral commitment, her spiritual beliefs, and her everyday behavior with her husband. And the question in this form would be appropriate if the client had already revealed that spirituality or religion were relevant to her.

4. *Express agreement with the client's spiritual beliefs or sensibilities when such self-disclosure could be therapeutic.* Here the therapist increases the intensity of the encounter by affirming and agreeing with the client on a spiritual matter. If a guilt-ridden client says, weakly, that God loves her, no matter what, the therapist can reply with stronger words and more emotion, "I agree that God loves you more than you will ever know." A therapist who believes in an afterlife can assent when a grieving father says that his son is with God now. Of course, the therapist must be able to agree authentically with the client. Without such commonality of belief, the therapist can still be sensitive and open up the conversation by asking the client to explore the meaning and power of a belief, say, in the possibility of a miracle from God to save a loved one's life, without appearing to hold the same belief.

5. *Articulate the client's dilemma without giving your own position.* With the parents who considered rejecting their gay son permanently (discussed earlier), I made a statement like the following: "I can appreciate the terrible dilemma you are in. On the one hand, you have your strong religious beliefs that homosexuality is wrong, and you wonder if you can be true to your beliefs if you keep your son in your life. On the other hand, you clearly have a profound love for your son and want to be there for him as long as you live. And that love is part of your religious values as well. This must be a heartbreaking situation for you." I said this to highlight the second part of the parents' dilemma, their commitment to their son, because that part of the struggle was not explicit in what they had said until then.

6. *Point out the contradictions between the client's spiritual beliefs, or between spiritual beliefs and clinical realities or moral issues.* For the couple with the gay son, the therapist might observe that the parents will have to choose

between two of God's teachings: how they see God's law on sexual behavior, and how they see God's law on parents' commitment to their children. This statement goes beyond laying out the dilemma; it suggests that the parents have to decide which of their competing spiritual beliefs will take priority. Or consider a client of mine, a born-again Christian woman who could not refuse to be involved with her ex-husband, who had become a Christian partly to keep her in his life. He told her that a real Christian would not turn her back on a man who cared for her. Although she disagreed with him, she could not cut off contact because he did not see the situation her way; he saw her as being selfish and un-Christian. I asked her to think about Jesus throwing the money changers out of the temple. Did she think that the money changers at that moment believed Jesus was doing the right thing out of love? She immediately saw the point and proceeded to disconnect from her toxic ex-husband. Of course, a therapist has to know a religious tradition well to make this kind of intervention. Wendell (2003) argues that therapists should know more about religion than they do before making more intense interventions that can cut clients off from their spiritual roots. More often than not, a therapist should refer clients to someone with the same faith tradition for this kind of challenging conversation.

7. *Challenge the client's way of handling spiritual beliefs on the basis of your own spiritual, moral, or clinical beliefs.* The key is to do this with a respectful yet firm "I" statement. For example, before ending the consultation with the parents who are heading toward rejection of their gay son and who want the therapist to change their son's sexual orientation, the therapist could say: "I appreciate how painful this dilemma is for you, and I am not living in your shoes. But before we finish this conversation, and since this may be the last time we meet, I want to give you a sense of how I feel about this kind of decision. Again, I cannot make the decision for you, but my own belief is that the highest calling we have from God is to be faithful to our children, even when they do things we believe are wrong. My own religious beliefs almost always lead me to come down on the side of maintaining family commitments rather than severing them." A therapist who does not have an explicit spiritual orientation could deliver the same message by staying at the moral level: that the right thing is never to reject one's child permanently. The strictly clinical level would not be strong enough for this kind of challenge, although mentioning the psychological and family toll of the decision on the adult son and the rest of the family might inform the moral and spiritual discussion.

The most intense forms of spiritual discourse are best reserved for extreme cases and require a good degree of empathic connection beforehand.

Most of the time, the spiritually sensitive therapist continues acknowledging and exploring the client's spiritual meanings and faith community, and how they connect to the clinical problem. Occasionally the therapist self-discloses or summarizes dilemmas. Even less frequently does the therapist set up the issues as requiring choice of one spiritual belief over another, and more rarely still does the therapist flat out challenge the way the client is resolving a spiritual–moral–clinical issue. But just as challenges are sometimes necessary in the clinical and moral realms, they may be necessary in the spiritual realm if we are to do our job as consultants and healers. But only if the therapist is prepared to swim in these deeper spiritual waters.

## CONCLUSION

As the healing art we call psychotherapy moves through its second century, its frontiers lie in tying together the disconnected threads of the human life: the genetic language of our bodies, the psychological language of our minds, the family systems language of our intimate bonds, the community language of our wider associations, the moral language of our personal and social obligations, and the spiritual language of our deepest connections and essential beliefs about the meaning and purpose of our common journey. Therapy that neglects any of these threads truncates the human experience. We are still in the early phases of exploring the work of the spirit in our consultation rooms and our communities.

## REFERENCES

Becvar, D. S. (1996). *Soul healing: A spiritual orientation in counseling and therapy.* New York: Basic Books.

Bergin, A. E. (1980). Psychotherapy and religious values. *Journal of Consulting and Clinical Psychology, 48*, 95–105.

Boszormenyi-Nagy, I. (1987). *Foundations of contextual family therapy.* New York: Routledge.

Browning, D. S. (1987). *Religious thought and the modern psychologies.* Philadelphia: Fortress Press.

Carlson, T. D., & Erickson, M. J. (Eds.). (2002). *Spirituality and family therapy.* New York: Haworth Press.

Doherty, W. J. (1995). *Soul searching: Why psychotherapy must promote moral responsibility.* New York: Basic Books.

Elkins, D. (1990, June). On being spiritual without necessarily being religion. *Association for Humanistic Psychology Perspective*, pp. 4–6.

Griffith, J., & Griffith, M. (2002). *Encountering the sacred in psychotherapy.* New York: Guilford Press.

Kaufman, G. D. (2004). *In the beginning . . . creativity.* Minneapolis, MN: Fortress Press.

Lambert, N. M., & Dollahite, D. C. (2006). How religiosity helps couples prevent, resolve, and overcome marital conflict. *Family Relations, 55,* 439–449.

Marks, L. (2004). Sacred practices in highly religious families: Christian, Jewish, Mormon and Islamic perspectives. *Family Process, 43,* 217–231.

Onedera, J. D. (Ed.). (2008). *The role of religion in marriage and family counseling.* New York: Routledge.

Shafranske, E. P. (Ed.). (1996). *Religion in the clinical practice of psychology.* Washington, DC: American Psychological Association.

Spilka, B., Hood, R. W., Hunsberger, B., & Gorsuch, R. (2003). *The psychology of religion: An empirical approach* (3rd ed.). New York: Guilford Press.

Stander, V., Piercy, F. P., MacKinnon, D., & Helmeke, K. (1994). Spirituality, religion and the family: Competing or complementary worlds? *American Journal of Family Therapy, 22,* 27–41.

Tan, S. Y. (1996). Religion in clinical practice: Implicit and explicit integration. In E. P. Shafranske (Ed.), *Religion in the clinical practice of psychology.* Washington, DC: American Psychological Association.

Walsh, F. (2008). Spirituality, healing, and resilience. In M. McGoldrick & K. Hardy (Eds.), *Re-visioning family therapy: Race, culture, and gender in clinical practice.* New York: Guilford Press.

Wendell, R. D. (2003). Lived religion and family therapy: What does spirituality have to do with it? *Family Process, 42,* 165–181.

Wieman, H. N. (1958). *Man's ultimate commitment.* Carbondale: Southern Illinois University.

Wieman, H. N. (1995). *The source of human good.* Atlanta, GA: Scholars Press. (Original work published 1946)

Wulff, D. M. (1996). The psychology of religion: An overview. In E. P. Shafranske (Ed.), *Religion in the clinical practice of psychology.* Washington, DC: American Psychological Association.

# Rituals and Spirituality in Family Therapy

## EVAN IMBER-BLACK

"I've been thinking, that maybe we should have a proper burial. For the baby, I mean. Just us, a few prayers, nothing more." Mariam had been thinking about it for a while. She didn't want to forget this baby. It didn't seem right, not to mark this loss in some way that was permanent. "What for? It's idiotic [he said]." "It would make me feel better, I think." "Then you do it," he said sharply. . . . One sunny morning that week, Mariam picked a spot in the yard and dug a hole. "In the name of Allah, and with Allah, and in the name of the messenger of Allah upon whom be the blessings and peace of Allah." . . . She placed the suede coat that Rasheed had bought for the baby in the hole and shoveled dirt over it.
—KHALED HOSSEINI, *A Thousand Splendid Suns* (2007, p. 86)

Throughout time and across cultures, humans make rituals. Whether to mark the small transitions in everyday life—opening the day, parting, reconnecting, sharing meals, closing the day; seasonal or annual transitions (e.g., birthdays, anniversaries, holidays)—or profound transitions on our path through life (e.g., birth, childhood, adolescence, committed partnering and parenting, grandparenting, aging, and death) rituals enable us to hold multiple and contradictory meanings, provide a container for complex emotions, shape relationships, express beliefs, create identity, heal losses, and celebrate life (Imber-Black & Roberts, 1998).

Rituals capture and reveal the required duality of human existence, anchoring us in the past and where we each come from in our families of origin, religion, and culture, while simultaneously leading the way to a transformed future. Continuity and change, constancy, and transformations are made possible through rituals large and small.

Because rituals touch us at the core of our humanity, spiritual meanings may be present in both formal religious traditions with centuries of history and in more secular, contemporary creative practices.

> When the Friedman family came to the Center for Families and Health at the Ackerman Institute for the Family, they were deeply mourning the loss of their daughter and sister, 25-year-old Esther, who had died of leukemia 2 months earlier. "We're most worried about our younger daughter, Malka—she seems to have no response about her sister's death," Mrs. Freidman remarked with confusion. Fifteen-year-old Malka insisted she was "just fine."
>
> Through his tears, Mr. Friedman said, "Ask her about her purse." On the floor next to Malka sat a grey metal lunch box. "This was Esther's—she took it everywhere," Malka told me. At first she protested, "It doesn't mean anything—I just like it." But when I urged her to reflect on the meaning of keeping this symbol with her in all of her daily activities, Malka became pensive. "It's like I have Esther with me, and at the same it reminds me that she is gone." And for the first time since her beloved sister's death, Malka began to weep. Without intentional planning, this religious Jewish adolescent had created a daily ritual capable of connecting her to Esther's life while quietly acknowledging her loss.

## ELEMENTS OF RITUAL

Rituals comprise six elements, each capable of carrying relational, cognitive, emotional, and spiritual significance.

### Symbols

All rituals have symbols capable of expressing multiple meanings (Imber-Black, 2005; van der Hart, 1983; Whiting, 2003). As we found out more about Esther's lunch box, we learned that Esther eschewed fashion. Using a metal lunch box to carry her belongings was her way of turning her back on contemporary culture, while making a personal statement about utility and pragmatics. When Malka appropriated her sister's lunch box, however, she decorated it with small reminders of Esther—flower stickers, painted birds, words from Hebrew songs. In so doing, she transformed this symbol, making it at once a connection to her sister's daily life, an emblem of what her sister loved, and a beautiful item for an evolving teen to carry. Thus, one symbol could hold and express Esther's life, and Malka's loss and ongoing development.

### Symbolic Actions

Rituals include symbolic actions, which also are capable of holding and expressing multiple meanings (Whiting, 2003). Symbolic actions may involve words, movement, behaviors, placement of people, dance, art, and music. Malka first decorated her sister's lunch box in a symbolic action that served to connect her to her sister's passions. Then she carried the lunch box with her in all of her daily activities, keeping the memory of her sister close.

### Structured Parts

Rituals include knowable, reliable structures (Whiting, 2003). It is this aspect of ritual that may connect us to what has gone before, to familiar traditions and history. The structured parts of a ritual anchor us to our past, whether that is our personal past or that of our family of origin, community, culture, religion, or humankind. Religious practices, daily customs, annual and repeated holidays, favorite foods that reappear, reiterating life-cycle traditions, are all examples of structured aspects of rituals. They remind us of where we have come from and help to shape who we are in the present. For Malka, using her sister's lunch box in much the same way as Esther had used it exemplifies this structured part of what became a daily ritual.

### Open Parts

To stay alive for us, rituals must make room for spontaneity and change. The open parts of our rituals enable adaptations to new life, individual development, changing relationships, altered beliefs, and loss. The new, the novel, the never before experienced in a ritual moves us into the future. Malka did not simply use her sister's lunch box in the form in which she inherited it. She decorated it with important facets of Esther's life, so that it could hold deeper aspects of her sister's memory. She transformed the lunch box from a routine and pedestrian item to a talisman. "It's like I take in the best of Esther, and become more me at the same time," Malka remarked. This open part to the ritual eased Malka's redefinition of herself—no longer a younger sister to Esther, but now her parents' only living child.

## Special Time

Rituals, unlike mere routines, occur in special time. This may be daily, such as a prayer before a meal; weekly, such as Shabbat; annually, such as an anniversary or a holiday; or uniquely, to mark a life-cycle transition, such as a wedding, commitment ceremony, or funeral. Knowing when a ritual will occur allows for both a period of preparation and a period of reflection and change after a ritual has occurred. I discovered in speaking with Malka that part of the ritual of carrying Esther's lunch box, indeed, involved special time. Every evening, when she returned from school and just before the family gathered for supper, Malka parted with the lunch box, carefully placing it on her dresser. And each morning, just after morning prayers, she retrieved it for her daily outings. As I explored this with Malka, we all discovered that when Malka spent time out of the house, she wanted to carry the lunch box. "I feel my sister's spirit in our house—we have lots of photos and keepsakes that help us all. But when I am out of our home, separate from our family, that's when I want to keep Esther in my heart."

## Special Space

Rituals occur in special space. This may be in a house of worship, a cemetery, a place in nature, a favorite room in a home; at a dining table; or on a prayer rug. When we enter this space, we know we are in ritual space. For Malka, this space was the world outside her home, mostly school and the homes of friends. In getting to know the family, I learned that for Mrs. Friedman, the special ritual space to mourn her daughter was the cemetery. This created a dilemma for her: According to religious law, she was not supposed to return to the cemetery until a year had passed. Acknowledging the necessary, open parts of rituals and her need for spiritual connection, Mrs. Friedman said, "It's just a rule I have to break. When I feel the need, I go to the cemetery."

# ENABLING THE SPIRITUAL ASPECTS
# OF RITUALS IN THERAPY

The six elements of ritual are all capable of responding to the spiritual needs of individuals, families, and communities. Although seldom trained to address the spiritual longings of our clients, we therapists simply need to listen, and they will let us know. Also, following such listening with a few simple questions often leads people to develop just the rituals they need.

Twenty-eight-year-old Maria came to therapy with her two nephews, Joseph, 12, and Anthony, 11. Maria had become the kinship foster mother of the boys 6 months earlier, following the death of their mother Tonia from AIDS. The boys' father, Maria's brother, was in prison for selling drugs. Maria brought the boys to therapy to establish their new home together. The therapy proceeded well along two interwoven tracks. The first was a structural family therapy, aiding Maria to establish herself as the parent. The boys came to accept Maria, both following her rules, and accepting and returning her affection. The therapy also honed in on reestablishing a relationship with the boys' father through letters and visits. The second aspect of the therapy centered on the terrible loss of their mother, and involved storytelling and sharing memories, while lifting the stigma that the boys felt because their mother died of AIDS.

The therapy seemed quite successful and was drawing to a close when Joseph began a session greatly upset. "I just want to know one thing—where *is* our mother?" Both Maria and the therapist were momentarily confused, because Tonia's death had been such a vital focus of the work. Then Anthony explained. "In 2 weeks it will be our mother's birthday. Kids at school are telling us to get flowers, to go to the cemetery, but our mother isn't in a cemetery—so where is she?" he asked emphatically. Maria quietly explained that their mother had been cremated, but that in the turmoil immediately following Tonia's death and her brother's imprisonment, the ashes were lost. Tonia's death had been marked by a Mass, but there was neither a burial nor a placement of ashes. Work that had been done in therapy to remove the shame that Joseph and Anthony had experienced was poised to be undone, as their schoolmates teased and ridiculed them, telling them that no ashes were kept because their mother died of AIDS.

The therapist worked first to normalize their experience. "There are lots of times when people don't have a grave to visit—think of families with soldiers who are missing in action. Or maybe their loved one is buried across the country or overseas," she said. The boys could relate to what the therapist was telling them, because their own grandmother was buried in Italy. "On our grandmother's birthday, Mom used to cook a special meal that she said Grandmother always made on birthdays. She played our grandmother's favorite music from the opera. We all loved eating those meals. Our mom would dance and cry. She would be happy and sad at the same time," Joseph recalled.

"Since there isn't a cemetery to visit, and no one knows what has become of your mom's ashes, how would you like to mark her birthday?"

their therapist asked. That question was followed by a flurry of conversation between Joseph and Anthony. "We need to make a cross," Joseph said with determination. "We have to decorate it—our mom loved yellow roses and pink carnations," added Anthony. Borrowing from the familiar ritual marking their Italian grandmother's birthday, Joseph chimed in, "Let's cook her favorite foods and play the music she loved." In the space of 20 minutes, and with no one saying the word "ritual," the boys planned a powerful ritual to mark their mother's birthday, to further their mourning and celebrate her life. Together with their therapist and aunt, they determined that in the following family therapy session, they would build the cross and paint it. They showed up with photos of their mother and family to share. Through continued conversation during this very active session, they decided that they would keep the cross at home in a closet and bring it out to their living room on two occasions—their mother's birthday and the anniversary of her death.

When their mom's birthday came, they did all the things they had planned. They moved the cross with special ceremony into the living room, cooked and ate her favorite foods, listened to the music she adored, and told stories of their mother's courage when she was ill. Although not a part of their prior planning, they spontaneously decided to light candles. "Just as our mother would in church," said Anthony.

Maria surprised them, spending her hard-earned money on yellow roses and pink carnations. During the ceremony, she shared the food but largely remained silent in the critical role of witness.

"When the boys started planning this with you, I was afraid it would make them too sad," Maria said in the next therapy session. "But they were happy and sad, and afterwards, they each seemed peaceful."

Using the previously discussed elements of ritual—symbols (the handmade and decorated cross); symbolic actions (cooking, eating, music, storytelling); special time (their mother's birthday and death anniversary); special space (their living room); structured parts (a cross like one they would find in a cemetery on a grave); and open parts (the last-minute decision to light candles)—these young boys were able to create a deeply meaningful ritual. They felt spiritually connected to their mother, to their extended family in Italy, to their church, and to the human experience of healing.

## GUIDING THE SPIRITUAL ASPECTS
## OF RITUALS IN THERAPY

In addition to careful listening and facilitating families' own discovery of spiritual meanings through rituals, therapists may also guide people by building on what they may already be doing or offering new ideas. The Friedman's youngest child, Chaim, age 8, sobbed in therapy that he missed his sister Esther, and revealed that he was crying a lot in school. Chaim was becoming increasingly isolated, because other children were beginning to tease him. His teacher, not trained to deal with such a loss, responded by telling him to leave the classroom and "pull himself together." As their therapist, I searched within the family for a small ritual to help him. Each family member, except Chaim, was carrying a small reminder of Esther to give them comfort—Malka had her lunch box "purse"; the mother wore Esther's earrings; the father carried a worn out photo of Esther when she was well. I suggested that Chaim might want to carry some small item to remind him of Esther to comfort him, especially at school. "When you feel especially sad at school, you can secretly touch this item, and it will give you comfort," I told Chaim. The other family members immediately chimed in, suggesting possible items he might carry. In the next session, Chaim showed me a small key chain that had belonged to Esther. "I keep it in my pocket. If I start to feel sad, I rub it. I haven't been crying at school, and I feel close to Esther," Chaim told me.

## AUTHENTIC AND MANIPULATIVE RITUALS: THE RITUALS OF SEPTEMBER 11, 2001

Authentic rituals are generated by individuals, families, and communities. They may be deeply anchored in a people's history or created suddenly to respond to extraordinary circumstances. But the very same elements that adhere to authentic rituals can be used by governments, media, corporations, and religious hierarchies to shape manipulative rituals. Here symbols and symbolic actions are chosen to express a singular and predetermined meaning, often with an intention to exploit emotions and gain political or commercial advantage. Special times and spaces, rather than being chosen by families, communities, and cultures, are selected by sociopolitical hierarchies. The balance of structure and spontaneity is erased in favor of a highly scripted event, with little or no room for the unexpected. Participation in such manipulative rituals usually leaves people feeling dissatisfied and spiritually empty.

The many rituals created in the wake of the tragedy of September 11, 2001, provide a glimpse of this duality. Immediately, after the towers fell, the rituals began. "Missing" posters went up all over Manhattan, forming heartbreaking mosaics (Sella, 2001). Most were portrayals of the missing person in a prior joyful ritual—a wedding, a birthday. For many, as time went on, the word "missing" was struck, replaced by "please pray for." These posters quickly became a spontaneous interactive ritual as strangers wrote messages, placed flowers, or tied ribbons in solidarity with mourners (Imber-Black, 2003b). On the first Friday following September 11, 2001, people across the United States lined streets to light candles, a collective symbol of light and warmth. Of note, no government designed or initiated this ritual. Rather, it arose spontaneously and spread through the Internet, followed by media reports.

The Jewish New Year, Rosh Hashanah, was coming. I reached in to my own ritual history and spiritual life, baking challah for my family as I had every year of my adult life. Slowly kneading the resistant dough, I reflected on the symbolic action my husband and I had practiced for the past two decades. We carried special honey from our international travels each year, imparting a sense of sweetness from another culture to our own. How, I pondered, would any of us be able to experience sweetness this year? Reaching for hope, I placed my 4-year-old granddaughter, Josie's, hands on the dough to shape the Jacob's ladder climbing skyward. Only then did I experience a sense of tomorrow, of potential and possibility, even in the midst of our terrible grief.

Millions of people far from the attacks reshaped old rituals and created new ones to address the enormity of loss.

A young girl's bat mitzvah was scheduled for September 15th. The Brotman family struggled with the dilemma of creating an authentic ritual capable of expressing loss, healing, and celebration. With no coaching from adults, this bat mitzvah girl lit a candle and spoke of the victims of September 11, 2001. She donated part of her gifts to relief efforts. A temple member gave her an additional gift to make up for gifts of those who were not able to travel. Barbara Brotman captured the contradictions this ritual was able to hold: "For her bat mitzvah, my daughter got a dichotomy: Life is wonderful/life is unbearable. We gave [our blessing] in the raw awareness of the parents whose blessings came to naught that day" (Brotman, 2001, p. C1).

As many of us began to work with families who had lost loved ones, I became aware of their struggle to escape contrived or manipulative rituals. The city of New York offered small urns of anonymous dirt from Ground Zero; most families found these to be without meaning. The media generated a pain-inducing "6-Month Anniversary." In the broader American culture, we do not mark "6-Month Anniversaries," but we do in a made-for-TV commercial world. Children who lost parents were given lunch with sports stars and sent to Disneyland, with much media hoopla and the confounding message that profound loss earns one a trip to an amusement park.

In contrast with these inauthentic rituals, the Garcia family created an authentic ritual to address the terrible reality that their loved one Frank, a security guard, was among the missing dead.

"We have no body to bury," Mrs. Garcia told me with tears streaming down her face. "At first I thought that meant we couldn't have a funeral. But my niece said, "Let's put all of what he loved in a coffin—his guitar, his plant watering can, copies of the music he wrote, and stories of the tricks he played on all of us." At first, their priest hesitated. "I told him, 'This is our way to send his spirit to heaven,' and then he agreed."

The first anniversary of September 11, 2001, exemplified the struggle to create and maintain authentic rituals, and to prevent these from being swept aside by manipulative rituals. The day was a mixture of meaningful rituals capable of holding our grief and honoring memory, coupled with pseudopatriotic displays intended to facilitate a march to war. President Bush declared September 11, 2001, to be "Patriot's Day." This banal name for an essentially unnamable event led some towns to hold parades and picnics. Families coming to Ground Zero were instructed to bring only roses and sunflowers that would later be gathered into a permanent bouquet. But many rebelled against this government-scripted procession, carrying instead their loved ones' favorite flowers and holding their photographs aloft. Nearly half of those who lost family members stayed away from the public ceremony, preferring to organize their own private ritual far from the glare of cameras.

The manipulative rituals of September 11, 2001, raised political interests over emotional and spiritual needs. Some communities fought back. In March 2002, New York City announced it was taking the firefighters away from the World Trade Center site. Black firefighters, previously unacknowledged by the government or media, responded with a series of authentic rituals, at once emotional, spiritual, and political. Under the banner of the Vulcans and Vulcanettes, they rallied and successfully fought the city edict. In an intergenerational ritual designed to protect the lives of surviving children, African American and Caribbean firefighters promised, "The needs that your father might have met, we will meet them." Finally, each person at the gathering wrote a small note—to a lost family member, to God, to themselves. Each note was tied to a balloon and blessed by their chaplain.

As a united community, they set the balloons aloft (Imber-Black, 2003b; Diane Smith, personal communication, November 1st, 2001).

The ongoing clash of political manipulation and spiritual imperatives was evident once again in the 2007 rituals of September 11. Without consultation, New York City officials decided to move the ceremony away from Ground Zero. What was hallowed ground for those who never recovered loved ones was about to become commercial real estate. The outcry of relatives resulted in moving a portion of the ceremony back to Ground Zero for one last year. The speaking role of presidential candidate Rudolph Giuliani in the government-designed ritual upset many people. Tiring of the public ceremony, a grassroots organization, *www.myGoodDeed.org* began to urge people to do a compassionate act for others to commemorate September 11, 2001 (Kleinfeld, 2007), whereas another, *9/11 Families for Peace*, comprising many families who had lost a family member, honored their loved one through nonviolent initiatives (National Public Radio, *www. theworld.org*, September 10, 2007; see also Perry & Rolland, Chapter 20, this volume).

Eight months after the September 11, 2001, attacks, a small village in Kenya first learned of the tragedy from a Masai man who had been in the United States. On June 3, 2002, the members of the tribe created a ritual to express their own pain and their spiritual connection to the victims and their families. In a sacred ceremony, they blessed 14 cows to be given as a gift to the people of the United States. One of the men said, "The cow is almost the center of life for us. It's sacred. . . . You perform rituals with it" (Lacey, 2002, p. A6). It's easy to imagine that these cows might have come to a children's park in the United States, furthering a sense of international support and connection in the wake of September 11, 2001. Instead, this authentic and deeply spiritual ritual was rejected by the United States government, which refused to accept the cows.

## WHEN THE SPIRITUAL CONTEXT OF LIFE-CYCLE RITUALS IS OVERWHELMED BY MATERIALISM

Life-cycle rituals carry the possibilities of bringing us close to the sacred and mysterious parts of human existence, including birth, growth, sexuality, love, and loss. Many life-cycle rituals originate in spiritual contexts. Every religion has rituals to mark people's movement through life—rituals to celebrate the birth of children, adolescent rites of passage, marriage, and death (Cohen, 1991). Contemporary Western culture has secularized many of these rituals, while also maintaining some religious and spiritual elements. Such rituals exist on a precarious tightrope, embedded in original religious contexts while simultaneously expressing current social and cultural values.

Beginning in the 1980s, a decade known for material display, and continuing to the present, many life-cycle rituals have been trivialized and stripped of their spiritual and relational potential. Popular magazine articles about weddings focus on expensive gowns, gourmet caterers, and silk chair coverings, with no mention of the deeper meaning of commitment or the profound changes in family relationships that a wedding should hold. For many families, bar mitzvahs have become theme parties, replete with costumes, boat trips, and baseball memorabilia. Connections to the spiritual meaning of the ceremony or its developmental possibilities for the entire family are minimized. Funeral directors offer "drive-through funeral visiting," where mourners view a coffin on a computer screen and head quickly back to work, obviating any celebration of the life now gone or the opportunity for comfort and healing for survivors (Imber-Black & Roberts, 1998).

The focus on the material over the spiritual in many contemporary life-cycle rituals is no more evident than in the contemporary transformation of the Latina coming-of-age ritual, *quinceañera* (Alvarez, 2007). Originally a celebration of primarily upper class Latin Americans to mark their 15-year-old daughters' passage to womanhood, the *quinceañera* has been adopted across social classes by Latino immigrant families in the United States. In many Latin American countries, when a girl turns 15, or *quince*, she is considered to have crossed the threshold from girl to woman. Whereas most families would mark this special birthday, only very wealthy families create parties not unlike debutante balls in the United States. Often the *quinceañera* contains a trip to the church altar and a blessing by a priest or minister, but this religious aspect mostly takes a backseat to a fantasy of becoming a princess for a day.

Similar to weddings and bar mitzvahs, whole industries have sprung up in response to the demand for this ritual in the United States—consultants, expos, and a magazine called *Quince Girl*. In 2007 Latino immigrant families will spend over $400 million on this ritual, including many poor and working-class families who will go into debt to give their daughters gowns, limousines, caterers, and cakes resembling those for a wedding. Undocumented migrant workers may spend hundreds of dollars, equal in impact on the family's resources to the tens of thousands spent by a well-to-do family. In Mexican families, community members often share the costs of a *quincea-*

*ñera*, thereby symbolically sharing the support of a girl's ongoing development, but other Latino groups have not adopted this custom.

Family therapists who work with families in advance of a life-cycle ritual are in an important position to help families examine the values that such rituals may hold and express. As critics in the front row of the theater of social change, we often hear of emerging trends from families with whom we work, well before these trends make the 6 o'clock news. We have the privilege and responsibility to help families challenge the powerful impact of popular media, advertising, and consumerism; the politics of class; and the empty display of money and circus-like atmosphere that many life-cycle rituals have become. Simply asking engaged couples what they want their wedding to *mean*, or inquiring of families about to engage in a rite of passage ritual for an adolescent what *beliefs* they hope to impart in the ceremony has the potential to refocus people on the powerful developmental, relational, and spiritual elements available in these rituals. Raising questions about an ethnic ritual, such as *quinceañera*, requires special sensitivity on the part of the therapist, coupled with awareness of the ritual's historical and sociological context. As Alvarez (2007) notes, this ritual carries the possibility of uniting a community, creating a sense of continuity in a new land that may bridge many national boundaries (see Falicov, Chapter 8, this volume). The aim in therapy is to examine with families how to participate in such transformed rituals without being overwhelmed by the demands of a material society.

## CONNECTING FAMILY AND COMMUNITY WITH RITUALS

Shortly after the death of Esther Friedman, and while the family was observing Shiva, the traditional week of mourning in Judaism, the community began planning a ritual in her memory. A special bride's chair would be named in Esther's honor. This chair was to be lovingly handmade and auctioned to raise money for brides who could not afford a wedding. "This is the way of our community," said Mr. Friedman. "And it is true *tzdakah* (charity)—no one is ever allowed to know that a bride was helped." And then he added, "I'm anticipating this ritual with trepidation. Esther so wanted to be a bride. But I know when I see that chair, I will see her spirit." The family agreed that this ritual would be bittersweet, holding their sadness and joy. "She was such an important part of our community—people just loved her. They've never done this for anyone else. It really tells you who Esther was, not just to our family, but to everyone who met her," Mrs. Friedman commented. "For me, that chair will hold the wedding she didn't live to have, and the bride who gets to sit in it will be touched by Esther, I know."

Communities that create authentic rituals unleash the spiritual experience of being united with that which is more encompassing than our individual lives and separate families. Every June in Jarratt, Virginia, members of the African American community get together to clean the graves of their ancestors. Uniting from many different churches, they spend the day visiting several cemeteries. As one woman, Virginia Ampey, told me, "Who we are today is because of our ancestors—we stand on their shoulders. And so we must take care of them." The community members search for plots that are 60 or more years old, because these graves most likely have no one to take care of them. A community elder has the responsibility of telling others how to find the graves of great-great grandparents, making sure that this vital connection is maintained. This elder teaches his or her children in the next generation to carry on this holy obligation. After the graves are cleaned, candles are lit by the community members. "Our ancestors surely see the light," Virginia Ampey said, "and we leave with a sense of peace and serenity like no other" (personal communication, Virginia Ampey, November 20, 2007).

Community rituals often express healing and celebration via an intricate threading of memory and hope. Such rituals may be a singular occurrence, such as the dedication of the bride's chair. Or they may involve a permanent memorial to be visited and revisited. The Vietnam War Memorial in Washington, D.C. is frequented by families and friends who lost men and women in that war. They make what has been deemed "pilgrimages" to the Wall, where they search for their loved one's name and make rubbings to bring back home. This ritual is repeated daily by thousands of individuals, connecting personal loss with a much larger community of mourners.

The Names Project, a ritual memorializing those who have died of AIDS, comprises individually hand-sewn $4'' \times 6''$ panels connected together in a gigantic quilt. Each patch represents a person who has died of AIDS, and each is created lovingly and with care by family and friends to express essential aspects of the person who died. The quilt arose from another ritual, a memorial marking the murders and commemorating the lives of San Francisco mayor George Moscone and Harvey Milk, the first openly gay supervisor on the city council. In a spontaneous outpouring, mourners covered the walls of the Federal building with placards bearing the names of those who had died of AIDS. The placards tore loose with wind and rain, but people stood for hours reading the names. Quilt originator Cleve Jones said, "Let's take all of our individual experiences and stitch them together to make something that has strength and beauty" (Ruskin, 1988, p. 9) And so the quilt was born.

The Names Project quilt began as a ritual in the gay community. It quickly spread to include those who have died of AIDS from other communities, and serves as a vibrant reminder that grief has no boundaries.

When the quilt is shown, a ceremony is held in which tens of thousands of names are read aloud as the quilt is unfurled in a symbolic action of connection and uplift. Choosing a quilt for this community healing ritual mirrors the community endeavor of quilt making, connecting those who grieve with one another. Such connection countermands the isolation that so many people with AIDS and their families have experienced. A quilt symbolizes the warmth and caring that becomes available when survivors connect with one another, affirming life even in the face of awful death. This quilt, a painfully unfinished ritual that is now too large to be displayed completely, reminds us of the magnitude of our loss (Imber-Black, 2003a).

The Clothesline Project of the Cape Cod Women's Agenda is devoted to helping women recover from abuse. Women create hand-decorated T-shirts and hang these from a clothesline in a community display. Although each T-shirt is different, their communal and public presentation connects and empowers the women. The exhibit includes ringing gongs, peeling bells, and blowing horns in a symbolic action showing how often a woman is assaulted, raped, and murdered (*Ms. Magazine*, 1991, p. 95). The contradiction of regaining power in the midst of servitude is evident in these hand-painted depictions of violence hung with irony on a clothesline. The Clothesline Project uses a ritual to remind us of a relational and spiritual imperative: It is our joint responsibility to protect the most vulnerable among us.

Unlike family rituals, communitywide rituals involve witnesses. The Vietnam Memorial Wall is visited by multitudes of people who did not lose a person in the war, but who want to give witness to the tragedy and keep the memory alive long after the last relative who knew a soldier is gone. When the AIDS quilt is displayed, we go to see it to bear witness to the thousands of lives lost. When we visit Yad Vashem, the Holocaust Memorial, we affirm our own responsibility to stand up against evil. Through these public rituals, we confirm, we testify, we open what may have been kept secret. And through the powerful experience of joint witnessing we are changed.

# SWEET APPRECIATION: RITUALS CELEBRATING
# A LIFE AND TRANSCENDING A DEATH

Thanks in old age—thanks ere I go,
For health, the midday sun, the impalpable air—for life, mere life,
For precious ever-lingering memories, . . .
For gentle words, caresses . . . for sweet appreciation
—WALT WHITMAN, "Thanks in Old Age"

In 2003, I met a couple in the Center for Families and Health. Married 18 years, and with a young son, they came to "work on their marriage." But the husband had Stage IV colon cancer, and there had been no conversations about his impending death. Rusty was a musician, composer, and comedian; Alison was an actress. His illness and our work together became the crucible for breaking years of mutual silence and healing the wounds of alienation.

A metaphor, "Sweet Appreciation," from a poem by Walt Whitman, set to music by Rusty, shaped a series of rituals. Our clinical team heard about some of these rituals in the therapy. Some members were honored to help shape, participate in, and witness them. As the couple's estrangement ameliorated, Alison organized a surprise. This first "Sweet Appreciation" ritual, held at a favorite New York theater artists' café, involved singers who adored Rusty, performing and recording the best of this dying man's work. "I know it added months to my life," he told me. "More important, it gave me a sense of meaning, that what I've created will live after me."

I visited Rusty during his final hospitalization. Friends and family were holding a vigil next to his room in "Sweet Appreciation." They played his music and told stories of his life. Each in turn was able to say good-bye. They called his memorial "Sweet Appreciation II."

As sometimes happens in therapy, our team at the Ackerman Institute was touched by this man and his wife and son long after our work ended. We needed our own healing rituals. For my part, whenever I present this work, I play Rusty's music for the audience. Everyone hears "Sweet Appreciation" and I feel my connection to them. Last year, we named our clinic for Rusty in a celebration, "Sweet Appreciation III." This ritual melded two communities—the Ackerman Institute comprising therapists, students, and alumni, and the theater arts community that loved this man.

In my dedication, I said: "What does it mean to give a name? For all of us, without our knowing it at the time, our first experience in life of a loving relationship is when we receive our name. Naming a baby confers hopes and dreams and imagination for a life not yet lived. And when we name a building, or a program, we connect the very essence of a person who is no longer with us with all of those who will come tomorrow. The act of naming is a profound act, one that braids exquisite strands of memory into a tapestry of healing."

Whenever I visit a place that carries a person's name, I grow curious and I ask, "Who was this person?" And so I anticipate a 12-year-old boy whose father is dying of cancer, asking me, "Who was Rusty?" And I will answer, "He was a man I knew, and 3 months before he died, he sat in my office with his young son and spoke words that many sons wait their whole lives to hear from their fathers when he said, 'I am so proud of you. Do you have any idea how proud I am of you and how much I love you?'"

And I imagine a wife close to losing her husband turning to me and asking, "This man your clinic is named for—who was he?" And I will tell her the story of a man in the final stage of his life who told me, "I'm here to make my marriage better. I'm here to repair old hurts. I'm here to learn new ways to be together."

I picture an adolescent, angry that her parent is dying, saying to me with belligerence, "So who was this guy?" And I will tell that teen of the last time I saw Rusty—he was in a hospital bed, his wife stroking his arm, his son by his side—and the most important thing he had to tell me, with that special pride of legacy in his voice, was that his son had starred in a school performance the night before, that friends had videotaped it for him, and that he had a soul-satisfying peek at what would live after him.

And I see a husband, at first trying to conceal all of his deep feelings engendered by a life-shortening illness, asking me, "Just who was this fellow?" And I will speak of a special man, a man who learned it was OK to be directly angry, even at the one person who was taking care of him; a man who, together with his wife and our team, shaped a sacred space where truth could be spoken; a man cherished by his family and who, by his own example, helped those he loved to move gently toward his life's end.

And I envision family therapy trainees wondering, "Who is Rusty?" I will say to those trainees, "He was a man who, no matter how his physical body deteriorated, showed up at Ackerman with his wife every Tuesday afternoon for 6 months. He came to transform, he came to reveal, he came to give and receive the gifts of relationship. And if you are lucky in your career, you'll get to work with a man like this and his family."

My team and I learned anew through this work and these rituals that death ends a life but not a relationship. Such work is, in essence, deeply spiritual.

## CODA

The spiritual possibilities in rituals may come unexpectedly, connecting a multiplicity of generations unknown, uniting us with memories seemingly not our own, and offering relationships that transcend death.

In 2005, my husband, Lascelles Black, adopted Humanistic Judaism. Our loving friends and family spoke, witnessed, embraced his decision. Fred Silverstein, 88 and husband of our dear friend and colleague Olga Silverstein, stood and wrapped Lascelles in the small tallis given to Fred by his parents 75 years earlier at his bar mitzvah. And for a brief moment, these two secular Jews were cloaked in centuries of history, meaning, ethics, knowledge, turmoil, suffering, and joy.

Fred Silverstein died in 2006. His tallis remains with Lascelles, symbol of a man whose deep convictions and delightful contradictions we dearly loved.

## REFERENCES

Alvarez, J. (2007). *Once upon a quinceañera: Coming of age in the USA*. New York: Viking.

Brotman, B. (2001, September 18). Amid sorrow, a celebration of the future. *The Chicago Tribune*, p. C1.

Cohen, D. (1991). *The circle of life: Rituals from the human family album*. San Francisco: HarperCollins.

Hosseini, K. (2007). *A thousand splendid suns*. New York: Riverhead Books.

Imber-Black, E. (2003a). Ritual themes in families and family therapy. In E. Imber-Black, J. Roberts, & R. Whiting (Eds.), *Rituals in families and family therapy* (rev. ed., pp. 49–87). New York: Norton.

Imber-Black, E. (2003b). September 11th: Rituals of healing and transformation. In E. Imber-Black, J. Roberts, & R. Whiting (Eds.), *Rituals in families and family therapy* (rev. ed., pp. 333–344). New York: Norton.

Imber-Black, E. (2005). Creating meaningful rituals for new life cycle transitions. In B. Carter & M. McGoldrick (Eds.), *The expanded family life cycle: Individual, family and social perspectives* (pp. 202–214). Boston: Allyn & Bacon.

Imber-Black, E., & Roberts, J. (1998) *Rituals for our times: Celebrating, healing and changing our lives and our relationships*. Lanham, MD: Jason Aronson.

Kleinfeld, N. (2007, September 2). As 9/11 nears, a debate rises: How much tribute is enough? *The New York Times*, pp. A1, A25.

Lacey, M. (2002, June 3). Where 9/11 news is late, but aid is swift. *The New York Times*, pp. A1, A6.

*Ms. Magazine* (no author; no title) (1991, July/August), p. 95.

Ruskin, C. (1988). *The quilt: Stories from the NAMES project.* New York: Pocket Books.

Sella, M. (2001, October 7). Missing: How a grief ritual is born. *The New York Times Magazine,* pp. 48–51.

van der Hart, O. (1983). *Rituals in psychotherapy. Transition and continuity.* New York: Irvington.

Whiting, R. (2003). Guidelines to designing therapeutic rituals. In E. Imber-Black, J. Roberts, & R. Whiting (Eds.), *Rituals in families and family therapy* (rev. ed.). New York: Norton.

# Meditation and Relational Connectedness
## Practices for Couples and Families

### JERRY GALE

> Healing . . . complicates the system by opening and restoring connections
> among the various parts–in this way restoring the ultimate simplicity
> of their union. . . . The parts are healthy insofar as they are joined
> harmoniously to the whole.
> —WENDELL BERRY (1977, p. 137)

In the past 30 years, meditation has established a major foothold in Western culture. From scientific research, popular press, spiritual and religious communities, and countless workshops, millions of people in North America have practiced meditation in one form or another. Most research and clinical applications have been individually focused. There is clear evidence of the benefits of meditation for individuals (e.g., stress reduction [Kabat-Zinn, 1990, 2003]; borderline personality disorder [Linehan, 1993a, 1993b]; emotion regulation [Baer & Krietemeyer, 2006]; depression [Segal, Williams, & Teasdale, 2002]; Coffman, Dimidjian, & Baer, 2006]; anxiety disorders [Roemer, Salters-Pedneault, & Orsillo, 2006]; posttraumatic stress disorders [Tirch & Amodio, 2006]; anger [Bankart, 2006]; eating disorders [Tirch & Amodio, 2006]; and psychological well-being [Brown & Ryan, 2003; Brown, Ryan, & Cresswell, 2007]). There is also clear evidence the physiological (muscular, respiratory, heart, neurological, and hormonal) benefits of meditation (Siegel, 2007). There is also abundant literature on how meditation facilitates a spiritual state of being (see, e.g., Boccio, 2004; Gross & Muck, 2003; Wachholtz & Pargament, 2005).

## MEDITATION AND RELATIONAL CONNECTEDNESS

More recently researchers and clinicians have started to address the relational benefits of meditation. Recent studies have demonstrated how mindfulness practices improve romantic relationships (Barnes, Brown, Krusemark, Campbell, & Rogge, 2007), facilitate the communication and regulation of emotions (Wachs & Cordova, 2007), and enhance relationship satisfaction (Carson, Carson, Gil, & Baucom, 2007). Another study (Block-Lerner, Adair, Plumb, Rhatigan, & Orsillo, 2007) suggests that mindfulness-based practices help couples cultivate empathy for one another. Gehart and McCollum (2007), showing how the Buddhist concept of suffering can reorient our understanding of problem-free mental health, discuss how mindfulness practices help change our relationship to suffering (including abuse, divorce, rejection, and loss).

Western cultures' focus on the individual has limited appreciation of the interpersonal aspects of meditation for relationship change and the value of involvement in a community of shared beliefs and practices (sangha; Hanh, 2003). Typically, meditation and contemplative practices are presented as an individual activity for internal change. This chapter offers specific practice applications to strengthen and repair relational connectedness in couples and families.

Although many of these practices are adapted from Buddhist traditions, it is important to note that Buddhism represents a philosophical orientation with a rich and intricate psychology of mind. The classical Buddhist text Abhidhamma presents a detailed taxonomy of the mind and states of consciousness, as well as antidotes to various distresses. Written over 2,500 years ago, it has application to human distress regardless of one's religious views. As noted by Tirch and Amodio (2006), most of the current clinical meditation models "target secular aims based on scientific grounds even if inspired by Buddhist sources" (p. 102). The practices presented in this chapter are for clients of all faiths and beliefs, and do not espouse a particular religious perspective.

It is my premise that what is common in all forms of meditation and contemplative practices—for individuals, for two or more persons, or for groups—is an experience and enhancement of relational connectedness (see

Flemons, 1991; Verela, 1976). Even in Zen practices of emptiness, there is a relational encounter of self and no-self, such that completion is achieved in the relationship of connection–separation, both within and between people (Flemons, 1991).

This perspective of relational connectedness is common to various theoretical frameworks, including systems theory (Bateson, 1979, 1987), the biopsychosocial model (Engle, 1992), and various postmodern discursive theories (Bakhtin, 1981; Davies & Harré, 1990; Shotter, 2003). Gregory Bateson (1987) explicitly notes that we are not "bounded by the skin" (p. 319), and that the individual mind is immanent in "pathways and messages outside the body," such that it is part of a larger Mind, which is "comparable to God" (p. 467). John Shotter (2003) states how our lives might change if "we were to treat ourselves more as 'participant parts' of a larger, ongoing, dynamic indivisible realm of living activity" (p. 461).

Experiencing relational connectedness is a felt response that is difficult to express in words. It is an experience and state of Being that can transcend time, space, and language. One's sense of self can be expanded and opened in ways that change the very nature of identity and relationship with others. The array of problems, fears, and disconnects that lead to narrow meanings of identity can be transcended. Poetry is often an effective medium to express this state of Being. Consider the words of the 13th-century poet Rumi (Barks, 1995, p. 28):

> When you are with everyone but me,
>> you're with no one.
> When you are with no one but me,
>> you're with everyone.
> Instead of being so bound up *with* everyone,
>> *be* everyone.
> When you become the many, you're nothing.
>> Empty.

Even when words leave one with an uncertainty of meaning, poetry (and meditation) invites new possibilities for profound experiences and relationships. Rumi's poem suggests possibilities for being in relationship while letting go a reified, bounded-self holding fears and cravings.

As noted earlier, many specialized meditation programs can help clients with specific issues. More generally, mindfulness practices help therapists and clients to find calm centering, balance, and focus (Boccio, 2004; Goldstein, 1983; Hanh, 1975). They can facilitate a positive climate for therapeutic change and growth when used in or between sessions:

- Therapists can practice meditation in their personal lives and before challenging sessions.
- Clients can be encouraged to practice meditation between sessions, particularly before and after stressful interactions.
- Therapists and clients may start or end sessions with 5 minutes of silent meditation, deep-breathing, or contemplative exercises.
- Therapists can facilitate interactive meditative practices in sessions with couples and family members.

## THEMES AND INTERACTIVE EXERCISES FOR COUPLES AND FAMILIES

The following six themes and interactive exercises are directed toward couple and family relationships. They are offered to orient readers to a few of many useful ways to bring meditation into family and couple therapy. They promote the following aims: (1) to reduce emotional reactivity and defensiveness between members or partners; (2) to facilitate intimacy and deep listening with another; (3) to help families heal and reconnect after loss; (4) to help clients find reconciliation with family members; (5) to offer practices that help couples and families embrace spirituality in their lives; and (6) to initiate meditation and relational aspects for the therapist. Various individual meditations (e.g., breathing, mindfulness, and relaxation practices) are also very effective and complementary to the interactive meditations offered.

In offering the following practices, it is relevant to note that the experience of performing them is different than the words used to explain them. The words used to describe them only point to an activity. The instructions (offered as suggestions) are not the practice, nor do they need to be followed prescriptively. Consider each practice as an invitation for your clients to explore with their partners or family members new ways of interacting and experiencing one another, as well as strengthening relational connectedness.

### Reducing Emotional Reactivity and Defensiveness between Family Members

Couple and family interactions can come to an impasse when partners or members experience intense emotions that override cognitive functioning and communication (e.g., problem-solving abilities, prior agreements, and viewing multiple perspectives). When this emotional state dominates the person's perceptions and actions, in turn, it can lead the partner or other family members to react with a heightened emotional response, or retreat into a defensive mode. This cycle can become self-reinforcing and challenging to interrupt as each person's view become absolute in its opposition to the others.

One practice to reduce emotional reactivity in couple and family sessions is the *stop exercise*, from the teachings of the Armenian Greek mystic G. I. Gurdjieff. This practice requires first eliciting the clients' agreement that whenever you (the therapist) say "stop" they immediately stop their words and actions at that precise point, no matter what they are discussing. Midsentence and midgesture, each person is to stop and freeze in his or her position, until you say "continue." During this 1- to 3-minute pause of movement and sound, each person is to reflect for a few moments on his or her situation and interactions.[1] When you say "continue" the couple/family member can resume their exchange. The "stop–continue" sequence can be presented numerous times. It is best to practice this first with the clients in nonemotional discussions, helping them learn to use the periods of silence/inaction to reflect on their own feelings and thoughts, as well as on others. At times this can be a playful practice and, over time, one that the clients themselves can do outside sessions (with the person who leads stopping his or her actions/words as well).

A second practice for emotional reactivity is *witnessing emotions*, a shared sitting practice I developed for couples (and families). It is best to present this practice first during a nonreactive time. Similar to an individual mindfulness practice of noticing one's own emotions, this exercise invites each person to share verbally with the other(s) his or her experience of an emotion. Following is an example of how this practice can be presented.[2] Deliver this in a slow manner, timing your words to the partners' response to one another. Not every question posed below needs to be asked, nor does every question require a response. Do allow time for the person to respond verbally and report his or her experiences.

> "I would like the two of you to sit facing each other. Pat, you can go first with describing your emotions. Kim, sit silently observing Pat. Pat, your eyes can be open or closed, whichever is easier for you. Begin by describing your present emotional state and how you feel. What thoughts arise? Notice what parts of your body are relaxed and what parts might feel tension. Reflect a moment on yourself and your partner, and notice what thoughts arise? Tell Kim what thoughts and sensations arise.

"Now recall a time you felt a particularly strong emotion. Remember that event in as much detail as you can. Notice how the emotion arises in your body. Where do you feel it? What color is it? Does it move? What are the boundaries of the feelings and the emotions? As you feel the emotion in your body, what thoughts or stories arise? Do the stories suggest particular ways you should respond? Notice how the experience of the emotion and the story change. Notice the beginning and end of each wave of sensation. Notice how your thoughts move. Notice how emotions present a particular way to view the world and see others. Pat, tell Kim what you notice. Notice how it feels talking about the emotions. Can you see the space within the awareness? Can you witness the emotion and your response independent of your watching? How do you feel as you watch yourself experience the emotion and stories that are evoked? As you observe the emotion, send love and compassion to the feelings. See how much you can saturate the emotional field with love and compassion. What do you experience now? Reflect a moment on yourself and Kim and what thoughts arise. Bring the experience to a close and find a place of comfort for yourself.

"Kim, please share with Pat your observations of what you heard and observed with Pat."

When the partners finish this practice, they can switch roles. Depending on the comfort level of the couple, this practice can last from 2 to 10 minutes. Be sure to keep the time balanced for the couple.

A third meditation for emotional reactivity is *smiling meditation for embracing and transforming negative emotions* (Hanh, 2003, p. 26). This meditation uses affirmations and is presented to the partners (or family) as they sit together. They can practice this in session and also do it at home. Although it is good to maintain a continued practice of this meditation, it is also a good practice to use in the midst of an emotional exchange to bring calmness to partners and a new beginning to their conversation.

1. Breathing in, I am aware of my body. Breathing out, I smile to my body.
2. Breathing in, I am aware of pain in my body. Breathing out, I smile to the pain in my body.
3. Breathing in, I am aware of pain in my mind. Breathing out, I smile to the pain in my mind.
4. Breathing in, I am aware of the feeling of fear in me. Breathing out, I smile to the feeling of fear in me.

5. Breathing in, I am aware of the feeling of insecurity in me. Breathing out, I smile to the feeling of insecurity in me.
6. Breathing in, I am aware of the feeling of sadness in me. Breathing out, I smile to the feeling of sadness in me.
7. Breathing in, I am aware of the feeling of anger in me. Breathing out, I smile to the feeling of anger in me.
8. Breathing in, I am aware of the feeling of jealousy in me. Breathing out, I smile to the feeling of jealousy in me. (Hanh, 2003, p. 26)

These exercises may be combined in couple therapy, for instance, with Scheinkman's (2008) integrative model. They are useful for highly reactive family-of-origin interactions, for instance, in conjunction with Bowen coaching methods (McGoldrick & Carter, 2001).

### Facilitating Couple Intimacy and Deep Listening with Another

*Tai Chi wrists* is adapted from the martial art of Tai Chi.

"Begin this practice in silence. Face your partner, about 2 feet apart, with one arm, either the right or left, but the same arm for both of you, raised. Have your corresponding leg slightly forward, your wrists, and the side of the hand where the little finger is, very gently touching the other person's wrist. The touch should be as light as possible while still being in contact. Relax your elbows and knees. Breathe. Allow your wrists and arms to begin inscribing a circle. Any size, direction, and speed of the circle's rotation are perfectly fine. As the circle movement continues, maintain silence and eye contact with one another. Relax into the movement and breathe.

"See if you can let the circle rotation move you. Allow the characteristics of being the leader or follower blur, such that both of you are simultaneously leading and following. Even let go the distinction between these actions, such that the rotation of the wrists has no beginning and no end, no initiator and no follower. As you relax even more, let the circle move you and notice whether you can continue the movement without using muscles. Just relax your elbows and knees, and breathe. When not using muscles, it is possible to do this activity for a while without experiencing fatigue. You may notice the movement changing speed or direction. As you maintain eye contact with your partner, notice how the rest of your body feels. Allow the movement to find its own closing point, independent of your thoughts, and come to a rest. Thank your partner."

Following the activity, invite the couple to talk about their experience. Were there moments that one's sense of discrete individual boundary with the other person blurred? Were there moments of leaderless movement? If the activity was difficult, what was difficult? Depending on the couple's response to the activity, you can try variations. For example, instead of both partners trying not to lead one another, designate one person as the leader and the other as the follower. Switch roles, or even have them both be the leader or the follower simultaneously. What do the partners notice in their relationship when they take on different roles of directing?

When couples experience a strong connection in doing this practice, you can explore other ways they can maintain or deepen bonds in their lives. This can include physical contact and spiritual connections, such as shared values, rituals, and/or involvement in a faith community. If at times one partner experiences a profound spiritual connection with the world, or a heightened state of awareness or flow (Csikszentmihalyi, 1990), how can the partners also sustain connection between them? When they are physically apart, how can the partners sustain relational connection across distances?

Loving kindness practices, taught by many Buddhist teachers, cultivate nonjudgmental and nonattached love and compassion for other beings (Salzberg & Kabat-Zinn, 1995). The following practice, *cultivating loving kindness for your partner*, begins with the partners sitting comfortably facing one another in silence.

> "With eyes half open, maintain a relaxed gaze upon one another. Try to see the whole field of the person without focusing on any one aspect. Maintain a calm and mindful state of mind. If at times you notice the experience of judgment or dislike, repeat 'loving kindness' silently to yourself during these moments. Begin to see the person in front of you as you have known him or her over time. Notice the different images and characteristics of who the person is and who he or she has been over the years. Consider even who the person was before you knew him or her. Notice different images, memories, stories, and emotions that may arise as you gaze at your partner. Recall different moments and experiences of love, joy, appreciation, and peace you have felt with this person. You may notice spreading warmth with this awareness. Hold these feelings and pause, noticing your own response to these sensations and perceptions.
>
> "Recall the challenges, difficulties, and suffering your partner has experienced at different times of her or his life. Recall the difficult times you have shared together. Extend your thoughts to your heart region and, from your heart, feel love, compassion, and warmth for this

person and for your relationship. Cultivate an engaged equanimity with this embrace. Imagine a golden thread connecting your heart to the other, send your love and joy to the other person's heart, and be open to feel the love and joy the other person is extending to you. Notice the warmth and connection that arises with this practice. Breathe into it and relax. When you finish, share your experiences with your partner."

A third practice to facilitate intimacy, attentiveness, and deep listening is *mirroring*, adapted from improvisational theater (Gale, 2004). This activity, conducted in pairs (*A* and *B*), can be fun for children, as well as adults.

"Begin by facing one another. Person *B* initiates with a slow movement. Person *A* mirrors this movement. Movements should be slow to help the partner keep up. It is important to keep attention on your partner and not plan ahead for what you might anticipate. Without talking, Person *B* at any time can begin following Person *A*, who then becomes the initiator. This shifting can occur at any time; hence, it is important to keep focus on each other. If at times you lose connection with your partner, slow down and breathe. You can even mirror each others breathing. When you are both ready to finish, bring the movement to a close and share with each other the experience."

Although this practice can be quick and fun to heighten mindful interpersonal awareness, when extended into a slow, dance-like movement there can be a profound experience of intimacy, connection, and timelessness.

## Helping Families Heal and Reconnect after Loss

Loss of a loved one can be devastating. Emotional suffering can foster family conflict and cutoffs; social isolation; and loss of purpose, meaning, and connection. Following are two ritual practices to help couples and families to heal and reconnect. They are especially valuable when members haven't participated in a funeral or memorial service, or if they haven't supported each other through the loss experience. Both practices invite them to discuss meaning and purpose in life, reestablish routines that honor self and others, and transform lost bonds into ongoing spiritual connections (see Walsh [Chapter 4], and Imber-Black [Chapter 12], this volume).

The first practice, *creating a family remembrance site*, is a shared ritual, adapted from ancient Hindu and Buddhist traditions, establishing a sanctuary, or altar, in the home to honor and remember deceased family members. Invite all family members to participate in creating a dedicated site, such as a room, a garden, or a place that has special meaning for them. Everyone can be encouraged to contribute in some way, by sharing pictures, personal items, flowers, incense, candles, drawings, readings, and anything else someone sees as related to the deceased person. A family tree, artistically drawn by members, can show the relationships and significance of the deceased person in the immediate and extended family across generations (Hanh, 2003; McGoldrick, Gerson, & Petry, 2008).

Help family members plan a time for a shared ritual of remembrance at their created site and discuss what they want to include. Invite them to consider topics that encompass the past, present, and future, and connect the deceased with ancestors and others who have died, with all who survive, and with those who are to come. Participation could include stories of the deceased person (noting characteristics shared by other family members), key events in his or her life, experiences that shaped this person's life, and legacies for survivors and the future. Moments of silent meditation, recitation, and music can also be incorporated.

The second practice, *mindful and honoring eating ritual*, helps family members engage in what typically is a mundane activity, yet experience it in a new way. Often with the loss of a loved one, one may experience a dulling of senses and an emptiness of relational connection and purpose in the world. This practice invites not only a reengagement with the world and ordinary activities but also suggests ways we can honor and embrace the memories and legacy of a loved one. This practice can introduce a ritual that honors and embraces relational connections across space and time, linking survivors with those recently deceased, and with ancestors across the generations.

Bring an apple for each family member.

> "As you hold your apple, take a moment to really consider the fruit in your hand. Use all of your senses. Notice the smell, weight, texture, and shape. Be aware of thoughts, images, and sensations. As you experience this apple, consider its history and the countless events and actions that transpired to bring this apple to your hand today. The many stages of how an apple grows: from germinating seeds that establish roots, mature into a larger plant, grow flowers and give rise to the fruit. The many actions and people involved to bring the apple to your table. Acknowledge and offer appreciation to the fruit for being with you at this time. Eat the fruit very slowly, chewing each mouthful 10 to 20 times. Notice the taste and texture as you chew and swallow. Notice how both taste and textures change as you chew. Continue to contem-

plate the apple. Consider the multiple generations of trees coming to life, bearing fruit, dropping seeds, and producing new generations leading to the apple you are eating. Consider future apples growing from these seeds. Consider the relationship of this apple, in your hand, to all apples over the generations.

"Consider the miracle of what needed to happen for each tree to grow: for the proper balance of sun, earth, and water, all leading to this precise moment of connection and experience. Take a moment to appreciate how the nutrients of this apple are now being metabolized and integrated within your body. How you are benefiting from the many generations that have produced this apple. Consider how the energy of this apple will contribute to your future actions. Consider how other events and people also contribute to your actions and sense of meaning. How do you honor and give acknowledgment to these other events and people? Consider the legacy of an apple tree and its generational influence. Sit for a few minutes with these thoughts and sensations."

When finished, invite the couple or family members to discuss their experiences. What other thoughts, images, and sensations did they notice? This practice can be done at other times by the couple or family, and with other food items. An honoring ritual can be made of this activity. You can also invite participants to take the apple seeds and plant them.

### Helping Clients Find Reconciliation with Family Members

*Beginning anew: the practice of reconciliation and renewal,* adapted from Hanh (2003), is a practice for two or more persons. The premise is to view every social encounter as a revitalization of the relationship. There are three steps, which include sharing appreciation, expressing regret, and expressing hurt and challenges. The steps require each person to consider carefully and select what words to express. Sharing appreciation requires a close attentiveness of the partner to discern and express positive attributes. Too often, positive attributes of another person pass by the observer quickly and without awareness, such that they are seen but unnoticed, and words of acknowledgment are thereby left unspoken. Often, there is no mindfulness, attention, or reflection on the other's positive behaviors. In the second part, expressing regrets, each person acknowledges his or her words and actions that have caused harm or suffering to the other. As Hanh notes, this requires "humility and the willingness to let go of our own pain and pride" (p. 119). This activity also requires careful reflection on one's own actions. For the third step, each person expresses his or her own hurt. With attention to both what one says and how one says the words, the expression of hurt needs to be communicated with mindfulness and love, and without blame or critique.

In helping clients with this practice, it may be useful to record the discussion for playback and review. At times, what we think and intend to say may be very different than how we present our words. Tone, facial expression, timing, and particular word choices can suggest different meanings. Likewise, there are times when we think we are hearing what another person is saying, but our thoughts are adding nuance and reading alternative meanings into the words. It can be helpful to watch the videotape of the interaction and discuss what each person sees (Gale, Odell, & Nagireddy, 1995). This witnessing also presents a mindfulness practice for family members to carefully attend to their communication, as well as the consequences of their actions.[3]

A second interpersonal meditation is *mediation for compassionate listening*, which offers a *mantra* (affirmation) that family members can recite to one another (Hanh, 2003). This affirmation can be written out and given to the clients to use when they are having a difficult time listening to one another. It can be read silently or aloud, with deep breathing. At times, it may be helpful for the couple to read aloud together.

1. Breathing in, I know that I am breathing in. Breathing out, I know that I am breathing out. . . . In. Out.
2. Breathing in, I calm my body. Breathing out, I smile. . . . Calm. Smile.
3. Breathing in, I know I have suffered. Breathing out, I smile with compassion. . . . My suffering, Compassionate smile.
4. Breathing in, I know you have suffered. Breathing out, I smile with compassion. . . . Your suffering, Compassionate smile.
5. Breathing in, I know we both suffer. Breathing out, I want us both to have a new chance. . . . Our suffering, a new chance.
6. Breathing in, I listen. Breathing out, I hear. . . . Listening. Hearing.
7. Breathing in, I hear your bitterness. Breathing out, I embrace you in my heart. . . . Bitterness, Embrace you.
8. Breathing in, I hear your wrong perception. Breathing out, I do not burn with anger. . . . Wrong perception, not burning.
9. Breathing in, I know I have made you suffer. Breathing out, I am sorry. . . . You suffered. I am sorry.
10. Breathing in, I open my heart. Breathing out, in my heart there is room for you. . . . Opening my heart, Room for you.
11. Breathing in, I want to be happy. Breathing out, I want you to be happy. . . . My happiness, Your happiness.
12. Breathing in, I see us happy. Breathing out, that is all I want. . . . Our happiness, Is all I want. (Hanh, 2003, pp. 22–23)

The next practice is *letters in the wallet reminder*, adapted from Hanh (2003). Similar to the previous practice, this one invites the couple or family members to begin composing their own affirmations. To set the stage for this practice, you might tell them:

"When we are emotionally distraught in a relationship, there is a tendency to blame the person we think has hurt us. Strong emotions can cloud our view of another, and blind us to other qualities of the person, as well as to other aspects of the relationship. As negative thoughts and emotions arise, they tend to cloud our view of that individual, and block out awareness of positive experiences and memories. Even the stories arising in our minds can work to justify and strengthen negative characterizations. It can be very useful to have a 'bell of mindfulness' to remind us, in the midst of difficult emotions, 'to keep love and compassion alive in us and to help us refrain from uttering condemning and harsh words and from acting out of our anger' (Hanh, 2003, p. 121). [The therapist might sound a small bell ('inviting' it, but not 'striking' it) at difficult moments in a therapy session.]

"To continue, I want you to write down some statements that you can use anytime you feel strong emotions and judgment about another person: 'Dear one, I suffer and I want you to know it.' And on another sheet of paper, write, 'Dear one, I am doing my best. Please help' (Hanh, 2003, p. 120). As you write down these statements, notice your internal responses. What feelings, images and thoughts arise? Share these with your partner. Do particular people or events arise as you think of these statements? With your partner, take a few moments to share what it would mean truly to tell someone that you are suffering, and that you want their help. Keep both of these statements in your wallet, and whenever you feel rising emotions and a critical mind, take a moment to read both statements. If you want, share them with the other person. Either way, use these moments to breathe and carefully consider how you are suffering in this moment, and how to bring peace and compassion to yourself.

"Next, I would like you both to consider a specific person with whom you at times feel angry and cut off. This could include one another. Notice how your thoughts and emotions change when you think of this person. Now take a moment to consider how you have suffered from this split. Look in your heart for forgiveness and compassion for this person. Consider how healing can occur to reconnect you to this person. As you meditate on this, attend to your own thoughts, images, and inner stories of what you can do. Breathe into and let pass any critical and judgmental thoughts that arise. When you are ready, write words from your heart for reconnecting to this person. Write whatever statements or phrases you want as a reminder of the positive connection you have for this other person. Keep these letters in your wallet to use whenever you need to remind yourself, or to share with the other person. Now take a few moments and discuss this activity with your partner." [4]

## Initiating Practices to Help Couples and Families Embrace Spirituality in Their Lives

All of the meditation practices in this chapter cause one to depart from viewing the individual as a discrete and monadic identity; rather, one sees each person as connected to a larger ecology of existence and meaning. Meditation practices provide a pathway for people to experience this relational connection both within themselves and with all others, from intimate relationships to kin and community networks, as well as to larger systems of which they are a part. This relational perspective also invites a relational understanding of accountability in terms of being sensitive and responsive to moment-to-moment interactions and how each person participates in meaning making. Each action and utterance is generative and opens up possibilities of meaning and response, both interpersonally and in the broader ecology. A mindfulness-based practice combined with loving kindness can open up *all* activities (even the mundane) and all relationships to be fresh, pristine, and miraculous. Regardless of whether one is sitting by the beach, washing dishes, or driving to work; whether one is happy or sad, in a house of worship or shoveling cow manure, one can appreciate the uniqueness of the situation and one's participation in the context.

*Genealogy of the ordinary* is adapted from several meditations from Tarthang Tulku (1977). This practice can be done in any setting, including at home, walking outdoors, pulling weeds, sweeping the driveway, riding in a car, and the like. This exercise invites each person to consider ordinary objects from past, present, and future perspectives. Often mundane objects that we pass are either ignored or viewed from a critical perspective (that it's dirty, has a chip in it, has fading color, etc.). With this meditation, each person is to consider the history of the object and how it came to be in its present location, and what the future of the object might entail. This can be practiced in session with any item in the office. Help people engage all of their senses and imagination to tell a rich and detailed account of the object, and to find appreciation and value in the item. Following is an example of how family members could do this practice in the car.

Although this can be done anytime, taking a family trip or being stuck in traffic are opportune times. Everyone in the car can do this practice, although the driver must be responsive to changing traffic situations. In this oral activity, each person, one at a time, shares his or her emerging thoughts. Instructions are as follows:

"As you gaze out the window of the car, notice any object that attracts your attention. It may be a flower, a tree, a mound of dirt, a sign, trash, another vehicle or driver, a building, a person walking, automobile exhaust rising, and so forth. As you contemplate the object, consider the historical events and actions, both human and environmental, that have played a part in the object's creation and placement at this location at this time. If it is a manufactured item, consider the people and events involved in producing the object. If its origins are organic, consider how it came to be created and how it developed. If it is trash, consider what the object was prior to being tossed away and its relationship to the people who held it. Regardless of what the entity is, consider the natural beauty of the item. Consider all that needed to happen over time and space for you to be aware of this object at this precise moment. Consider the future of the object and what it will be like over time. Notice how change is inevitable. Consider other times you may have seen but not noticed this object. How might you respond next time you see this object?"

A loving kindness meditation can also be incorporated into this practice.

## Initiating Meditation and Relational Aspects for the Therapist

In conducting all of these practices, it is important to consider the therapist's participation in the process. The therapist is an active strand in these relational tapestries. It is most valuable for therapists to have their own mediation practice. Segal, Williams, and Teasdale (2002) noted that their mind–body stress reduction (MBSR) program to prevent relapse of client depression achieved improved results when instructors maintained their own meditative practice. Additionally, therapists can benefit from meditation in other ways, including nonjudgmental mindfulness, calmness, responsiveness to their inner feelings and thoughts, and improved concentration (Carlson & Brown, 2005, have developed a scale for assessing mindfulness). Compassion can also be cultivated through meditation, and there is evidence that self-compassion helps therapists take better care of themselves, as well as improve therapeutic relationships. (Neff, 2003a, 2003b, 2004, has developed an assessment for examining self-compassion.[5])

It is also important that the therapist practice meditation to better determine when and how best to incorporate these practices in sessions. Otani (2003) warns that "like hypnosis and other clinical techniques, the use of meditation without proper training is unethical" (p. 104). Concern about possible contraindications for meditation is noted both in traditional Buddhist texts and in clinical publications (Germer, Siegel, & Fulton, 2005; Otani, 2003). Meditation can bring up emotionally charged states that the person may not be prepared to manage. Linehan, who developed dialectical behavioral therapy (DBT), has stated that "extended meditation practice is contraindicated for many patients with severe psychopathology" (cited in Welch, Rizvi, & Dimidjian, 2006, p. 123). In most Eastern traditions, meditation is taught by a teacher with extensive experience, who can closely monitor and guide the novice's experiences. Therefore, it is important for therapists to be knowledgeable about meditation principles and cautions, to assess client vulnerability, and to guide meditation experiences carefully in and between sessions.

## CONCLUSION

In closing, I want to mention the expanding frontier at the intersection of meditation, neuroscience, relational connectedness, and spirituality. Siegel (2007) presents strong evidence that our brains have social circuitry, such that a sense of connectedness is crucial for well-being. Siegel also suggests that meditation can have direct influence on our brains and even change neural functioning. Recent publications (Edwards, 2008; Fishbane, 2008; Walker, 2008) present examples of how neuroscience, couple therapy, and meditation work together to facilitate therapeutic change. This relational perspective is a crucial aspect of therapeutic work with couples and families, and a framework that can bring healing in our world.

## NOTES

1. If you have introduced other individual mediation practices to clients, such as deep breathing, then this is a good time for clients to engage briefly in their practice.
2. For this practice, and others, I present the mediation as if I am talking to the clients. Quotation marks signify the segments of what I might say to the clients.

3. Through having therapists conduct discourse analysis of their own therapy, I have found that they develop increased mindfulness in their interactions (Gale, 1996, 2000).

4. A variation of this exercise is to have the couple jointly compose a commitment letter of peace. This statement includes pledges for both persons or groups (see Hanh, 2003, pp. 134–136).

5. This assessment is available at *www.self-compassion.org.*

## REFERENCES

Baer, R. A., & Krietemeyer, J. (2006). Overview of mindfulness- and acceptance-based treatment approaches. In R. A. Baer (Ed.), *Mindfulness-based treatment approaches: Clinician's guide to evidence base and applications* (pp. 3–30). Amsterdam: Academic Press.

Bakhtin, M. M. (1981). *The dialogical imagination* (M. Holquist, Ed.; C. Emerson & M. Holquist, Trans.). Austin: University of Texas Press.

Bankart, P. (2006). Mindfulness, compassion, and wisdom: Working with anger. In M. G. T. Kwee, K. J. Gergen, & F. Koshikawa (Eds.), *Horizons in Buddhist psychology: Practice, research and theory* (pp. 75–84). Chagrin Falls, OH: Taos Institute Publications.

Barks, C. (1995). *The essential Rumi.* San Francisco: Harper.

Barnes, S., Brown, K. W., Krusemark, E., Campbell, W. K., & Rogge, R. D. (2007). The role of mindfulness in romantic relationship satisfaction and responses to relationship stress. *Journal of Marital and Family Therapy, 33*(4), 482–500.

Bateson, G. (1979). *Mind and nature: A necessary unity.* New York: Bantam Books.

Bateson, G. (1987). *Steps to an ecology of mind.* Northvale, NJ: Jason Aronson.

Berry, W. (1977). *The unsettling of America: Culture and agriculture.* San Francisco: Sierra Club Books.

Block-Lerner, J., Adair, C., Plumb, J. C., Rhatigan, D. L., & Orsillo, S. M. (2007). The case for mindfulness-based approaches in the cultivation of empathy: Does nonjudgmental, present moment-to-moment awareness increase capacity for perspective-taking and empathetic concern? *Journal of Marital and Family Therapy, 33*(4), 501–516.

Boccio, F. J. (2004). *Mindfulness yoga: The awakened union of breath, body and mind.* Boston: Wisdom Publications.

Brown, K. W., & Ryan, R. M. (2003). The benefits of being present: Mindfulness and its role in psychological well-being. *Journal of Personality and Social Psychology, 84*, 822–848.

Brown, K. W., Ryan, R. M., & Creswell, J. D. (2007). Mindfulness: Theoretical foundations and evidence for its salutary effects. *Psychological Inquiry, 18*, 211–237.

Carlson, L. E., & Brown, K. W. (2005). Validation of the Mindful Attention Awareness Scale in a cancer population. *Journal of Psychosomatic Research, 58*, 29–33.

Carson, J. W., Carson, K. M., Gil, K. M., & Baucom, D. H. (2007). Self-expression as a mediator of relationship improvements in mindfulness intervention. *Journal of Marital and Family Therapy, 33*(4), 517–528.

Coffman, S. J., Dimidjian S., & Baer, R. A. (2006). Mindfulenss-based cognitive therapy for prevention of depressive relapse. In R. A. Baer (Ed.), *Mindfulness-based treatment approaches: Clinician's guide to evidence base and applications.* (pp. 31–51). Amsterdam: Academic Press.

Csikszentmihalyi, M. (1990). *Flow: The psychology of optimal experience.* New York: Harper & Row.

Davies, B., & Harré, R. (1990). Positioning: The discursive production of selves. *Journal for the Theory of Social Behavior, 20*(1), 43–63.

Edwards, M. (Ed.). (2008). *AFTA Monograph Series: Neuroscience and family therapy: Integrations and applications.* Washington, DC: AFTA.

Engel, G. L. (1992). The need for a new medical model: A challenge to biomedicine. *Family Systems Medicine, 10,* 317–331.

Fishbane, M. D. (2008). "News from neuroscience": Applications to couples therapy. In M. Edwards (Ed.), *AFTA Monograph Series: Neuroscience and family therapy: Integrations and applications* (pp. 20–27).

Flemons, D. G. (1991). *Completing distinctions: Interweaving the ideas of Gregory Bateson and Taoism into a unique approach to therapy.* Boston: Shambhala.

Gale, J. (2004). Experiencing relational thinking. *Context, 75,* 10–12.

Gale, J. (1996). Conversation analysis: Studying the construction of therapeutic realities. In D. Sprenkle & S. Moon (Eds.), *Family therapy research: A handbook of methods* (pp. 107–124). New York: Guilford Press.

Gale, J. (2000). Patterns of talk: A micro-landscape perspective. *The Qualitative Report, 4,*(1/2). Available online at *www.nova.edu/ssss/qr/qr4-1/gale.html.*

Gale, J., Odell, M., & Nagireddy, C. (1995). Marital therapy and self-reflexive research: Research and/as intervention. In G. H. Morris & R. Chenail (Eds.), *The talk of the clinic* (pp. 105–130). Hillsdale, NJ: Erlbaum.

Gehart, D. R., & McCollum, E. E. (2007). Engaging suffering: Towards a mindful re-visioning of family therapy practice. *Journal of Marital and Family Therapy, 33*(2), 214–236.

Germer, C. K., Siegel, R. D., & Fulton, P. R. (2005). *Mindfulness and psychotherapy.* New York: Guilford Press.

Goldstein, J. (1983). *The experience of insight: A simple and direct guide to Buddhist Meditation.* Boston: Shambhala.

Gross, R. M., & Muck, T. C. (Eds.). (2003). *Christians talk about Buddhist meditation, Buddhists talk about Christian prayer.* New York: Continuum.

Hanh, T. N. (1975). *The miracle of mindfulness: An introduction to the practice of meditation.* Boston: Beacon Press.

Hanh, T. N. (2003). *Creating true peach: Ending violence in yourself, your family, your community, and the world.* New York: Free Press.

Kabat-Zinn, J. (1990). *Full catastrophe living: Using the wisdom of your body and mind to face stress, pain and illness.* New York: Delacorte.

Kabat-Zinn, J. (2003). Mindfulness-based interventions in context: Past, present, and future. *Clinical Psychology: Science and Practice, 10*(2), 144–156.

Linehan, M. M. (1993a). *Cognitive-behavioral treatment of borderline personality disorder.* New York: Guilford Press.

Linehan, M. M. (1993b). *Skills training manual for treating borderline personality disorder.* New York: Guilford Press.

McGoldrick, M., & Carter, B. (2001). Advances in coaching: Family therapy with one person. *Journal of Marital and Family Therapy, 21*(3), 281–300.

McGoldrick, M., Gerson, R., & Petry, S. (2008). *Genograms: Assessment and intervention.* New York: Norton.

Neff, K. D. (2003a). The development and validation of a scale to measure self-compassion. *Self and Identity, 2,* 223–250.

Neff, K. D. (2003b). Self-compassion: An alternative conceptualization of a healthy attitude toward oneself. *Self and Identity, 2,* 223–250.

Neff, K. D. (2004). Self-compassion and psychological well-being. *Constructivisim in the Human Sciences, 9*(2), 29–37.

Otani, A. (2003). Eastern meditative techniques and hypnosis: A new synthesis. *American Journal of Clinical Hypnosis, 46*(2), 97–108.

Roemer, L., Salters-Pedneault, K., & Orsillo, S. M. (2006). Incorporating mindfulness- and acceptance-based strategies in the treatment of generalized anxiety disorder. In R. A. Baer (Ed.), *Mindfulness-based treatment approaches: Clinician's guide to evidence base and applications* (pp. 52–74). Amsterdam: Academic Press.

Salzberg, S., & Kabat-Zinn, J. (1995). *Lovingkindness: The revolutionary art of happiness.* Boston: Shambhala.

Scheinkman, M. (2008). Multi-level approach: A roadmap to couples therapy. *Family Process 47*(2), 197–213.

Segal, Z. A. M., Williams, J. M. G., & Teasdale, J. D. (2002). *Mindfulness-based cognitive therapy for depression: A new approach to preventing relapse.* New York: Guilford Press.

Siegel, D. J. (2007). *The mindful brain: Reflections and attunement in the cultivation of well-being.* New York: Norton.

Shotter, J. (2003). Real presences: Meaning as living movement in a participatory world. *Theory and Psychology, 13*(4), 435–468.

Tirch, D., & Amodio, R. (2006). Beyond mindfulness and post-traumatic stress disorder. In M. G. T. Kwee, K. J. Gergen, & F. Koshikawa (Eds.), *Horizons in Buddhist psychology: Practice, research and theory* (pp. 101–117). Chagrin Falls, OH: Taos Institute Publications.

Tulku, T. (1977). *Time, space and knowledge: A new vision of reality.* Oakland, CA: Dharma Press.

Verela, F. J. (1976, Fall). Not one, not two. *Coevolutionary Quarterly,* pp. 62–67.

Wachholtz, A. B., & Pargament, K. I. (2005). Is spirituality a critical ingredient of meditation?: Comparing the effects of spiritual meditation, secular meditation, and relaxation on spiritual, psychological, cardiac, and pain outcomes. *Journal of Behavioral Medicine, 28*(4), 369–384.

Wachs, K., & Cordova, J. V. (2007). Mindful relating: Exploring mindfulness and emotion repertoires in intimate relationships. *Journal of Marital and Family Therapy, 33*(4), 464–481.

Walker, G. (2008). Mind-ecologies. In M. Edwards (Ed.), *AFTA Monograph Series: Neuroscience and family therapy: Integrations and applications* (pp. 8–19). Washington, DC: AFTA.

Welch, S. S., Rizvi, S., & Dimidjian, S. (2006). Mindfulness in dialectical behavioral therapy (DBT) for borderline personality disorder. In R. A. Baer (Ed.), *Mindfulness-based treatment approaches: Clinician's guide to evidence base and applications* (pp. 117–142). Amsterdam: Academic Press.

# Healing from Relational Trauma
## *The Quest for Spirituality*

### MARY JO BARRETT

Trauma interrupts emotional, psychological, spiritual, sexual, and/or intellectual development, and chronically or acutely impinges on a person's ability to cope or function. Most of the clients that I work with have been traumatized by physical and/or sexual violations. My career has been dedicated to helping my clients heal from these violations and from their debilitating symptoms, and developing specific interventions to interrupt dysfunctional sociopolitical, familial, and intrapsychic patterns. This work led to the creation of the Collaborative Stage Model (Trepper & Barrett, 1990). In 1992, we began conducting exit and follow-up interviews with our clients. As they left the program, we asked them what they believed had changed in their lives and to what they attributed this change. We then followed up 6 months and 1 year later, again asking whether they had maintained their changes and, if so, to what they attributed their changes in retrospect. Fortunately, we have been able to interview some clients as long as 20 years after they left the program. What they told us has changed my life and my treatment of trauma.

## LOVE AND KNOWLEDGE

A Soul met an angel and asked: "By which path shall I reach heaven
quickest—the path of knowledge or the path of love?" The angel
looked wonderingly and said, "Are not both paths one?"
—OLIVE SCHREINER (in Keen, 1994, p. 93)

The stories our clients told us about what they believed created the change
in their lives revolved around two themes: love and knowledge. First, they
believed that their own desire, will, and internal spirit created the change.
Generally, they reported that in their souls they had made the following
discoveries: "In the depth of my bones . . . [I felt that] I had [changed] and
that I could change"; "Therapy was a process of getting myself back, not
changing who I am but reconnecting with my spirit"; "I learned to love
myself again"; "I came to remember that I deserved to be happy"; "I started
to value myself and other people around me." They had tapped into a reser-
voir of self-love.

They also told us that the meaning of the world and what they believed
about people had changed—especially finding out that everything was not
black or white, good or evil. The clients told us of the following personal
discoveries:

"I began to see that the whole world and everybody in it were not dan-
gerous."
"We began to treat members in our families like we were being treated
in the program, with respect and care."
"We learned that there were good people out there who wanted and
could help."
"I started to see more beauty where there used to be only gray."
"Everyone was not good or evil; there is a middle ground."
"The therapy renewed my faith in mankind. I just kept meeting more
and more people who cared and took the time for me."
"There was a time when I thought everyone would hate me for what I
did. What I learned is that they hated what I did but not me."

What they told us is that being in a treatment program changed their view
of the world and the people in it.

People want ways to bring meaning into their lives to provide access to the
world of faith and meaning; a time to experience awe. Awe helps us to find the
faith to move forward. (Hammerschlag & Silverman, 1997, p. 8)

Good treatment of trauma provides faith and meaning.

The second theme of change was knowledge. Clients felt that they had become aware of their recurrent patterns and had discovered new methods of coping, functioning, and interacting. It was clear that many aspects of therapy—from the practical insights to psychoeducational processes—gave them new knowledge about how to deal with the world. They reported that they learned communication skills, how to create safe boundaries, and how to relieve their anxieties or to struggle with their addictions. At the same time, many clients said that they were changing on a deeper level. They felt that they were regaining the essence of who they were. As they were learning skills, methods of communicating, ways of coping with their pain and rage, they were simultaneously discovering new meaning about their world and the individuals in it. They learned through both the cognitive-behavioral techniques utilized and the practice of mindfulness integrated into their treatment and lifestyle.

The Buddha says that clinging is the cause of pain, and that ignorance is the cause of clinging (Dick Olney, cited in Moore, 1996, p. 24). One of the first steps in seeking healing is learning. We first have to learn how negative emotions and behaviors are harmful to us, and how positive emotions are helpful. And we must realize how these negative emotions are not only very bad and harmful to one personally but also harmful to society and the future of the whole world. That kind of realization enhances our determination to face and overcome them (His Holiness the Dalai Lama, in His Holiness the Dalai Lama & Cutler, 1998, p. 38).

As the clients learned more about people, patterns, and self, they clung less to damaging old beliefs about themselves and the world around them. It became clear that the process of change had tapped a divine spark in the majority of clients we interviewed. They had realized a source of goodness and caring that moved them to act on principle, to do what is right for themselves and for others. They had learned through the psychoeducational techniques and their healing relationships with the therapists, their family members, and others in their groups that their negative self-judgments were hurting themselves and others, both physically and spiritually. We spent many conscious moments helping clients see how hurting others was also damaging to themselves. Christianity, Judaism, and Islam all teach that each of us is created in the divine image. What we helped clients learn was that when evil thoughts, feelings, and/or behaviors arise, this becomes an opportunity to behave "God-like," as a "creator" instead of a "reactor." This does not necessitate a belief in God. It requires a desire to feel and to be different. Our integrative treatment approach had enabled clients to envision the world and themselves differently.

The more open I was to clients, the more I heard. The change of spirit was happening simultaneously as their behaviors changed. But as they talked and I listened, it became clear that this change of spirit came from the meaning and value they experienced in relationship to the treatment teams. The healing from trauma is a quest for spirituality. This quest reflects a deep need for meaning and value.

I began to look at my work with my colleagues through a different lens. By no means did we throw out the vast base of knowledge we had accumulated through the years. Nor did we abandon our bag of tools/interventions. We began to add a new perspective. We added the belief system that becoming spiritually aware of ourselves would invite into our relationships an energy that would help our clients resist their usual hurtful behavior. After talking with more than 600 clients, we began overtly to introduce a spiritual discipline into our day-to-day practice, both personal and professional. As with any other body or mind faculties, the spiritual sense is a faculty that must be developed and maintained. I realized I had to focus regularly on these spiritual moments in both my professional and personal life. I approached this shift as I approach anything else: The clients had told us that therapy provided meaning and human value and connection; then I set out to understand how this happened, so that I and the therapists I train could provide meaning, value, and connection more consistently (Siegel, 2007).

## INTEGRATING SPIRITUAL MEANING AND VALUE INTO TREATMENT

When individuals are abused, as children or as adults, by someone in a position of power over them and to whom they are attached, the result is a traumatic interruption on many levels. Here we focus on the level of spirit. Each story is different, but all clients report that the abuse has forever changed them and altered how they see the world. When individuals are abused, they experience a loss of trust, innocence, and peacefulness. They begin to see the world as dangerous, and there is a heightened awareness of the presence of the evil inclination. They become acutely aware of their vulnerability in the universe, and they no longer feel powerful. They have split into the judge and the judged. They have lost their sense of self-determination. They are burdened with a sense that what they do or who they are does not have much value or influence in their world.

The Dalai Lama states, "True spirituality is a mental attitude that you can practice at any time" (His Holiness the Dalai Lama & Cutler, 1998,

p. 300). When we view spirituality as the Dalai Lama does, we see that when the spirit is violated, then the mental attitude that is practiced afterward is one of fear, anger, pain, self-judgment, and/or self-blame. Our task then becomes helping clients practice a spiritual attitude of self-acceptance, helping them "wake up from the bad dream that they are incomplete or insufficient or lacking something," or that they are damaged goods. (Olney, in R. Moore, 1996, p. 4).

It was no accident that at the same time I was involved in the follow-up study, I was in the midst of my own personal and professional crisis. I had come to realize that I had been vicariously traumatized. I had not been damaged physically or sexually, and not by family members. Yet I had a damaged spirit. My happy, optimistic, energetic, divine spirit was gone. Rabbi Alan Miller describes internal spirituality as a Godliness: "The term God is rather the name we give to the interpersonal process of growth and creativity that takes place naturally among men and women striving towards authentic fulfillment" (quoted in Hirsh, 1994, p. 4). I had found in my life that I was no longer moving toward this process of growth and creativity. I had lost many of my essential beliefs that had brought me to this profession and to my specialty in trauma. My view of the world had changed. I no longer believed that people are basically good. Rather, I had become afraid of the evil inclination. I felt certain that it was more powerful than the human desire to be good. I was no longer as clear about the meaning of life. As a clinician, I could view this as depression, but I knew in my soul that it was a crisis of spirit. An existential crisis is very different than a situational depression. Day after day, moment after moment, my work with survivors and offenders had taken me down the road of the most evil and painful human experiences. Just like the clients I work with, I had been changed forever—changed through the process of listening to them and being compassionately there for them in their most painful narratives. Of course, having a dying spirit made me more empathetic to my clients' stories about their loss of spirit, but it was destroying me and my family.

I was suffering from *compassion fatigue* (Barrett, 2008; Figley, 1995), which I define as the depletion and subsequent symptoms that we experience as the result of passionately and compassionately giving of our energy in the service of care. We are all complex mechanisms that operate on energy: physical, emotional, intellectual, spiritual, and sexual energy. To operate our lives as clinicians, mothers, fathers, lovers, friends, daughters, sons, and siblings, we use energy on all five of these levels. I had spent the last 15 years using up my energy without replenishing, and now I was running on empty. I came to the realization that something must change radically for me. Like any good clinician, I made an assessment and tried to determine the symptoms, and the function of each of these symptoms.

At the same time that I was becoming increasingly aware of my painful loss of spirit and my symptoms of compassion fatigue, I was also hearing, through the interviews, stories of renewal. It was serendipitous: The path of renewal for my clients would also become the path of renewal for myself.

## CONSCIOUS SPIRITUALITY

The task before me was how to rebuild my spirit so that I would be spiritually available to my clients. The next step would be how to teach others the importance of conscious spirituality. Our clients need us to communicate with a vocabulary that offers hope, inspiration, and comfort. How do we develop hope and inspiration, then convey this to others?

I believe that change happens in stages. The Collaborative Stage Model (CSM) that we have developed in working with trauma is a three-stage model (Trepper & Barrett, 1990). Moving unconscious knowledge to consciousness also happens in stages. Because it has proven successful to organize treatment in these stages, it was helpful for me to think about these three stages when organizing my own plan for spiritual renewal. Stage 1 is the introduction to the concepts of spirituality and the need [fwl]for spiritual connection within ourselves and between people. Stage 2 is the active integration of these ideas into the program and into their lives. Stage 3 is consolidation and celebration of the positive changes, with commitment to continue on a spiritual journey.

### Stage 1: Creating a Context for Change

There is an interesting story about P. D. Ouspensky, a student of the great Middle Eastern mystic L. I. Gurdjieff.

> Ouspensky had several turbulent nights in a row, taking a mind-altering drug, then spending intense hours trying to unravel the mystery of the meaning of life. He would sometimes think that he had found the answer, but in the morning he was unable to remember it. One night, he had the idea of writing down what occurred to him. Sure enough, when he woke up in the morning, no matter how hard he tried, his nighttime revelations eluded him. When he remembered that he had written the answer down in his notebook, his excitement was palpable. Expecting to read a long and complicated expla-

nation, what he found were these four words: THINK IN OTHER CATEGORIES. (Dick Olney, in R. Moore, 1996, p. 3)

This was the first stage of spiritual renewal for me. I had to begin to "think in other categories." I had to become aware of what constrained me from experiencing myself and the world around me at any given moment. The first steps were to slow down, step back, and observe. My life, personal and professional, like that of so many others, had become so busy and filled with routine that I had lost much of my sense of awe and the time to discover beauty. I had to create a context where there would be opportunity for spiritual growth. The Buddhists speak of "practice." I needed to create space in my life where I could practice a new attitude toward life, toward the world, and toward self. First, I formally acknowledged the need for a shift in my spirit. I began to discuss with the important people in my life the changes necessary to rekindle my passion for humanity.

I knew I needed love and knowledge to be able to change. I asked for help. I asked colleagues, friends, and loved ones to support me on this journey and to participate in any ways that they found comfortable. Many people close to me had commented on numerous occasions that I was different, that I had lost my spirit. It appeared that I was the last to discover my dwindling spark. They were all quite supportive of this quest. They shared their own stories and offered support. I realized I needed knowledge, so I began to read and take courses. I read about different cultures' paths toward spirituality. I explored Native American traditions, as well as Zen and Kabbalistic philosophies of spirituality and meditation (e.g., Berg, 1993). I also read outside the field of family therapy, delving into the many disciplines that have struggled for decades with the issue of spirituality. There was much literature to read. I only skimmed the surface. Once I got over the shame of my narrow lenses and my ignorance of the fields of transpersonal psychology and humanistic psychology, I gleefully feasted on newfound sources of knowledge. The work of Ken Wilbur and Dick Olney were particularly great influences. Wilbur helped me make sense of the role of mysticism in psychology and how consciousness works on a continuum. His writings on Eastern and Western views of personal growth truly began the integration process for me. Wilbur (1991) writes in *Grace and Grit*:

> According to the mystics, when we go beyond or transcend our separate-self sense, our limited ego, we discover instead a Supreme Identity, an identity with the All, with universal Spirit, infinite and all pervading, eternal and unchanging. As Albert Einstein explains: "A human being is part of the

whole, called by us Universe; a part limited in time and space. He experiences himself, his thoughts and feelings as something separated from the rest—a kind of optical delusion of his consciousness. This delusion is a kind of prison for us, restricting us to our personal desires and to affection for a few persons nearest us. Our task must be to free ourselves from this prison." Indeed, the whole point of meditation or contemplation is to free ourselves from the "optical delusion" that we are merely separate egos set apart from each other [and] from eternal Spirit, and to discover instead that, once released from the prison of individuality we are with all manifestation, in a perfectly timeless and eternal fashion. (p. 18)

Through my consultations with Olney, I came to recognize the importance of experiencing one's own sense of beauty. Olney's *self-acceptance training* is simply defined as "experiencing myself as I am without the inhibitions of self-judgement, self-criticism, or self-evaluation. It is not a goal, but an attitude toward life which one can come back to again and again" (Moore, 1996, preface).

Dick Olney often said:

You are not your body. You are not your name. You are not your thoughts. You are not your emotions. You are not your memories. You are not the content of your consciousness. You are the unspeakable. That which cannot be named. If you name it you turn it into one more concept. A better question than "Who am I?" is "What am I?" What you are is life! You are carrying the gift of life. You are a fire that has been burning for millions of years. You are your ancestors. (Moore, 1996, pp. 28–29)

As I studied, it became clear to me that I had become deeply imprisoned in my own "optical delusions," and what I needed was to be on the path to freeing myself. I discovered that my journey had to involve vehicles to the unconscious. This meant providing an environment for meditation, peaceful sleep, celebration of life, and prayer. Everyone's context for spiritual renewal is unique, but there might be some common elements. Years after I had renewed my spiritual practice, I was having a conversation with my rabbi about spirituality and psychotherapy. He gave me an article that discussed the different needs that can be met through prayer and attempted to answer the question, "Why do people pray?" In an article entitled "How Can Reconstructionists Pray?" I discovered that what I was doing in my office was a form of prayer. Prayer is not necessarily an appeal to God, nor is it merely asking another source to do something for us. It is an opportunity to go inside ourselves, alone or in community, and call upon our own desire and resources to create change. It is the time to look inward and draw upon our own creative, moral energy to create this positive force outside of ourselves. Prayer is a vehicle to "think in other categories" (Moore, 1996, p. 4) in order to unravel the mystery of life. Much of the work that was necessary to rekindle my spirit and free me from the prison I had built around myself came through different forms of prayer. It can be a form of meditation, a form of appreciation, a form of awareness of our universal membership in humanity.

I had successfully changed my environment to include the elements of prayer in my life on a regular basis. These elements seemed to summarize how spirituality works in the treatment of trauma. In fact, my own personal work and our treatment had incorporated all these elements:

• *Spiritual discipline.* We need to discipline ourselves to focus regularly on creative, beautiful, and sacred encounters, developing and maintaining a regular practice of stepping back and noticing spiritual moments as they occur—or remembering those moments.

• *Meditation.* We all live at a very rapid pace. We can learn to welcome the opportunity to slow down to remember what has deeper meaning, beyond our daily distractions.

• *Connection.* This is an opportunity to leave our spiritual isolation. Through either connection with others or connection with our own sense of value and power, we can focus on and perhaps express what is really important to us.

• *Celebration.* Moments of celebration, like laughter, can transport us beyond ourselves, beyond ego, beyond self-judgment.

• *Support.* Renewal is enhanced by the support of a caring group. There is often a tangible power when the energy of a group is focused in a mutual direction.

• *Rededication.* It is easy to lose perspective, to miss the forest for the trees. We all get so wound up in a situation that we lose sight of who we are and what we stand for. We need a method that draws us out of ourselves and restores the larger picture.

• *Acknowledgment of need.* Most of us are raised to think that we have control of our lives; therefore, we are responsible for what happens to us—both good and bad. It is necessary to acknowledge our vulnerability. Removing our defenses can move us to the honest self-awareness we require to get past our personal obstacles.

It also became clear that what the clients had been telling us in our follow-up interviews was that therapy and their relationships with us had been part of their getting out of prison. We had incorporated these elements into our therapy. By defining prayer this way, we had been praying for 25 years with clients and had not even realized it. By having meaningful connections with others, the clients had experienced themselves as part of the greater universe, not just seeing themselves as their body, name, thoughts, memories, and consciousness, but something more.

Stage 1 of the Collaborative Stage Model revolves around three primary goals:

1. To provide safety for clients in treatment and in relation to the team, and in moving toward safety in their lives.
2. To provide an environment where clients can begin to tell their story about all aspects of their lives, through family, individual, and group modalities.
3. To acknowledge clients' need for change and commit to the program.

When consciously integrating spirituality into trauma treatment, we keep these same three goals. First, it is essential to provide an environment where it is safe and accepted for clients to discuss their need and desire for spiritual and moral behavior, as well as their views of it. Next we want to hear their current beliefs about people, good and evil, meaning, and relationships; what role religion currently plays in their lives; and what they think the future holds for them. Finally, how do they see therapy being helpful in this domain? Are there specific behaviors or topics about spirituality they want to integrate in their program? It is useful in Stage 1 to teach about the helpfulness of a mindfulness practice. In this stage, we discuss the neurobiological phenomena of trauma and how a mindfulness practice can heal the "trauma mind."

In my own life, Stage 1 consisted of learning about spirituality, defining it, then creating a plan for spiritual practice. It became clear to me that this practice is an essential part of healing from trauma. This awareness developed during the interviews, and I decided to introduce this element of connection and spirituality more overtly into Stage 1 of the treatment program.

At our Center for Contextual Change, all therapists have made a conscious effort to create a physical environment that is more conducive to spiritual discipline. We have the capabilities to provide appropriate music and aromatherapy, as well as candles, footstools, headrests, pillows, and so forth. This allows the client to design his or her own context for spiritual awareness. From the start, we share with them that we have discovered from talking with our clients that elements of spirituality have been helpful to integrate into treatment, such as rededication, celebration, or meditation. When appropriate, we share with our clients the research as it relates to the brain (van der Kolk, McFarlane, & Weisaeth, 1996; Solomon & Siegel, 2003). We discuss their definitions of spirituality and morality, and how it may feel for them to integrate these into their treatment program. It is common for us to integrate their use of prayer or their religion into sessions. As might be expected, there are questions and discussions about our views of spirituality. Our answers are direct. We share the information we have received from past clients, refer them to the literature, and discuss the personal nature of each person's journey. We are available to guide but not to direct them or to instruct them on how to be spiritual. Simply put, "We are here to guide you, through the sharing of information and by example, in how to transform your negative reactivity to positive, proactive shifts toward yourself and one another."

We not only work with those who have suffered abuse but also with offenders, whenever possible. Many offenders "have found God" in jail. We see this not as an answer—that they are "saved" and "cured"—but instead as a pathway for understanding their abusive behavior and stopping future abuse. In other words, how do they really live a God-filled life?

We introduce language that helps all our clients begin to understand, identify, and discuss the internal conflict of good and evil. Clients who have been traumatized understand this language instinctively. Many have already identified this conflict. We use their language for identifying this struggle: evil inclination, Satan, the dark side, or the evil part. We might help them by introducing them to the Parts Model of Richard Schwartz (1995).

## Stage 2: Challenging Patterns and Expanding Realities

Stage 2, the active integration of these ideas, involves learning the patterns that constrain us from creating harmony in our lives; it also entails practicing new methods of being proactive that produce expanded realities. On one level this means considering the following questions: What are the patterns in my life that produce violent behavior or behaviors that are self-abusive? What are the patterns that keep me in an abusive relationship or keep me reacting to the world as a victim? What are the constraints that stop me from changing these patterns? Then, together, in family, individual, and/or group modalities, we explore alternative behaviors, and create new behavioral and neurological pathways, cognitions, and feeling patterns that help clients expand their repertoires beyond victim–perpetrator, from negatively reactive to positively proactive.

We have discovered that the absence of spiritual connection is a variable that allows people to abuse themselves and others. During Stage 2 we introduce active alternatives for bringing spiritual connection into clients' lives. The CSM explains when to utilize cognitive-behavioral techniques, such as Dialectical Behavioral Therapy (Linehan, 1993), or EMDR (Shapiro, 1997), which we actively use in our trauma treatment. These approaches also integrate mindfulness methods as cornerstones of their interventions.

In my own quest, this meant utilizing the knowledge I acquired in Stage 1 and applying this knowledge into a conscious program of practice. It meant interrupting daily patterns of disconnection and expanding practices of connection. In practical terms, it can be understood in terms of input and output. I tried to find a balance between putting out positive and negative energy into the environment, and also between putting out too much positive energy and not putting positive energy into my body, mind, and soul. I had to practice changing patterns in every realm of my life. I began an active ritual of meditation; I gave up caffeine in order to sleep uninterrupted. I began, with my colleague, the Self-Care Exchange, a weekend retreat for professionals, at a spa. I began asking for help and support on a regular basis. I tried to change on every level: how I treated my soul, my body, my friends, my family, my colleagues, and strangers. It takes a great deal of energy to be mindful. When I lived a life that had ignored my spirit, most of my energy had been sapped. Using energy to replenish energy made more sense than using energy to deplete or to maintain the status quo.

> Performance, health, and happiness are grounded on the skillful management of energy.
>
> —JIM LOEHR (2003, P. 5)

As if I were an elite athlete, I designed a training program for myself. I had performed at intense high level for an elongated period of time without a period of true recovery. Dick Olney named his treatment model Self-Acceptance Training, "because you constantly have to be [practicing] to accept yourself, moment by moment. You can never do it once and for all" (in Moore, 1996, p. 5). I have found that training oneself to be mindful of one's spirit, in and out of therapy, is also a moment-by-moment endeavor. The Dalai Lama and many of his followers involve themselves in rigorous training to reach virtuous states of mind—compassion, tolerance, caring, and so forth—as many athletes also train rigorously, with equal time spent in recovery and in performance. I began practicing a formula of energy practice. I evaluated how much energy I used throughout the day and replenished myself energetically on a regular, frequent basis.

Engaging in training or a method of bringing about inner discipline within one's mind is the essence of spiritual life, an inner discipline that has the purpose of cultivating these positive mental states. Thus, whether one leads a spiritual life depends on whether one has been successful in bringing about that disciplined, tamed state of mind, and translating that state of mind into one's daily actions. (His Holiness the Dalai Lama & Cutler, 1998, p. 309)

In Stage 2 of treatment, we actively teach methods to discipline the mind to bring about positive mental states toward oneself and each other. It is imperative that the clinician practice his or her own discipline and communicate this value system moment by moment in the therapy room. This practice comes easily to us as family therapists. We are strength-oriented, relational, discipline-minded, solution-focused, and strategic—all the necessary concepts for spiritual practice. Another strength of family therapists is our action-oriented and involved approach with our clients. This stance allows clients to experience us as human beings and puts us in a collaborative position. Consequently, if we are involved in spiritual practice, then our clients will experience us as spiritual beings and, we hope, allow us to accompany them in their spiritual quest. In *Healing Ceremonies*, Hammerschlag and Silverman (1997) discuss the importance of genuine human contact in the process of healing: "True healing only occurs when both participants (physician and patient) are connected in pursuing the common goal of healing. This connection promotes healing and should be expressed. This partnership also works both ways and affords the physician with the opportunity to grow and to become reenergized" (p. 13). As Albert Schweitzer commented, "Patients carry their own doctor inside. They come to us not knowing that truth. We are at our best when we give the physician who resides within each patient a chance to go to work" (cited in Hammerschlag & Silverman, 1997, p. 16).

Indeed, this is Stage 2, giving that healer inside the chance to go to work. By providing the context, the supportive relationships, the mentor, and techniques, individuals, families, and groups of people can practice spiritual healing. Being the mentor for spiritual practice is an essential ingredient:

"I watched how my therapists handled everybody and everything. How they talked to the judge, how they talked to the attorneys, and how they talked to each other. They were always the same, firm but respectful. I learned a lot from watching them."

"We had some pretty good fights during therapy but I knew he [the therapist] still liked me. I guess I learned how to fight fair during those times."

"I always felt special, not like I was the favorite, but more like I was a
good person."
"Everyone I met at the Center, and I met a lot, were all good people. I really learned a lot about how to treat people from them—
particularly in group."

Teaching clients to experience liberation from negative judgment through
expressive techniques such as art, movement, poetry, music, and/or journal-
ing can help to create a sense of comfort and help them to behold the wonder of their lives. Helping them practice prayer, meditation, self-hypnosis,
and creative imagery can provide relief from their emotional, spiritual,
or physical pain. Once they experience some relief in the office, they will
desire that relief and want to practice on their own. People are involved
daily in altering their consciousness through hurtful and addictive patterns
by abusing food, alcohol, drugs, sex, and power. I want to help people alter
their consciousness in nonabusive ways. I do believe that we can become
addicted to balance in our lives. It becomes a natural form of altering our
consciousness.
    As Dick Olney pointed out,

Every time you experience liberation from your self-image you will feel a lack
of tension, a wonderful sense of open space. You can just rest in that sense of
comfort and ease. Each time you feel that way it becomes easier to recall. You
have had an experience that can give you some comfort, even when you slip
back into the bad dream. (in Moore, 1996, p. 28)

    I want to help provide our clients with relief from their traumas. Dur-
ing our interviews, over 80% of clients commented on the relief they experienced during sessions:

"I knew there would be times when we would all be fighting and hating
each other, but I could also count on the times we would remember
why we had all stayed together through all of this shit."
"Sometimes, my therapy sessions would be the only time I would feel
good all week."
"I use to feel like such a loser because of all the things I did to my wife
and kids. It was amazing the first time I ever saw the light in my
soul."
"I remember the first time I saw my evil side; I was scared but I knew
it was it. While I was doing the imagery I was aware for the first

time that I could fight him with another side of me. I remember I left the office smiling."

"I remember the first time I learned to meditate and I saw Susie; she was always the friend who could make me smile. I still bring up Susie's image while I am mediating, and it is 5 years later."

"In one session I literally felt my heart break when I was talking about the abuse; I learned an imaging exercise to put it back together. I have mended that damn thing more times than I'd like to remember."

The techniques we teach are borrowed from many practices. The clients try out different options and practice what fits them. We want our clients to feel the power of their spirit. These are people who have felt powerless, disconnected, and out of control in their lives. We want part of the treatment to enhance their sense of power: "When you believe yourself to be powerless in determining your destiny, you fail to thrive. . . . Choice is the greatest power you have. Believing you can influence your destiny makes a difference at every level of your being" (Hammerschlag & Silverman, 1997, p. 16). It is important to remember that the clients I am speaking of are all victims and/or perpetrators of trauma, many court mandated, many on probation, crossing all racial, religious, and ethnic groups and from different socioeconomic and educational backgrounds. Spirituality is universal, and it helps us be aware of our unity.

## Stage 3: Consolidation

In Stage 3 of the treatment model we consolidate changes the clients have made through the program, design relapse prevention, and ritualize their gains through ceremony and celebration. We also celebrate the relationships they have made within and outside the program.

When I refer to consolidation of my spiritual journey it is something entirely different. The journey is never-ending; it is constantly evolving. Our clients' change also continues to evolve; it does not stop once they leave therapy.

There is a form of consolidation each and every time we practice. One can end a spiritual experience with a ritual, whether that is a mindful awareness of feeling good or noticing beauty, or summarizing in our mind what opportunities are available to continue spiritual practices. Noticing these opportunities is a constant rededication to the commitment to live a moral and spiritual life.

I am constantly rededicating my professional life to finding ways to provide opportunities for spiritual growth with my clients. I agree with Hammerschlag and Silverman (1997): "People want ways to bring meaning into their lives to provide access to the world of faith and meaning. A time to experience awe. Awe helps us to find the faith to move forward. Ceremonies can help provide a way to get in touch with courage and inspiration in order to find healing" (p. 3). In the consolidation stage of working with clients' spiritual quests, we acknowledge all that we have learned about meaning. We commit ourselves to trying to use those moment-by-moment opportunities presented to us to live a moral and spiritual life. Through ritual and ceremony we rededicate ourselves to the process of this quest. We bring ceremony into the sessions. We celebrate the hard work of healing. We celebrate the existential shifts that have been made from violence to nonviolence, from victim–survivor to beyond survivor. We celebrate the behavioral changes, as well as the deep changes within each person's heart. By Stage 3 of treatment clients are committed to a way of life that integrates behaviors that lead to healing, not further suffering. Clients remembered some of their consolidating rituals:

> "During one of the last sessions we looked into a crystal ball, and everyone in our family looked [into it] for ways that we could possibly hurt each other again. Then we imagined alternatives to help each other get out of the angry places. When some of those times came up, sometimes we would start laughing because we remembered the crystal ball."
>
> "In one of the last sessions, I was about 18, and I remember imagining what it would feel like when I fell in love and was safe. I carried that image with me for almost 10 years. When it happened, I knew it, because I had felt it once before."
>
> "We always ended the group with music and a special affirmation. I started doing that with my kids, a peaceful bedtime ritual."
>
> "My parents renewed their vows after therapy ended. We took pictures. I remember feeling like I had a new beginning."
>
> "It was unbelievably sad to say good-bye. It was like leaving an entire group of best friends, but I felt free at the same time. I knew I would always be connected to them and that I could always get help when I needed it."

Lise, who had been in treatment as a teenager, wrote this poem when asked about her experience.

*My Life's Renewal*

I spun out of control
Losing sight of all hope
My family turned away
And my soul bent over in pain
Feeling neglected and betrayed
My mind overflowed with rage
My behavior became unpredictable
The ability to dream, now fictional
Saturated with anger
I put myself in danger
Behaving shamelessly
Ignoring any authority
I had collapsed
I thought no one was watching until someone caught me
They helped me to see
That I could become free
With some dedication
And spiritual application
I learned to grow
Away from the pain I had known
Able to appreciate life
With more positive insight

When I hear these lines, I know that they are about spirituality. The quest for spirituality is an ongoing process, but when you experience a spiritual moment, you have no doubt that your spirit has been touched. As the Dalai Lama affirms:

> That is what I call basic spirituality—basic human qualities of goodness, kindness, compassion, caring. Whether we are believers or nonbelievers, this kind of spirituality is essential. As long as we are human beings, as long as we are members of the human family, all of us need these basic spiritual values. We must still find a way to try to improve life for the majority of the people. Ways to help them become good human beings, moral people, without any religion. Education is crucial. Instilling in people a sense that compassion, kindness are basic good qualities. (His Holiness the Dalai Lama & Cutler, 1998, p. 307)

The spiritual quest during the trauma recovery happens in stages. First, in a safe environment, is acknowledging how the trauma has impacted your spirit, acknowledging how you have changed, and rekindling the desire to reconnect spiritually with self and other. Second is designing the personal training program that will re-create the proactive energy that lies within all of us. During this stage comes the spiritual practice that will take our personal vibrations and continue to build energy. Finally, we have the commitment to ongoing spiritual practice—commitment to continue doing something different, building on compassion, morality, and kindness toward self and humanity.

To conclude, I share this meditation with you. Our clients agree that it is helpful to punctuate endings with ritual. It can be useful to end sessions, stages of treatment, supervision sessions, or staff meetings with such a ritual. As you read each line, pause, breathe, and reflect on its meaning for you:

> May I be at peace
> May I come to know the beauty of my own true nature
> May my heart remain open
> May I be whole and healed.
> And may we all bring healing into the world for the highest good
> Whatever that may be.
>
> —Unknown

## REFERENCES

Berg, P. (1993). *Kabbalah for the layman* (Vol. 1). New York: Kabbalah Learning Center.

Figley, C. (1995). *Compassion fatigue.* New York: Brunner/Mazel.

Hammerschlag, C., & Silverman, H. (1997). *Healing ceremonies.* New York: Perigee Books.

Hirsh, R. (1994, Spring). Spirituality and the language of prayer. *The Reconstructionist*, pp. 1–6.

His Holiness the Dalai Lama, & Cutler, H. (1998). *The art of happiness.* New York: Riverhead Books.

Keen, S. (1994). *Hymns to an unknown God.* New York: Bantam Books.

Linehan, M. (1993). *Cognitive-behavioral treatment of borderline personality disorder.* New York: Guilford Press.

Moore, R. (Ed.). (1996). *Walking in beauty: A collection of psychological insights and spiritual wisdom of Dick Olney.* Mendocino, CA: DO Publishing.

Schwartz, R. C. (1995). *Internal family systems theory.* New York: Guilford Press.

Shapiro, F. (1997). *EMDR: The breakthrough "eye movement" therapy for overcoming anxiety, stress, and trauma.* New York: Basic Books.

Siegel, D. (2007). *The mindful brain.* New York: Norton.

Solomon, M., & Siegel, D. (2003). *Healing trauma.* New York: Norton.

Trepper, T., & Barrett, M. J. (1990). *Systemic treatment of incest: A clinical handbook.* Bristol, PA: Taylor & Francis.

van der Kolk, B., McFarlane, A., & Weisaeth, L. (Eds.). (1996). *Traumatic stress: The effects of overwhelming experience on mind, body, and society.* New York: Guilford Press.

Wilbur, K. (1991). *Grace and grit.* Boston: Shambhala.

## SUGGESTED READING

Das, S. (1997). *Awakening the Buddha within.* New York: Broadway Books.

Levoy, G. (1997). *Callings: Finding and following an authentic life.* New York: Three Rivers Press.

Miller, A. (1990). *Banished knowledge.* New York: Anchor Books.

Moore, T. (1994). *Soul mates.* New York: Harper Perennial Library.

Moore, T. (1996). *The education of the heart.* New York: HarperCollins.

Redfield, J. (1993). *The Celestine prophecy.* New York: Warner Books.

Staub, J. (1996). *Connecting prayer and spirituality.* Wyncote, PA: Reconstructionist Press.

Weil, A. (1997). *8 weeks to optimum health.* New York: Knopf.

Wolin, S. J., & Wolin, S. (1993). *The resilient self.* New York: Villard Books.

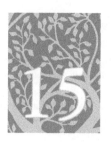

# Healing from Refugee Trauma
## *The Significance of Spiritual Beliefs,*
## *Faith Community, and Faith-Based Services*

### HUGO KAMYA

The challenges of addressing trauma among refugee populations require that all who are involved in their care gain a deeper understanding of the role of faith in refugees' healing process. This chapter explores the interface of faith-based services, pastoral counseling, and clinical practice, and suggest ways of tapping spiritual resources in therapy through linkages with faith communities, the practice of prayer, and the use of metaphors. I offer clinical illustrations from my therapeutic work with Mot, a young refugee, one of the "Lost Boys" from Sudan.

## FAITH IN THE CONTEXT OF COUNSELING
## AND THERAPY

Mental health and social service practitioners who work with refugees need to consider ways to draw upon spiritual resources in their efforts to foster healing and positive adaptation. Over the past century, spiritual matters have been seen as the province of faith-based professionals trained in pastoral care and counseling. *Pastoral care* is the "broad, inclusive ministry of mutual healing and growth within a congregation and its community through the life cycle" (Clinebell, 1984, p. 26). Pastoral care attends to the spiritual and ethical wholeness of the person, of groups, and of the wider system (Doehring, 2006). It involves helping acts directed toward healing, sustaining, guiding, and reconciling of troubled persons whose distress concerns ultimate meanings and concerns (Clebsch & Jaeckle, 1975). This care also supports individuals and communities who suffer exclusion and oppression within or outside faith structures.

*Pastoral counseling* is a faith-based clinical practice that seeks to help individuals, couples, and families in spiritual and emotional distress. It is intentionally directed toward helping people find the hope and the courage to act in behalf of their own good. For Hunter (1995), pastoral counseling is an art anchored in a field whose primary metaphors are health and healing.

Gerkin (1984), proposing a hermeneutical approach, sees pastoral counseling as the supportive and affirming presence of individuals and communities during times of crises and transitions. The pastoral counselor is both a listener to stories and a teller of stories. Such practice involves attending to each person's worldview as a living human document of pain and healing that may also illuminate the nature of religious experience. Gerkin gives special attention to the recovery of religious meaning as the central concern of such counseling. Therefore, he seeks to address the authenticity of one's worldview that must be interpreted and reinterpreted to bring about wholeness in an evolving narrative. Gerkin highlights the context of "story" when counseling the individual or working with the community. This way of approaching faith in practice has much in common with Michael White's (1995) narrative approach to therapy.

Despite the longstanding barrier between the field of mental health and pastoral care, there is growing recognition that a bridge is needed to address the psychosocial–spiritual needs of clients in therapy. I am fortunate that my own training and practice, initially in pastoral care and counseling, then in clinical social work and family therapy, have enabled me to cross this bridge and see the possibilities for bringing faith usefully into practice by therapists who have not had faith-based training.

Using faith is like what some theologians have described as a "leap into the dark." This leap in therapy with refugee populations invites clinicians to enter into what White (1995) describes as "re-membering" and "re-authoring" of lives, with compassion for refugees' suffering and conviction in their potential to overcome it and to construct meaningful lives.

There are many ways in which refugees can experience renewal and healing through involvement in faith communities, and through prayer, exploration of metaphors, ritual and hope, and the telling and retelling of their stories both in therapy and in their communities. I frame this discussion around the clinical conversations I have had in my therapeutic work with Mot.

## THE REFUGEE EXPERIENCE: THE STORY OF MOT

Mot was one of the many refugee children from Sudan who came to be known as the "Lost Boys" (a term they disliked, because they didn't think of themselves as lost). The United Nations Office of Refugees and Resettlement contracted with a church-based social service agency in Boston and agencies in other parts of the United States to provide a wide range of services for their resettlement and adjustment. This social service agency refers refugees with serious adjustment difficulties to therapists in private practice in the community, such as myself. Mot, who lives with a foster family, was referred to me for therapy because of his increasing belligerence and behavior problems at school.

The story of Mot captures the crisis of faith, God, and healing in his life. Mot is a 19-year-old young man who comes from the Sudanese Dinka tribe, and who spent days roaming the devastated war fields in southern Sudan. During that time he crossed several rivers, and several times he was chased by wild animals. He also spent days hiding from various warring groups, often without any food. He ended up crossing into northern Uganda and finally settled into the refugee camp at Kakuma in Kenya. His is a story of great pain and suffering, dotted throughout with the following questions:

"Why did this happen to me?"
"What about my brothers and sisters? What happened to them?"
"Why did the gods do this to us?"
"Why do brothers kill each other?"
"How can I forgive them as we have been taught by *Deng*?" (*Deng* is a spirit God in the indigenous spiritual tradition of the Dinka tribal group.)

These questions are essentially spiritual, as well as psychological and therapeutic challenges. They speak to important issues in the faith and self-understanding of the life of Mot and, indeed, all other refugee children who have seen and been wounded by so much evil. They question and search for answers as they attempt to make meaning of their lives. In their struggle to deal with the psychological impact of these events, they try to make sense of senseless atrocities.

In fleeing from their country, these refugees have had to overcome the trauma of war, persecution, torture, and inhumane treatment. Their sense of basic trust and security has been shattered. Their struggle also includes trying to understand themselves in the context of challenges faced by most immigrants in adaptation to a new life in a foreign land far from home (Akhtar, 1999; Coll & Magnuson, 1997; Kamya, 1997). The migration process involves multiple losses, including loss of kin and social support systems, identity, belief systems, and status (Falicov, 2002). Separated from familiar and cherished people, places, and possessions, refugees often go through prolonged transitions and must begin to build new, reconfigured identities and lives, learning new customs, language, norms, and values. Host societies present challenges of loneliness and alienation. African refugees and Muslims, in particular, often face racism and discrimination. In short, immigrants, and especially refugees, experience varying levels of physical, psychological, sociological, emotional, and spiritual/religious rootlessness.

Asylum seekers, who arrive in the United States without prior legal refugee status, must also endure many months of living in limbo and on the margins of society (Tribe, 2005). They often experience profound isolation and despair; many contemplate suicide. Unable to work legally, most pass long days and nights alone in rooming houses or homeless shelters; some are held in cells in prison-like detention centers, a terrifying and retraumatizing experience. With their immigration status unclear and precarious, asylum seekers face the threat of deportation and return to the unsafe environments, persecution, or torture they fled. Their faith beliefs and practices are all the more essential to sustain their efforts to persevere and not succumb to memories of terror, ongoing insecurity and powerlessness, or hopelessness about the future.

Refugees desperately need to tap resources that meet their ongoing spiritual needs. Falicov suggests that practitioners ought to assist them in finding faith communities that attend to their needs. Faith communities offer a sense of belonging and connection. Faith communities also provide a link and continuity to the lives of refugees and immigrants. The celebrations of rituals within these faith communities build the links or the transitions toward a sense of coherence (Falicov, 2002). Faith-based communities provide the texts and the historical contexts within which to understand the complexity of life for refugees and immigrants.

## FAITH IN ACTION

The burgeoning literature on refugees and immigrants addresses their psychological, emotional, and physical well-being. Very little, however, attends to the spiritual and/or religious dimension and the rootlessness they commonly experienced. For many, their experience of community and belonging is often best lived out in their beliefs and faith. Healing from refugee trauma involves tapping spiritual wellsprings to strengthen and rebuild this sense of community and connectedness.

My work with refugees has increased my understanding of faith's role in my interactions with them. Many of their questions underscore the importance of finding God when faced with the apparent absence of God in their lives. And, for so many, faith is tied to the communities from which they are now severed. I am becoming increasingly aware that using faith in the care of refugees is about accompanying them and listening to their stories with compassion.

## FAITH COMMUNITY AS EXTENDED FAMILY AND SPIRITUAL HOME

To define *community of faith*, one must take into account the varied meanings of community. As Whitehead and Whitehead (1993) propose, psychologically, *community* refers to a special quality of solidarity that people experience in relationships. Sociologically, it signifies a style or structure of group life. Therefore, a *community of faith* can be defined as a form or style of life characterized by a sense of solidarity, with shared values and goals. Healing or transformation, therefore, must be understood in the context of the community of faith.

A faith community can also be seen to function like an extended family for immigrants and refugees. Falicov (2002) writes about the physical and psychological extended family that immigrants experience. For most refugees, the physical extended family is distant, and loved ones may be deceased or dispersed with forced migration. Belonging to a faith community involves refugees in a new type of kinship network that provides physical, psychological, and spiritual connection; comfort; and support.

Faith communities provide practical assistance in meeting basic needs. They meet psychosocial–spiritual needs by serving as "translocal communities" (Ortner, 1997), inviting participation into a "community of mind" anchored in shared faith beliefs. When congregations reach out to refugees, it is important that they not only invite them in but also learn about and gain appreciation for their religious and cultural background. Immigrants may feel alienated from a faith community that seems too foreign to their own spiritual experience, or they may feel they must hide or deny essential aspects of their spiritual life to be accepted. For instance, many who come from African cultures combine indigenous faith beliefs and practices with

Christianity or Islam (see also Falicov, Chapter 8, this volume). When there is common ground in values and practices, with respect for differences, the faith community can become a spiritual home for immigrants and refugees and also link them with their family, cultural, and spiritual heritage.

My work with refugee youth from the Sudan has heightened my own valuing of community and its importance to their sense of belonging, connection, and courage. In turn, these attributes have helped them to make meaning and re-story their lives. I have listened to the pain and frustration as refugees' stories have opened to greater and deeper layers of connection for themselves and their families. They have talked about various communities that have brought them closer to themselves and to their own deliverance from the tragedies in their lives. Many have spoken about worship and the connection to people and rituals that their faith services have inspired in them.

In addition to encouraging participation in a faith community, clinicians can tap spiritual resources in the practice of therapy. The use of prayer and metaphor deserves attention when therapy draws on people's faith to attend to their needs. In the next sections, I will discuss prayer and metaphor in relation to my work with Mot.

## PRAYER AS A FORM OF COMMUNION AND HEALING

Across cultures and religions, most people turn to some form of prayer in the face of adversity (see Walsh, Chapter 1, this volume.) The value of prayer for health, well-being, and healing has been well documented (Dossey, 1993; Koenig, McCullough, & Larson, 2001). For refugees and immigrants, prayer is a major spiritual resource, both within communal services and in personal practice. On a number of occasions, Mot has spoken about the value of prayers and rituals in worship services in which he has participated. Raised in southern Sudan, he has taken refuge in the recitation of Christian *mantras*, or repetitive prayer and chanting, a common practice among the southern Sudanese Christians. This exercise has often created a centering practice for Mot, in which he is able to recollect himself when he is overwhelmed or flooded with painful wartime memories. He has discussed with me his ability to say certain words and phrases that he repeats to himself as a way of finding comfort, such as *waare, imani* (which translate to river, peace). His prayers have been a mix of traditional chants that call on the spirits of the air, *Deng , Dayim,* and *Mani,* who are called upon in war to defeat those "who hurt us," and the Christian vocal prayer beseeching a saving God who defeats evil. In my work with Mot, I have sought to understand with him how he uses prayer to express his faith, his work, and his life as a religious person. When Mot utters prayer, he experiences various transformations, some of which reveal new identities and life possibilities.

For Mot, prayer has carried with it a power that offers him protection from evil and misfortune. Prayer has also strengthened Mot's conviction and determination to overcome his life difficulties. At times, his prayer has also been a form of admission of his vulnerability and an assertion of some sense of control over his life. When Mot has used prayer to connect to his existence, I have also observed his wish to enter into communication with and willingness to surrender to something larger than himself. Thus, as he shares with me his use of prayer, it has become an opportunity for us to explore his growth in awareness of his own condition. It has also become a way of connecting to others, such as family members and friends, whom he cannot touch or reach at this time in his life. Mot feels their spiritual presence as he mentions them in his prayers. His prayers have been both vocal and silent. In vocal prayer, he has openly prayed for loved ones left behind or for those who have died or been killed. Remembering them in prayer has been a way of honoring them.

As well as a sense of connection, refugees also speak at times about their sense of disconnection from loved ones and from protective communities. Mot has often talked about "those people who lied to me," referring to families that took him in as he trekked south to escape the killing fields of Sudan. He recalls many occasions when people offered to take him in and others but ended up abusing them, making them do hard manual labor to earn their upkeep. He often talks about living with a sense of betrayal and with the suspicion that no one really cared. That leads him to question whether God can be completely trusted.

While prayers seeking deliverance and protection tend to preoccupy the life of refugees and immigrants who come to me, other prayers acknowledge with gratitude God's presence and role in taking away their troubles. Many refugees have talked about being created by God and owing their very existence to God. The belief in a caring and loving God often helps to sustain them in their tribulations. Therefore, it has been important to ask about their perception of God and God's willingness to step in when life becomes difficult. Such a sense of hopefulness is no more clear than in Mot's own words:

"Sometimes, we crossed the same river two or three times to escape being noticed by the enemy. We kept running. We did not know who we were running away from. We could not trust anyone. It was very scary. Some of the children belonged to the enemy, and they reported on us.

We were too scared to sleep at night. We wondered what would happen to us. We hated them and I suppose they hated us. We hoped God, who created all of us, would save us from danger. And God did!"

Aylward Shorter (1975), an anthropologist and a priest who worked in Africa, in his book *Prayer in the Religious Traditions of Africa*, notes the work of Fran Heiler, who observed prayer as a communication and as a communion of the social human relations. For Heiler, prayer is an awakening into one's consciousness. It is a dimension of life that transcends and reinterprets every social relationship and social experience. It is also seen as serving a number of social purposes, whether uttered formally or informally.

Shorter outlines 15 recurrent themes in African prayer, subsumed under four major categories: relational themes, situational themes, purposive themes, and universal themes. One relational subtheme is that of divine governance: In God's master mind, God both protects and challenges. Mot's words echo this both/and paradox, revealing a sense of despair regarding the challenges, yet also a sense of hope in God's protection and provision. In working with Mot, I have invited him to share prayers and intercessions in his own life. Listening to his prayers, I have heard some of Shorter's themes. Together, we have delved into the wishes his prayers express, the values they hold for him and the direction toward which they point. I have also wondered with him about the commitments his prayers are making in these utterances. What has become increasingly clear to us in our work together is the interconnectedness of these utterances for him with the community in his life. Some prayers have been about naming some of his fellow travelers on his escape journey in repetitive utterances. Above all, I have also begun to notice how much his current situation is related to other people in his life, the purpose and meaning in his life and, ultimately, his own commitment to greater hopes for his life.

Clinical work with refugees is about exploring ways of connecting (Kinzie, 2001). Prayers offer one important way to reconnect refugees and immigrants with loved ones left behind. Prayers invoke relational themes in which refugees and immigrants also connect with family members who have died, and with each other. Prayers are not just about intercession. They are also about honoring family members and the gifts they have given each other.

## METAPHORS AS CONDUITS OF HEALING

Metaphor is another useful tool as a spiritual resource for refugees and immigrants. Metaphor is also commonly used in faith-based community services.

Babits (2001) has described metaphor as holding "the inner edge of possibility." The use of metaphor can expand clinical possibilities. Metaphors often suggest more than one way of understanding reality. They provide new windows of understanding even as they leave a lot to interpretation. Metaphors are often alive and rich in meaning. For Babits, metaphor is "most readily associated with image . . . vision, which is our most developed sense, occupying a larger area of the cerebral cortex than any other" (p. 23).

Metaphors can be found in most faith traditions. They are also employed in different indigenous traditions. Several scriptural texts are laden with metaphoric pictures that seek to explain reality and mystery. The use of metaphors to reveal and hold complexity can be a valuable spiritual resource in therapy with refugees.

Meaning making is a crucial process for recovery and resilience, particularly in the wake of trauma and loss (Walsh, 2007). A key aspect involves efforts to gain a "sense of coherence" (2006) through new perspectives on senseless atrocities, unbearable suffering, and overwhelming struggles: to see them as comprehensible, manageable, and meaningful challenges. In clinical work with refugees, metaphors indeed can provide that "sense of coherence." Therefore, a careful exploration of metaphor is key to therapeutic work.

Metaphors also transcend polarized "either–or" choices in the lives of immigrants by offering a rich and complex way to understand the personal, family, and social transformations they experience and their capacity to find both/and solutions (Falicov, 2002, p. 2). For instance, viewing their new faith community as a "spiritual home" and "spiritual extended family" enables refugees to feel connected, without cutting off from their deep bonds with their family and culture of origin. As Falicov stresses, adaptation and well-being are fostered when immigrants and refugees can forge a bicultural identity, with roots in both worlds.

In my work with Mot, as with many other refugees and immigrants, I have used metaphor to provide a window of understanding into the plight in his life and the life journey ahead. Metaphors also offer him ways of using his faith to interpret important messages and assist him in holding on even when things seem impossible. Indeed, our work together has also been best understood through metaphor.

"A river flowing with joy" is one metaphor that Mot has used frequently to describe his wish in life. He has described many rivers he has crossed. "Most of these rivers were furiously angry at us. They swept everything that came their way. They carried off my cousin. We never saw him again. I would like to swim in a new river that flows with joy." These images speak about Mot's relationship to the ordeal he went through as he traveled to find a new home. He has often depicted his own sense of peace as "a river that flows with joy." Together we have explored this image and found ways to expand this imagery. I have asked him how the river gives to him—what soothing he feels as he imagines the river in his life. While he recognizes the turbulence that comes with the river, he also notices its calmness. Such ability to acknowledge goodness alongside tragedy has been very effective for Mot in managing moments of frustration in his life. Together we have sat with the pain of his situation and the helplessness that comes along with it. We have also been able to sit back and unpack the resilience, and the joy that comes with it. We have been able to embrace the complexity and the simplicity that this situation presents.

More recently, Mot has begun to expand the river metaphor to his ongoing life challenges. A river that flows with joy holds a sense of hope for him as he constructs a new life in the United States. When things have not gone well at his school, in his foster family, and in his community, Mot has talked about his "river letting him down" and his wish that things were better. Although he has been in the United States for 5 years now, he continues to describe his life as a "river that still flows in many different directions."

For my part in our work, I have wondered with him about other ways the river could provide more opportunities for healing. We have talked about water and its life-giving force. He has described how he walked miles in his little village to fetch water that was used in his home. He remembers how the river provided habitat for the fish that were food for his tribal group. The waters of the Nile also provided irrigation for their crops and farms.

We have also expanded the metaphor to seek new meanings of water and river in his life today. He now describes his life in the United States as a long river with "winding twists and turns." "Sometimes I like them," he says, "sometimes I hate them." Indeed, the river has become one way to unpack good days and bad days in his life.

Mot's use of metaphors is common among Africans to comprehend their world and their place in it, which are existential, spiritual matters. Many of them use figures of speech, because they speak to a core understanding unmatched in other, more concrete or factual ways of speaking. Often these figures of speech provide a window into their self-understanding and their core beliefs. Metaphors open up to greater and greater possibilities.

As Mot and others have talked with such rich imagery, I have also tapped into figures of speech that express my core beliefs, with the hope that I can connect to their core beliefs. In doing so, I have come to a happy realization that it is not just the figures of speech that matter but the very experiences that underlie them. My own life experiences and the attack on my family when I was a 10-year-old boy brought me face-to-face with a crack in the window, the result of a shot fired at my father as he escaped through the window. Over the years, what was once a literal crack became a metaphor for me. I have come to realize that what gives me hope is less about a particular figure of speech, the "crack in the window," which for me became a "ray of hope," but the events that surround that image.

As I have described elsewhere (Kamya, 2005), no event has been more hope filled for me than the crack in the window I noticed after armed men attacked our home, shooting at my father. I can vividly recall that each time I looked at that crack in the window I held some hope that my father was still alive and would return to us some day. Although it took many years for my prayers to be answered, the crack gave me a secret joy and expectation I so badly needed. It has continued to hold hope for me, both in my personal and professional life. It provides the passion to do the work and to hope against doubt, or even to carry hope for my clients who are in despair. My work with them has been one of "faithful companioning" (Schlauch, 1995) and faithful hoping as we all have sought to locate that "inner edge of possibility" within the metaphors we have consulted and, in the process, creating even more metaphors that have helped to ground us in our work.

## ACCESSING FAITH-BASED SOCIAL SERVICES

Faith-based services are provided by three types of faith-based organizations: (1) religious congregations; (2) national networks; and (3) free-standing religious organizations (Vidal, 2001). Faith-based organizations place particular emphasis on the integration or use of faith in the provision of services. Such approaches may range from the principles, philosophy, or theology that guide a belief system to the use of scriptural texts or writings that inform a particular faith.

Faith-based services are sometimes pitted against secular social services that do not claim faith as a tenet of the work they do. However, faith-based organizations in communities worldwide have deep historical roots that are closely linked to the cultural and social environment of the people. Indeed, the call to service and to care for the stranger is deeply rooted in the beliefs that condition any people's or society's effort to do justice to the less fortunate and ameliorate the most cruel aspects of the human condition.

Clinicians, including family therapists, ought to take seriously the contribution of religion in shaping these deep-rooted beliefs and the possibility that faith can transform the systems in which we live. Many refugees and immigrants are strangers in most communities. They are the outcasts, the poor, the ones in need, and often the lowly. When family therapy adopts what some liberation theologians call " a preferential treatment for the poor" or make serving the poor the hallmark of their practice, immigrants and refugees feel a sense of value and connection (Kamya & Trimble, 2002). This stance is not unlike that for social justice (see Perry & Rolland, Chapter 20, this volume). Family therapy expounds the tenets of social justice by engaging in a critical consciousness (Freire, 1973) with those who are served. Indeed, faith-based services challenge practitioners to enter into an act of love toward those they serve. Family therapy assists refugees and immigrants to name the multiple conditions of their lives, identify the limits imposed on them, and take action toward change.

## A CALL TO HOPE

The call to service is also a call to hope. Faith-based services engage this important spiritual resource for immigrants and refugees and their families. When hope is incorporated into clinical work with clients who struggle with trauma, therapists need to understand the meaning systems they bring to their self-understanding. Images of hope conjure up metaphors that can be useful in therapy. Hope can be seen as a life force that gives meaning in the face of meaninglessness. Powerful stories, folklore, gospel, music, and art are creative human efforts to translate—and transcend—past trials and traumas into meaningful experiences. Telling those stories in word, song, or picture can be evidence of both hope and change in the sense that there is striving for movement and possibility in oneself, and an effort to communicate it in a transformative way to others.

Family therapy in the context of faith evokes these images by delving into all that provides hope. In working with Mot, I find that hope is something created in relationship with something outside of ourselves (nature, supreme being or beings, people, animals, rivers, and all life). Hope also does not come from one person. It is given to another so that two or more people together create the hope between them. For Mot, this experience has been one of complex, faith-filled moments. It has been about putting together different parts of his fragmented past and gaining that sense of coherence, so he can look into a new future and his ability to author a new identity. This challenge has cast us into looking in those places where he can find solace and comfort, and find "wellsprings for healing and resilience" (Walsh, 2006; see Chapter 2, this volume).

When therapists work in the context of a faith-based philosophy or in partnership with faith-based organizations, immigrants and refugees can gain access to important resources for communal worship and programs for job training, language proficiency, and economic sufficiency. In Mot's case, the faith-based social service agency provided just that. Mot's participation in this faith-based community has helped him find different ways of connecting, all of which have brought him some degree of satisfaction in his life.

Family therapy can draw on these faith-based resources to access a community's sense of hope, its resilience, and the will to survive and strive toward a greater sense of agency.

## CONNECTION WITH ANCIENT SPIRITUAL TRADITIONS AND ANCESTORS

Therapists can also attend to resources of refugees that are rooted in the traditional beliefs of their particular group. For many African immigrants, belief in both natural and supernatural worlds is very strong. As worshipers, refugees and immigrants invoke and pray to various spiritual powers. It is important for family therapists to acknowledge that, for many, mystical powers do exist. This belief in divine and spiritual beings translates into a commitment to worship in varied forms, which can be a valuable resource as long as they sustain a sense of connection, purpose, and meaning.

Another way to reconnect immigrants and refugees to their community and loved ones is to invoke the connection to ancestors and the spirits of the dead. Among the Baganda of Uganda, the living dead, who are believed to dwell around homesteads, are considered to be benevolent spirits. These spirits are invoked in times of trouble or despair. Family therapy can explore with immigrants and refugees the stories that surround such ancestors and use them to assist clients in overcoming their troubles. Remembering them serves to reconnect and to honor all involved and to foster healing.

## FAITHFUL COMPANIONING

Kaethe Weingarten (2000) writes powerfully about our role as witnesses in the helping process and the importance of being empowered participants (see also Weingarten, Chapter 18, this volume). In my work with Mot, I have continually labored to understand the role I play with him as I witness his story of suffering and resilience. My "faithful companioning" compels me to stand in solidarity with him as he negotiates the various aspects of his life, understands his ability to survive his ordeals, and moves forward to build a new life now.

As I continue my work with him, I have come to appreciate the fact that faithful companioning must be done with great humility. I have come to a better understanding that he has more to give to this journey than I could ever offer him. Faithful companioning is accepting that Mot is inviting me into his sacred space as a witness to his journey. Mot's story can offer family therapists a valuable way to work with immigrants and refugees, and to tap the abundant spiritual resources that faith communities and faith-based services can provide.

## REFERENCES

Akhtar, S. (1999). *Immigration and identity: Turmoil, treatment and transformation.* Northvale, NJ: Jason Aronson.

Babits, M. (2001). Using therapeutic metaphor to provide a holding environment: The inner edge of possibility. *Clinical Social Work Journal, 29*(1), 21–33.

Clebsch, W., & Jaeckle, C. (1975). *Pastoral care in historical perspective.* New York: Jason Aronson.

Clinebell, H. (1984). *Basic types of pastoral care and counseling.* Nashville, TN: Abingdon Press.

Coll, C. G., & Magnuson, K. (1997). The psychological experience of immigration: A developmental perspective. In A. Booth, A. C. Crouter, & N. Landale (Eds.), *Immigration and the family: Research and policy on U.S. immigrants* (pp. 91–131). Hillsdale, NJ: Erlbaum.

Doehring, C. (2006). *The practice of pastoral care: A postmodern approach.* Louisville, KY: Westminster John Knox Press.

Dossey, D. (1993). *Healing words: The power of prayer and the practice of medicine.* New York: Harper.

Falicov, C. J. (2002). Ambiguous loss: Risk and resilience in Latino immigrant families. In M. Suarez-Orozco (Ed.), *Latinos: Remaking America.* Berkeley: University of California Press.

Freire, P. (1973). *Education for critical consciousness.* New York: Continuum.

Gerkin, C. (1984). *The living human document: Revisioning pastoral counselling in a hermeunetic mode.* Nashville: Abingdon Press.

Hunter, R. (1995). The therapeutic tradition of pastoral care and counselling. In P. D. Couture & R. J. Hunter (Eds.), *Pastoral care and social conflict* (pp. 17–31). Nashville: Abingdon Press.

Kamya, H. (1997). African immigrants in the United States: The challenge for research and practice. *Social Work, 42,* 154–165.

Kamya, H. (2005). African immigrant families. In M. McGoldrick, J. Giordano, & N. Garcia-Preto (Eds.), *Ethnicity and family therapy* (3rd ed., pp.101–116). New York: Guilford Press.

Kamya, H., & Trimble, D. (2002). Response to injury: Toward ethical construction of the other. *Journal of Systemic Therapies, 21*(3), 19–29.

Kinzie, J. D. (2001). Psychotherapy for massively traumatized refugees: The therapist variable. *American Journal of Psychotherapy, 55,* 475–490.

Koenig, H., McCullough, M. E., & Larson, D. (Eds.). (2001). *Handbook of religion and health.* New York: Oxford University Press.

Ortner, S. (1997). Fieldwork in the postcommunity. *Anthropology and Humanism, 22*(1), 61–81.

Schlauch, C. R. (1995). *Faithful companioning: How pastoral counseling heals.* Minneapolis: Fortress Press.

Shorter, A. (1975). *Prayer in the religious traditions of Africa.* Nairobi: Oxford University Press.

Tribe, R. (2005). The mental health needs of refugees and asylum seekers. *Mental Health Review, 10,* 8–15.

Vidal, A. (2001). Faith-based organizations in community development. Available at *www.huduser.org/publications/pdf/faithbased.pdf.*

Walsh, F. (2006). *Strengthening family resilience.* New York: Guilford Press.

Walsh, F. (2007). Traumatic loss and major disasters: Strengthening family and community resilience. *Family Process, 46,* 207–227.

Weingarten, K. (2000). Witness, hope and wonder. *Family Process, 39,* 389–402.

White, M. (1995). *Re-authoring lives: Interviews and essays.* Adelaide, Australia: Dulwich Centre.

Whitehead, J. D., & Whitehead, E. E. (1993). *The promise of partnership: A model for collaborative ministry.* San Francisco: Harper.

# Forgiveness and Spirituality
## *Elements of Healing in Relationships*

TERRY D. HARGRAVE
JANET FROESCHLE
YVETTE CASTILLO

"My father was a mean and cruel man. He didn't just molest me once, but on several occasions, always making me feel that it was my obligation to satisfy him and make him happy. He was never concerned about what it would do to me. It always made me feel dirty, used, and evil. There was a huge part of me that he was supposed to protect that he simply walked all over. He stole a good part of my life. How do I forgive something so evil that has caused me so much pain and grief?"

When we come to the therapeutic work with families and relationships, we are often shocked by the destructive nature and carelessness with which some members are used and injured by others. Stories like the one above from Cheryl, a 38-year-old woman and mother of three, make us as helpers cringe, and we feel the urge to shout out, "Do not forgive. Lock him away and throw away the key. He is evil." But, as is the case with many who come to us for therapeutic help, Cheryl had deeply rooted spiritual beliefs that impelled her desire to forgive her father, who had died 2 years earlier. She deeply desired to "finally set the past behind her."

Therapists and helpers may often prefer to separate life and relationships from spiritual beliefs. Yet in both therapy and spirituality, people often seek a pathway to access elements of peace, nurture, reconciliation, trustworthiness, and love. Most of the time in therapy this effort is directed toward psychological issues relating to self and relationships. Many people, however, see spirituality as having a direct impact on their beliefs and feelings about themselves, and how they behave in relationships. In short, clinicians often see clients who feel that the sense of self, relationships, and spiritual life are linked together and should be integrated.

In clinical practice we find that many people dealing with enormously painful issues carry a belief that humans are hurt by relationships and they are healed by relationships (Hargrave, 2001). The very relationships that carry the potential to injure in such heinous ways, as demonstrated earlier, also hold the potential to restore love and trust, and eventually lead to peace. This truth originally led us to think of using forgiveness as a therapeutic strategy in the late 1980s. At that time, forgiveness was only regarded as a spiritual or religious concept and found little support in the field of mental health (Hargrave, 1994). More recently, there has been a virtual explosion in the study of psychological issues and forgiveness (Sells & Hargrave, 1998). Clinicians and researchers have recognized the value and strength of spiritual resources that are available in the work of forgiveness. Our purpose in this chapter is twofold: First, we briefly touch upon some core elements of forgiveness from research and religious perspectives. Second, we present a useful relational framework and case illustrations for approaching forgiveness in clinical practice. We also discuss ethical concerns surrounding forgiveness interventions.

## THE CONCEPT AND VALUE OF FORGIVENESS

The subject of forgiveness is now well established in the psychological literature and research (Worthington, 2005). It has been consistently shown that unforgiveness increases stress in individuals, which further increases anger and hostility, and may have a negative impact on physical health (Toussaint, Williams, Musick, & Everson, 2001). Forgiveness generates positive emotions and reduces stress (Witvliet, Ludwig, & Vander Laan, 2001). Forgiveness has been shown to be effective in promoting relational repair and reconciliation in a variety of interpersonal relationships and situations involving relational transgressions (Baumeister, Stillwell, & Heatherton, 1994; Hargrave & Sells, 1997), couple problems (Fincham & Beach, 2002), personality issues that contribute to dysfunction (McCullough & Hoyt, 2002); and unresolved family-of-origin damage that causes continuing individual or relational distress (Hargrave, 1994, 2001). Forgiveness research has been applied to self-respect (Murphy, 2005); cultural contexts (Sandage & Williamson, 2005); and international relations (Staub, 2005; Cairns, Tam, Hewstone, & Niens, 2005; Hill, Exline, & Cohen, 2005). The literature clearly points to the potential of forgiveness as a powerful intervention on both interpersonal and intrapersonal levels.

Most theorists and researchers (e.g., McCullough, Pargament, & Thoresen, 2000) agree with Enright and Coyle (1998) that forgiveness should be differentiated from *pardoning* (a legal term), *excusing* (which implies that the offender had a good reason for the offense), *condoning* (which implies justification for the offense), *forgetting* (which implies that the memory of the offense has simply decayed or dropped out of conscious awareness), or *denying* (which implies an unwillingness to perceive the harmful injuries that one has suffered. Most also agree that forgiveness is distinct from *reconciliation*, which refers to restoration of the relationship. As we see below, the work of forgiveness may—or may not—include efforts toward reconciliation.

It is possible to utilize the concept and intervention of forgiveness in therapy without connection to the spiritual, but doing so is difficult for many clients. Marty (1998), for instance, recognizes that forgiveness is the central theme in Christianity. This theme concerns a break in relationship between God and humans that must be repaired by humans seeking—and God granting—forgiveness. Many religious clients hold deeply to the belief that if God grants forgiveness, then they in turn are obligated to forgive others who have caused injury in human relationships. In this manner, clients see forgiveness as not only a way to heal relationships and their own hurts but also a spiritual obligation. This is consistent with Pargament (1997), who sees spirituality as the connection with the transcendent and the application of that transcendence to everyday life. For many clients who deal with relational pain or transgressions, forgiveness is an essential element of their healthy spiritual functioning, as well as healthy living. Therefore, as Worthington (2005) cautions, clinicians should not approach forgiveness without considering their clients' religious convictions.

Researchers differ in their definitions of forgiveness. Their positions, which guide varied practice approaches, can be seen as focusing on three aspects of forgiveness in intrapersonal and interpersonal healing processes: letting go of the pain caused by the injury, as well as the desire for retribution; rebuilding the relationship (reconciliation); and bearing with the relationship.

## Letting Go

Robert Enright, a leading forgiveness researcher, conceptualizes *forgiveness* as an intrapersonal process of replacing negative cognitions and affects with positive ones that have individual benefits (e.g., Enright, Gassin, & Wu, 1992; Enright & North, 1998; Enright & Fitzgibbons, 2000). Similarly, McCullough and colleagues (e.g., McCullough, 1997; McCullough, Fincham, & Tsang, 2003; McCullough, Sandage, & Worthington, 1997) have defined *forgiveness* as essentially a redirection of negative motivations (e.g., retribution) toward reconciliation. Worthington and collaborators (e.g., Exline, Worthington, Hill, & McCullough, 2003; Worthington, 2003; Worthington & Scherer, 2004; Worthington & Wade, 1999) view forgiveness from this internal frame of changing intentions toward a person who has caused harm from negative to positive. Likewise, DiBlasio (1998) views forgiveness as decision-oriented in releasing negative emotions and intentions toward the transgressor and concentrating instead on more positive emotions and intentions. Taken together, a common thread in these definitions of forgiveness involves *letting go* of the negative emotions in response to unjust or harmful treatment, deciding not to retaliate, and shifting toward positive intentions.

## Rebuilding the Relationship

Other researchers are much more concerned with the work of forgiveness from an interpersonal perspective. Baumeister, Exline, and Sommer (1998) and Exline and Baumeister (2000) emphasize the communication and connection between the relational parties that can result from the choice of forgiveness. Likewise, in his relational view of forgiveness, Hargrave has emphasized that forgiveness is based on a process of restoring as much love or trust to a relationship as possible after long-term damage or relational transgression (Hargrave & Sells, 1997; Hargrave, 2001). In these definitions, we see the common elements of *rebuilding relationship* as the offender and the injured person(s) seek to move past the destructive way to a more positive and constructive way that communicates both love and trustworthiness.

## Bearing with the Relationship

A third aspect of forgiveness extends beyond the concepts of *letting go* and *rebuilding relationship* to a concept of *bearing with the relationship*. This is mostly a religious precept, revealed primarily through Christian scriptures.

There is an expectation that because human beings are imperfect, forgiven offenders are likely to transgress again in relationships. The wronged individual is encouraged to continue patiently in the relationship, even bearing further instances of hurt or injustice, as the transgressor grows in trustworthiness. From this perspective, forgiveness is an ongoing process over time as transgressing individuals become more responsible and reliable in relationships. Consequently, at the minimum, the wronged individual gains peace of mind from having made every effort to resolve the hurt and repair the relationship. At the maximum, the wronged person and the transgressor are able to transform the once harmful relationship to one that is loving and trustworthy.

## Practice Application

These three concepts offer a good foundation for the integration of clinical methods and spirituality concerning the work of forgiveness. Forgiveness does involve letting go. An individual who has suffered harm or injustice has a right to treat the transgressor with enmity or to retaliate. In letting go, the wronged individual relinquishes the need for revenge and works to release the negative emotions associated with the hurt. The injured person may do this work individually in therapy and may—or may not—decide to reengage the transgressor directly.

Forgiveness can also involve relational repair if the injured person decides to reengage the offender in a mutual effort to build a loving and trustworthy future relationship. This requires an effort by the transgressor to recognize and admit to the wrong or hurt, with the genuine intent to do differently in the future. The person seeking to forgive makes an effort to understand the transgressor's background, life challenges, limitations, and development, while acknowledging his or her own relational faults. In this way, identification, communication, and reconciliation of love and trust can progressively be restored to the relationship.

A third aspect of forgiveness, in some religious teachings, involves bearing with the relationship, even though there may be repeated hurtful instances as the offender is gradually learning and growing in trustworthiness. Although this concept is only mentioned in the psychological literature, it has a substantial impact on the idea of forgiveness for some religious clients.

All three aspects of forgiveness have grounding in spirituality. In some ways, the process of forgiveness can be viewed as a progressively deeper spiritual experience. At the first level of letting go, forgiveness can be viewed as primarily a personal decision that benefits the wronged individual by reducing stressful negative emotions and avoiding harmful retaliatory behaviors. For the person who forgives, letting go has psychological and physical benefits, fosters resilience in moving on with life, and promotes well-being in other relationships (Walsh, 2006). At the second level of relational repair, forgiveness involves working toward relational reconciliation. It requires not only that the wronged individual do cognitive and emotional work, but also that the relational transgressor acknowledge and repair the harmful or unjust behavior. Finally at the third level of bearing with the relationship, forgiveness involves a commitment by the wronged individual to stay connected as the transgressor learns to be fully loving and trustworthy.

These three aspects of forgiveness are linked spiritually, but relational repair requires a mutual understanding and commitment to relational change. Bearing with the relationship requires the most spiritual commitment. In this way, we view these three aspects as building on one another and offering a deeper spiritual benefit the more they are integrated. However, a caution should be underscored: Bearing with a relationship should not be encouraged in therapy if there is a risk of recurring serious harm, as in violence or sexual abuse.

Forgiveness is complicated, difficult to define, and harder still to apply. The decision to forgive at each level is highly personal and subjective, and may vary depending on the significance of the relationship, the circumstances of the injury, and the severity of harm and future risk. All of these factors need to be taken into account in any therapeutic work.

## RELIGIOUS PERSPECTIVES ON FORGIVENESS

Although people turn to religion and spirituality for varied reasons, many seek a sense of reconciliation, peace, and healing between themselves and a higher being, as well as persons in their lives. In a secular clinical setting, it is important to understand these strivings and to help religious clients apply relationship to the transcendent in a meaningful way to the significant relationships and wounding experiences in their lives.

The elements of forgiveness as outlined earlier can be found in different faith traditions. Although it is not possible to convey here the complexity and nuances in various religious approaches to forgiveness, we note a few examples in Buddhism, Judaism, Christianity, and Islam to suggest various perspectives.

## Letting Go

Within the idea of letting go is the religious admonishment not to allow the injustice, hurt, or evil of a relational transgression to spiral into retaliation, additional damage, and vicious cycles of revenge. Central in Buddhism is the core tenet of compassion (Rye et al., 2001). While not excusing a transgression, Buddhism teaches compassion for the sinner. Buddhist teachings and practices aim to reduce negative and harmful emotions (Abbotts, 2002), and to let go of resentments and hatred to cultivate emotions that have a positive effect on individuals and their relationships. In Judaism, despite the ancient biblical injunction "an eye for eye" (Exodus 21:23), Jewish teachings avow the importance of reconciliation and forgiveness in family and community relationships (see Fishbane, Chapter 9, this volume). "Do not seek vengeance or bear a grudge against one of your people, but love your neighbor as yourself" (Leviticus 19:18; New York International Bible Society, 1978).

Christianity preaches letting go of transgressions and, moreover, offers God's forgiveness (for sins) of those who forgive. "Forgive and you will be forgiven" (Luke 6:37). "Be kind and compassionate to one another, forgiving each other, just as Christ God forgave you" (Ephesians 4:32; New York International Bible Society, 1978).

Islam is a whole life system, with guidelines for individuals, families, and their social, economic, and political systems (see Wolin, Taylor, Wolin, Raganathan, Saymah, and Zeyada, Chapter 5, this volume). The Islamic family and social system does not work well if its moral system is not in place (Ali, 2008). Forgiveness is important for two reasons:

1. Those who forgive and those who seek forgiveness will be rewarded by God in the life hereafter. Seeking forgiveness is a sign of humility, and forgiving others is a sign of magnanimity: "Whoever forgives and amends, he shall have his reward from Allah; surely He does not love the unjust" (Qur'an 42:40; Shakir, 2004).
2. Seeking forgiveness and forgiving others brings happiness in this life, improves relations with people, and enhances reputation and respect. Those who desire to be forgiven for their offenses—by others and by God—must learn to forgive others.

## Relational Repair

The primary idea in relational repair is movement toward restoring and reconciling love and trustworthiness in the relationship. Buddhist teaching and practices aim not only to foster inner peace and release negative emotions (Abbotts, 2002), but also to emphasize personal responsibility to achieve loving, harmonious relationships (see Gale, Chapter 13, this volume). In Judaism, there is the concept of *teshuvah*, or return: The offender not only repents of the wrong that has been committed but also returns to a right path of good standing in the relationship (Dorff, 1998). This requires atonement and correction in future actions. In Jewish observance, on Yom Kippur, the Day of Atonement, Jews fast and gather for prayer and ritual to atone for their sins in the past year and to remember loved ones who have died. Individuals also seek out family members, friends, or others they may have offended to acknowledge their hurtful actions and to ask their forgiveness.

Christianity also teaches this element of relational restoration in the concept of forgiveness. "If your brother sins, rebuke him, and if he repents, forgive him" (Luke 6:37; New York International Bible Society, 1978). In the story of the prodigal son, the older brother who stayed with his father is aggrieved and angry when the father forgives the son who strayed (Luke 15:11–32; New York International Bible Society, 1978). Among the teachings of repentance and forgiveness of the straying son and the father is the rebuke of the older son and inability to reconcile and enjoy the fruit of forgiveness (Marty, 1998).

In Islamic teaching, the concept of *safhu* means to turn away from sin or misdeed. Repentance is a necessary step for the offender to receive forgiveness and reward by God. "Take to forgiveness and enjoin good and turn aside from the ignorant. And if a false imputation from Satan afflict you, seek refuge in Allah; surely He is Hearing, Knowing" (Qur'an 7:199–200; Shakir, 2004). If there is repentance by the offender, it will bring a better bond between the two parties. However, forgiveness does not require repentance.

### Bearing with the Relationship

This is primarily a Christian precept. Christ is said to have been sent as a reconciling agent to the people of the world, who had a broken relationship with God due to sin. He takes on the punishment for the sin of humankind by experiencing crucifixion and death; "God presented him as a sacrifice of atonement, through faith in his blood. He did this to demonstrate his justice, because in his forbearance he had left the sins committed beforehand unpunished" (Romans 3:25; New York International Bible Society, 1978). Because Christ took the punishment for all humans, people now have the responsibility to repent and reconcile their relationships with God and live at peace with him. There is a recognition that humans do not live perfectly and are in need of continuing to strive toward eventual redemption and perfection. "Bear with each other and forgive whatever grievances you may have against one another. Forgive as the Lord forgave you. And over all these virtues, put on love, which binds them all together in perfect unity" (Colossians 3:13–14; New York International Bible Society, 1978). The Christian scriptures suggest that although we may suffer pain, rejection, and hostility in bearing with relationships, it will lead to individual growth and redemption.

In Islam, the concept of *ghafara* in forgiveness conveys the idea of bearing with faults or transgressions of others (Shakir, 2004), particularly within the family, even if some members cause a lot of pain by their wrongdoing: "Behold, among your spouses and your children are enemies unto you: so beware of them! But if you pardon [their faults], and forbear, and forgive—then, behold, Allah is Forgiving, Merciful" (Qur'an 64:14; Shakir, 2004).

## CLINICAL APPROACHES TO FORGIVENESS

Even with these religious teachings, it is not easy to let go of hurt and injustice. Most people hold a deep and abiding expectation of justice in human conduct with each other. Family therapists and, in particular, contextual family therapists (Boszormenyi-Nagy & Krasner, 1986) regard justice and trustworthiness as core expectations in healthy family relationships. When there has been a serious relational violation of love and trust, such as parental abandonment or spousal infidelity, the wounded person's emotional pain and sense of injustice can prompt *destructive entitlement*, an aggressive reaction to redress justified claims (Hargrave, 1994). Angry retaliation can further complicate the relational ledger with the initial transgressor, fueling escalating cycles of anger and retaliation. Furthermore, with the tendency of individuals to play out anger, resentment, manipulation, abuse, and threats with innocent parties, such as children (Boszormenyi-Nagy & Krasner, 1986), relational injustice can spiral out of control in an escalation of destructive actions harming others (Hargrave, 2001).

It is a natural tendency not to let go of injustice or hurt, but to move toward destructive entitlement (Hargrave, 1994). Several clinicians and researchers have suggested methods that can help individuals move toward letting go. Worthington (1998) has developed a pyramid model of forgiveness. In the first step, the wronged individual recalls the hurt or transgression and moves toward recognizing and resisting natural reactions of fear, withdrawal, or retaliation. The second step is to connect empathically with the wrongdoer by assuming that there is a reasonable explanation for the transgression, considering possible reasons or motivations, and/or recalling good experiences together. As one gains understanding of the offender as a person, and if the wrong is not an all-encompassing characteristic of the relationship, there can be a shift to a more positive outlook toward the transgressor. The third step is to make an altruistic gift of forgiveness: Even though the transgressor committed the wrong act and may not be deserving of forgiveness or a second chance, the forgiver offers the opportunity for reconciliation and restoration of the transgressor. The fourth step is commitment to the forgiveness as a point of focus. The fifth step is holding on to the idea of forgiveness in future relationships (Worthington, 1998).

Enright and Coyle (1998), with a similar focus on letting go, propose a developmental model of forgiveness. Starting with an uncovering phase, the wronged party examines his or her defenses, anger, and shame, thereby increasing awareness of the offense. Next, in the decision phase, the individual sees that anger and resentment are not working, and becomes willing and committed to attempt forgiveness as an option. In the work phase, the individual works to see the wrongdoer in context, gains empathy for the offender, and offers a "moral gift" of forgiveness. Finally, in the deepening phase, the individual seeks meaning in the process of suffering and may discover new purposes and realizations because of the injury.

Both of these models focus on cognitive restructuring and approach forgiveness in stages of an individual developmental process. Although there certainly is value in these approaches, the Hargrave model (Hargrave, 1994, 2001) is more relational and is neither developmental nor stage driven.

## THE WORK OF FORGIVENESS: HARGRAVE'S RELATIONAL MODEL

In Hargrave's relational model (outlined in Figure 16.1), the work of forgiveness fits into two broad categories of salvage and restoration, each with two stations, or foci of attention. *Salvage* involves the recognition that the individual or relationship (1) may be cut off through a choice of either relational party, (2) may be unavailable because the transgressor may now be dead, or (3) may carry the risk of further harm if the parties are still unloving or untrustworthy. In these cases, it is not possible or advisable for the harmed person to reconnect or restore the relationship. In the work of *restoration*, the victim has reason to believe that the relational transgressor will be, or has potential to become, loving and trustworthy in the future. In these cases,

| The Work of Forgiveness | | | |
|---|---|---|---|
| Salvage | | Restoration | |
| Insight | Understanding | Giving the Opportunity for Compensation | Overt Forgiving |

FIGURE 16.1. Hargrave's model of the work of forgiveness.

forgiveness is pursued, albeit cautiously, through a process of interactions that lead to a loving, restored relationship (Hargrave, 2001).

## Salvage

Salvage has two stations of work that assist the victim: insight and understanding. Insight enables the victim to identify and explore the systemic interactions by which he or she was harmed and learn strategies, boundaries, and new interactions that will protect him or her in other, future relationships or even in the relationship in which the damage occurred. In this way, insight allows the victim to pursue more loving and trustworthy relationships by preventing victimizers from taking advantage of common patterns that lead to destructive interactions. In addition, it allows to the victim to see his or her own destructive tendencies and correct them to achieve more loving and trustworthy interactions (Hargrave, 1994). In short, insight is the process of learning how to protect oneself from future injury and preventing oneself from taking destructive or retaliatory actions toward others.

*Understanding* in the work of salvage enables the victim to make human identification with the offender, recognizing that, most times, victimizers are damaging others because they were victimized and harmed. This is not intended to relieve, remove, or excuse irresponsibility on the victimizer's part. Rather, it humanizes the person who offended and traces the roots of the destructive behavior. Such understanding does not alleviate the victimizer's responsibility for the offense (Hargrave, 1994). The identification instead fosters the victim's realization that it is possible to experience damage and take responsible action *not* to follow the same destructive behavior as the victimizer. This identification in the station of understanding also has the common effect of reducing the amount of emotional pain felt by the victim.

The difference between salvage and restoration is profound and is primarily understood in terms of future interaction between victim and offender. In the work of salvage, there may never be a cause or opportunity for further interaction. Moreover, many individuals may decide not to reengage in a relationship with an offender. This choice should be respected by clinicians, and the person's courageous individual work to forgive should be honored. Loving and trustworthy actions are then directed to future relationships and tend to help the victimized individual work through old hurts and potentially destructive behavior.

### Restoration

The work of *restoration* brings the victim and offender back into relationship, with the intent to correct and transform destructive patterns from the past into future loving and trustworthy actions (Hargrave, 2001). In restoration, there are two stations that help clients pursue reconciliation and forgiveness. In giving the opportunity for compensation, the victim offers the offender the chance to make amends and rebuild trust that has been violated. The victim reenters the relationship gradually, increasing involvement that provides the offender with opportunities to act in trustworthy ways. If the offender shows trustworthiness in the new relationship, then this tends to ease the victim's painful memory of the past harm. In the station of overt forgiving, victim and offender usually come face-to-face, with the intent to address destructive behaviors overtly. Through the process of agreeing upon the nature of the destructive behavior or transaction, and the offender's acceptance of responsibility for the actions, along with the expressed intent to behave differently in the future, the victim and transgressor set the groundwork for future loving and trustworthy interactions (Hargrave, 1994).

It is important to reiterate that whereas it might be beneficial for people who have experienced destructive actions to pursue forgiveness, it is not essential or even wise always to pursue the relational work of restoration (Hargrave, 2001). The individual work of salvage can provide some healing of emotional pain from recent or past offenses and also promote future loving and trustworthy actions in other relationships. When a relational victimizer has died or is inaccessible, this provides a vital pathway for the victim in letting go of past damage and living more fully in the present. When the relational victimizer is still unloving or untrustworthy, the work of forgiveness through salvage allows the victim the power to draw healthy boundaries and not be exposed to further destructive actions, and to work on relationships that have a healthy balance of giving and receiving (Hargrave, 2001). In clinical work dealing with forgiveness, this distinction between salvage and restoration is essential if the victim is to be reasonably protected from future exploitation and serious harm.

## The Value of Forgiveness through Letting Go

Worthington's pyramid model, Enright and Coyle's developmental model, and Hagrave's category of salvage in the work of forgiveness model all give common directions on how an individual can proceed in the work of letting go. First, all three perspectives direct an honest look at how the wrong occurred and its effects on the injured person. This assessment clearly moves any natural reaction to withdraw, threaten, or be destructive to a cognitive level, where the individual has the ability to decide whether he or she will act destructively. Moving the reaction to a cognitive state and toward different actions also allows the individual to consider what course his or her spiritual or religious beliefs advise in terms of retaliation, anger, or threat. As we saw earlier, most likely the religious teaching will enhance the person's tendency not to be destructive.

Second, all three practice approaches encourage some kind of identification, empathy, or compassion toward the offender. This reminds the wronged party of the wrongdoer's humanness and frailty, while also connecting to the wronged party's own past or future mistakes in relationships. In religious terms, this perspective lends itself to helping the wronged party to realize that he or she is also in need of forgiveness for transgressions in life.

Letting go is not easy or hollow work toward healing and forgiveness. It is most often a sincere process of resolving intrapersonal turmoil and preventing a natural reaction toward destructive patterns of anger and retaliation. Engaging in spiritual contemplation, acknowledging the truth of the experienced wrong, then identifying with the wrongdoer are practical ways that an individual can gain intrapersonal healing.

### Case Example of Letting Go

Julia, a mother of three teenagers, described her family of origin as "crazy." "My father was a raging alcoholic and my mother never once confronted him on anything, because she was afraid that he would leave and she would be left destitute. My brother, my sister, and I were expected to lay low and ignore everything, just like our mother. The result was we were left to fend for ourselves." Julia recognized that her brother's alcoholism, her sister's financial irresponsibility, and her own raging anger were all related to the damaging childhood they shared, and she wanted to get resolution. "I am a deeply committed Christian and I take seriously the words of Jesus that if we don't forgive, the father in heaven will not forgive us. Besides, I know that it is the right thing to do, so I don't let my past get to me and damage my kids with my anger."

The spiritual injunction to forgive others is often cited by religious clients as a reason that they must reengage a harmful relationship of the past and let go of the issues. This was the understanding of Julia when she referenced the requirement to forgive her father and mother. In this case, the therapist used a story of Jesus in Matthew 12:38 to help Julia understand the difference between salvage and restoration in the work of forgiveness. "I agree with you that Jesus was all about the work of forgiveness and reconciliation, and I also take that injunction about forgiving seriously. But I also notice that in the stories about Jesus, he didn't necessarily take part in the relationships that were exploitive or that had a destructive intent. Julia thought for a moment and said, "No, but Jesus knew that some people were not trustworthy, and he was calling them on their stuff." The therapist continued, "Then I think that there is reason to believe that you can call your parents on their stuff, too, without being fearful that you cannot let go of how they injured you."

Through the next eight sessions of therapy, Julia and the therapist discussed her father and mother, and pinpointed the emotional pain and reactions that the destructive behavior caused. Through the process, Julia began to realize that even though her parents were responsible for the pain, she was able to move on from their actions and no longer felt the need to be a victim of the past. She found that as she experienced this emotional relief, she was able to let go of her anger toward the parents, but at the same time she recognized that she did not feel the need to engage them and expose herself to the same abusive patterns. In Sessions 9–12, Julia also began to take corrective measures to deal with her obsessive thought patterns and controlling behavior, which, she began to recognize, were coping skills that she had adopted in relationships to protect herself against others causing her emotional pain. In this case, forgiveness through letting go meant clarifying that reconciliation was not necessary, and that pursuing emotional healing and better relationships with others was possible.

## Relational Repair

Although religions teach that it is good to let go of wrongs done to you and not take revenge, there is also an expectation that the wrongdoer "repent" relative to the destructive behavior and that, upon repentance, the wronged party should then engage in a restored relationship. Although both the pyramid model (Worthington, 1998) and the developmental model (Enright & Coyle, 1998) give some direction regarding the wronged party's willingness to reengage in a reconciled relationship, neither sufficiently addresses the issue of repentance on the part of the wrongdoer. In our view, relational reconciliation is not possible without some evidence that the perpetrator accepts blame and accountability for the injury caused, then demonstrates trustworthy behavior (Hargrave, 2001).

In the Hargrave model, the work of restoration begins with the focus on giving the *opportunity for compensation*. In this station, the injured person allows the offender to rebuild trust in the relationship through acting in a trustworthy fashion. The therapist facilitates an open discussion of the relational violation, so that both partners can agree to work toward an improved relationship. In the therapeutic process, the person who experienced the hurt opens up to the relationship in small interactions, which do not demand intense conversations, to see whether the wrongdoer is willing to act in a trustworthy manner. If the wrongdoer handles these small interactions appropriately, the injured person then opens up in sequentially more complex interactions. In this manner, trustworthiness is demonstrated, and forgiveness is achieved gradually (Hargrave, 1994). Repentance is demonstrated not only in the wrongdoer's acceptance of guilt and accountability but also in his or her changed behavior (Hargrave, 2001).

In the work of restoration, repentance is also a factor in the last station of *overt forgiving*. Specifically, in an overt forgiving session, there should be an acknowledgment by the wrongdoer of the action that was a relational transgression (Hargrave, 2001). In addition, the wrongdoer should agree that he or she bears responsibity for the hurt and pain (Hargrave, 1994). In both stations, the opportunity for compensation and overt forgiving, the injured person holds the choice and ability to connect and commit to the future of the relationship but is encouraged to base this decision at least in part on a demonstration that the person who caused the pain takes responsibility for the wrong, has changed his or her behavior, and intends not to hurt the relationship in a similar manner.

## Ethical Considerations and Cautions

There is value in letting go of anger and gaining a sense of intrapersonal forgiveness of the offender. But reconciliation may not be not possible, advisable, or desired in every relationship that has been damaged. Furthermore, it would be unethical for a clinician to encourage a client to reenter a dangerous or abusive relationship (Hargrave, 2001). Relational repair is dependent upon the wrongdoer's willingness to change and to practice trustworthiness.

In cases in which the wrongdoer does not "repent," or is unwilling or unable to live differently, the injured individual is unsafe and should not proceed to reconcile the relationship (Hargrave, 2001). From a religious viewpoint, we also see that in the preceding traditions teaching that forgiveness in letting go is always desirable, but that forgiveness is relational repair that is dependent upon repentance and change by the wrongdoer.

### Case Example of Relational Repair

> Roger and Karen, in their 50s, had been married for 32 years, with two adult children and a grandchild living nearby. They described their relationship as perpetually unhappy. Karen complained, "From the moment we were married it always seemed that I was way down on his priority list, and the only thing that was really important was work. I always felt I was left alone to raise the family." Roger had his share of complaints about Karen also. "There was seldom any appreciation for what I was trying to do for us financially, and she always seemed more than willing to condemn me on my shortcomings as a husband." Despite their complaints, the couple most likely would have continued in their unhappy state had it not been for the discovery of Karen's 5-year sexual affair with one of her coworkers.

In cases such as this, where there is long-term relational irresponsibility, sorting out responsibility to move toward trustworthy reconciliation is difficult. Roger first insisted, "Karen needs to be crawling back to me on her hands and knees if she ever expects me to consider taking her back." Karen retorted angrily with statements like the following: "He left me alone all those years and totally ignored our marriage. Now he wants me to come crawling back to him? He deserves exactly what I've given him." Both felt justified in a position of anger, defensiveness, and destructive actions, but both also stated privately, in separate sessions, that they were not comfortable spiritually with their actions. Roger said, "Down deep I know that had I kept my priorities focused on God and my family, it would not have come to this." Karen likewise stated, "I know that carrying on this affair goes against everything I believe is healthy and spiritually right. I know that I am just defending it because I am fighting with God."

In this case, the therapist utilized the couple's spiritual beliefs as an impetus to pursue forgiveness with God as a precursor to forgiveness in the relationship. "Since both of you at different times have expressed discomfort with your actions and your relationship with God," the therapist said, "I wonder if you would be willing to outline a way for yourselves to get back into a healthy relationship with God?" When the partners agreed, the therapist asked them to outline on paper a short talk each would have with God to reestablish the type of relationship they wanted. The therapist stated, "Remember that this is only between you and God and does not involve your relationship with each other." After the couple outlined some thoughts, the therapist then had each spouse speak out loud his or her ideas as if God were present. Although the content of the talks varied, both included elements of repentance and sorrow for what had been done and the "hurt caused" by the actions. Both also included the language of asking God to forgive destructive actions.

The therapist used this initial repentance and request for forgiveness from God to start the partners on a path of discontinuing destructive actions toward one another. "If your desire is to stay connected to God through this process, then you need to be responsible for your own behavior and what you believe God would want you to do." They greatly reduced their angry outbursts and destructive accusations and demands. Karen also decided to put an end to the affair. After three more sessions, the therapist began suggesting that the model the couple used to reestablish a relationship with God was a method that could also be effective in reestablishing a relationship with one another. Using the Hargrave model of the work of forgiveness, the therapist alternately utilized a session of overt forgiving, then rebuilding trustworthiness through giving the opportunity for compensation. For instance, in some sessions they would talk through feelings associated with particular violations involving the affair, and Karen would overtly ask for forgiveness. In other sessions, the therapist would suggest specific ways to assist Roger in rebuilding trust in Karen.

> Roger and Karen continued in therapy for 6 months. Although progress in the relationship was very slow at first, both were willing to accept responsibility for their own destructive actions that put the marriage at risk. With that acknowledgment, and their expressed willingness to work on the issues that alienated them from one another, the partners began a journey to build trust into future interactions. This process was gradual, but by the end of therapy, both partners had forgiven the past and saw their relationship as more loving and trustworthy than it had been in years.

## The Value of Forgiving in Relational Repair

In many ways, forgiving through restoration is the epitome of what forgiveness is all about. It involves at least two people (or groups) coming together after some kind of relational trauma that may be very destructive and heinous, then resolving to move past the destruction and live in loving and trustworthy ways (Hargrave, 2001). From Judaism, Christianity, and Islam, we find this consistent message that God desires a loving, trustworthy, and right relationship with humans. Buddhism teaches the necessity of letting go of anger and destructive behavior, as well as compassion for the offender, to attain peace and relational harmony. From our clinical perspective, relational repair offers practical ways to pursue both intrapersonal and interpersonal healing as love and trust are rebuilt.

## Bearing with the Relationship

The primary idea of bearing with the relationship is recognizing that even when forgiveness and reconciliation have taken place, the parties involved are imperfect and may cause each other further hurts and pain. For example, the wrongdoer could be sincere about repentance or change but because of lack of personal growth, past habits, or injuries carried from other relationships, continue to make relational mistakes that result in pain for the partner who has previously forgiven him or her. From this perspective, forgiveness may also involve a commitment to continue in the relationship in spite of the additional relational wounds. This perspective, found primarily in Christian teachings, is not found in the mental health literature on forgiveness. As clinicians, we see some value to this "bearing with" process. It gives meaning and direction to the response to relational transgressions: Both parties—and their relationship—can grow stronger and more deeply spiritual because of the experience. We want to be clear that we do not advise this if the wrongdoer continually has disregard for the person he or she is hurting and makes no effort at either repentance or change. The concept of *bearing with* means that in the normal human experience, people are imperfect and will make mistakes that cause relational hurt. When the hurt, however, is chronic, and when the wrongdoer has little regard for those he or she hurts, the relationship cannot be regarded as loving or trustworthy.

It is important for us to reiterate that the three elements of forgiveness discussed in this chapter are appropriate at different levels, depending on the significance of the relationship, the situation and context of the violation, and the severity of the harm and future risk. The work of letting go is appropriate for most relationships. The work of relational repair is appropriate for some relationships. Bearing with the relationship is perhaps appropriate for even fewer relationships. The three issues—gaining intrapersonal relief from anger and resentment, reconciling a relationship that is both loving and trustworthy, and bearing with the imperfections of a changing relationship—must be held in balance. We understand that there are potential benefits to the religious idea of bearing with the relationship, but clearly we also see that this concept cannot be used as an excuse for an individual to continue untrustworthy or unloving abuse and pain. In other words, there is a limit to an offender's mistakes, damage, and lack of growth, and to the amount that should be borne by those who forgive.

## CONCLUSION

Forgiveness is inextricably linked with spirituality, because it brings forth the fundamental values of love, compassion, reconciliation, and relationship. It promotes a sense of individual peace, as well as furthering stronger and more intimate relationships. In this chapter we have sought to show that forgiveness is a consistent idea in the teachings of Buddhism, Judaism, Christianity, and Islam, as well as a growing area of research and practice in the mental health field. Through samples of these religious ideas and psychological/relational perspectives, we have drawn out some core elements, or aspects, of forgiveness that we have titled as follows: letting go, relational repair, and bearing with the relationship. Letting go promotes an individual and relational sense of compassion, peace, and perhaps even joy. Relational repair promotes resolution, intimacy, and trustworthiness. Bearing with the relationship promotes forbearance, patience, and kindness. Work at each of these levels requires sensitivity and clarity on the clinician's part; for the client, it requires courage and fosters individual, relational, and spiritual healing and growth.

## REFERENCES

Abbotts, A. (2002). Buddhism: Tibet. In J. Bowker (Ed.), *The Cambridge illustrated history of religions* (pp. 90–93). Cambridge, UK: Cambridge University Press.

Ali, M. A. (2008). *The importance of forgiveness in Islam.* Institute of Islamic Information and Education. Retrieved August 11, 2007, from *www.iiie.net/node/52*.

Baumeister, R. F., Exline, J. J., & Sommer, K. L. (1998). The victim role, grudge theory, and two dimensions of forgiveness. In E. L. Worthington, Jr. (Ed.), *Dimensions of forgiveness: Psychological research and theological perspectives* (pp. 79–106). Philadelphia: Templeton Foundation Press.

Baumeister, R. F., Stillwell, A. M., & Heatherton, T. F. (1994). How stories make sense of personal experiences: Motives that shape autobiographical narratives. *Personality and Social Psychology Bulletin, 20,* 676–690.

Boszórmenyi-Nagy, I., & Krasner, B. (1986). *Between give and take: A clinical guide to contextual therapy.* New York: Brunner/Mazel.

Cairns, E., Tam, T., Hewstone, M., & Niens, U. (2005). Intergroup forgiveness and intergroup conflict: Northern Ireland, a case study. In E. L. Worthington, Jr. (Ed.), *Handbook of forgiveness* (pp. 461–475). New York: Routledge.

DiBlasio, F. A. (1998). The use of decision-based forgiveness intervention within intergenerational family therapy. *Journal of Family Therapy, 20,* 77–94.

Dorff. E. N. (1998). The elements of forgiveness: A Jewish approach. In E. L. Worthington, Jr. (Ed.), *Dimensions of forgiveness: Psychological research and theological perspectives* (pp. 29–55). Philadelphia: Templeton Foundation Press.

Enright, R. D., & Coyle, C. T. (1998). Researching the process model of forgiveness within psychological interventions. In E. L. Worthington, Jr. (Ed.), *Dimensions of forgiveness: Psychological research and theological perspectives* (pp. 139–161). Philadelphia: Templeton Foundation Press.

Enright, R. D., & Fitzgibbons, R. P. (2000). *Helping clients forgive: An empirical guide for resolving anger and restoring hope.* Washington, DC: American Psychological Association.

Enright, R. D., Gassin, E. A., & Wu, C. (1992). Forgiveness: A developmental view. *Journal of Moral Education, 21,* 99–114.

Enright, R. D., & North, J. (Eds.). (1998). *Exploring forgiveness.* Madison: University of Wisconsin Press.

Exline, J. J., & Baumeister, R. F. (2000). Expressing forgiveness and repentance: Benefits and barriers. In M. E. McCullough, K. I. Pargament, & C. E. Thoresen (Eds.), *Forgiveness: Theory, research, and practice* (pp. 133–155). New York: Guilford Press.

Exline, J. J., Worthington, E. L., Jr., Hill, P. C., & McCullough, M. E. (2003). Forgiveness and justice: A research agenda for social and personality psychology. *Personality and Social Psychology Review, 7,* 337–348.

Fincham, F. D., & Beach, S. R. H. (2002). Forgiveness in marriage: Implications for psychological aggression and constructive communication. *Personal Relationships, 9,* 239–251.

Hargrave, T. D. (1994). *Families and forgiveness: Healing wounds in the intergenerational family.* New York: Brunner/Mazel.

Hargrave, T. D. (2001). *Forgiving the devil: Coming to terms with damaged relationships.* Phoenix, AZ: Zeig, Tucker, & Theisen.

Hargrave, T. D., & Sells, J. N. (1997). The development of a forgiveness scale. *Journal of Marital and Family Therapy, 23,* 41–62.

Hill, P. C., Exline, J. J., & Cohen, A. B. (2005). The social psychology of justice and forgiveness in civil and organizational settings. In E. L. Worthington, Jr. (Ed.), *Handbook of forgiveness* (pp. 477–490). New York: Routledge.

Marty, M. E. (1998). The ethos of Christian forgiveness. In E. L. Worthington, Jr. (Ed.), *Dimensions of forgiveness: Psychological research and theological perspectives* (pp. 9–28). Philadelphia: Templeton Foundation Press.

McCullough, M. E. (1997). Marital forgiveness. *Marriage and Family: A Christian Journal, 1,* 77–93.

McCullough, M. E., Fincham, F. D., & Tsang, J. (2003). Forgiveness, forbearance, and time: The temporal unfolding of transgression-related interpersonal motivations. *Journal of Personality and Social Psychology, 84,* 540–557.

McCullough, M. E., & Hoyt, W. T. (2002). Transgression-related motivational dispositions: Personality substrates of forgiveness and their links to the Big Five. *Personality and Social Psychology Bulletin, 28,* 1556–1573.

McCullough, M. E., Pargament, K. I., & Thoresen, C. E. (2001). The psychology of forgiveness: History, conceptual issues, and overview. In M. E. McCullough, K. I. Pargament, & C. E. Thoreson (Eds.), *Forgiveness: Theory, research, and practice* (pp. 1–14). New York: Guilford Press.

McCullough, M. E., Sandage, S. J., & Worthington, E. L., Jr. (1997). *To forgive is human: How to put you past in the past.* Downers Grove, IL: InterVarsity Press.

Murphy, J. G. (2005). Forgiveness, self-respect, and the value of resentment. In E. L. Worthington, Jr. (Ed.), *Handbook of forgiveness* (pp. 33–40). New York: Routledge.

New York International Bible Society. (1978). *New International Version of the Holy Bible.* Grand Rapids, MI: Zondervan.

Pargament, K. I. (1997). *The psychology of religion and coping: Theory, research, practice.* New York: Guilford Press.

Rye, M. S., Pargament, K. I., Ali, M. A., Beck, G. L., Dorff, E. N., Hallisey, C., et al. (2001). Religious perspectives on forgiveness. In M. E. McCullough, K. I. Pargament, & C. E. Thoreson (Eds.), *Forgiveness: Theory, research, and practice.* New York: Guilford Press.

Sandage, S. J., & Williamson, I. (2005). Forgiveness in cultural context. In E. L. Worthington, Jr. (Ed.), *Handbook of forgiveness* (pp. 41–55). New York: Routledge.

Sells, J. N., & Hargrave, T. D. (1998). Forgiveness: A review of the theoretical and empirical literature. *Journal of Family Therapy, 20,* 21–36.

Shakir, M. H. (2004). *The Holy Qur'an.* Elmhurst, NY: Tahrike Tarsile Qur'an.

Staub, E. (2005). Constructive rather than harmful forgiveness, reconciliation, and ways to promote them after genocide and mass killing. In E. L. Worthington, Jr. (Ed.), *Handbook of forgiveness* (pp. 443–459). New York: Routledge.

Toussaint, L. L., Williams, D. R., Musick, M. A., & Everson, S. A. (2001). Forgiveness and health: Age differences in a U.S. probability sample. *Journal of Adult Development, 8,* 249–257.

Walsh, F. (2006). *Strengthening family resilience* (2nd ed.), New York: Guilford Press.

Witvliet, C. O., Ludwig, T. E., & Vander Laan, K. L. (2001). Granting forgiveness or harboring grudges: Implications for emotion, physiology, and health. *Psychological Science, 21,* 117–123.

Worthington, E. L., Jr. (1998). The pyramid model of forgiveness: Some interdisciplinary speculations about unforgiveness and the promotion of forgiveness. In E. L. Worthington, Jr. (Ed.), *Dimensions of forgiveness: Psychological research and theological perspectives* (pp. 107–137). Philadelphia: Templeton Foundation Press.

Worthington, E. L., Jr. (2003). *Forgiving and reconciling: Bridges to wholeness and hope.* Downers Grove, IL: InterVarsity Press.

Worthington, E. L., Jr. (2005). Initial questions about the art and science of forgiving. In E. L. Worthington, Jr. (Ed.), *Handbook of forgiveness* (pp. 1–13). New York: Routledge.

Worthington, E. L., Jr., & Scherer, M. (2004). Forgiveness is an emotion-focused coping strategy that can reduce health risks and promote health resilience: Theory, review, and hypotheses. *Psychology and Health, 19,* 385–405.

Worthington, E. L., Jr., & Wade, N. G. (1999). The psychology of unforgiveness and forgiveness and implications for clinical practice. *Journal of Social and Clinical Psychology 18,* 385–418.

# Opening Therapy
# to Conversations
# with a Personal God

### MELISSA ELLIOTT

There is no completely open conversational space in therapy, just as there is no completely neutral therapist. Therapist and client are always opening and closing the doors to new places together, looking for that which has not been seen, listening for that which has not been heard, negotiating together the limits and the possibilities. I want to make the therapy space open enough for the most significant conversations to be heard and understood, and for the most significant others to be included in the construction of meaning, even when that significant other may be the Other, who is known by many names, whom some call God. If discourse is, as Bakhtin (1981) says, basically political, if story is made from many voices competing for space, then power is having space in the discourse. Justice, then, is when clients can tell their stories as they experience them.

The space that this justice would create for clients to speak of their experiences with a personal God can be limited both by *proscriptive constraints*—that this God-talk is not to be spoken of here, and by *prescriptive constraints*—that God can and should be spoken of here, but only in a certain way. The secular psychotherapy culture may influence a therapist to inadvertently impose proscriptive constraints, while the religious counseling culture may influence a therapist to inadvertently impose prescriptive constraints.

This is not to say that a therapist's choice to limit spiritual talk is always inadvertent. Some therapists say that they intentionally avoid discussing any religious topics with their clients: "That is the business of the priest, not the psychotherapist." And some clients say, "I prefer to deal with God's business in God's house."

However, most therapists recognize the significance of their clients' spiritual experiences and wish their clients could talk freely about them. This has been evident in many conversations with secular psychotherapists, pastoral counselors, and the multitude of therapists who, like myself, are influenced by both these cultures. Clients and participants in our research[1] have said that they want to have the option of including their spiritual experiences in therapy, and that they feel fragmented by attempting to delegate psychological and relational issues to conversations with their therapist, and spiritual issues to conversations with their religious leader. When I practiced in Mississippi, in a culture nestled within the southern Bible Belt, this was a relevant concern for many people I worked with in therapy. Almost every person there has, has had, or feels that he or she should have a personal relationship with God. Since then I have moved from Mississippi and now practice in more diverse settings, working with people who follow different spiritual paths. I continue to learn from clients when and how to include their spirituality in our therapy (Elliott, 2007). This does not mean that most therapies, in the South or elsewhere, should address spirituality; in fact, most sessions I have conducted had no overt spiritual content. It does mean, however, that as therapists we should clear our own obstacles, so that clients sense that the path is open to speak of their spiritual lives.

The therapy stories I tell here come from clinical work I did when I lived in Mississippi. I focus here on clients speaking of their relationship with a personal God. I have written elsewhere of such conversations with African American Mississippians (Elliott Griffith & Griffith, 1997) and with people of other faith traditions (Griffith & Elliott Griffith, 2002), conversations in which awareness of my ignorance afforded me appropriate humility and openness. The following vignettes are intentionally drawn from therapies with White Protestant Christians. This focus is founded in my desire to be open to surprise in the place where it is most difficult to open my eyes, within my home culture and my own tradition.

## THE ENTRAPMENT OF KNOWING

I first met Susan and her mother in my role as family therapy consultant to a panic disorders treatment program. Two years after this treatment, Susan returned, saying, "I'm in trouble again. I didn't want to go back to the panic disorders specialist, because he would not ever meet with me and my mama, but I knew that you would. I guess he thought I was too old for that, but what he doesn't understand is that Mama is the best support that I have, the only one who really knows. Anyway, I get the feeling he thinks I should see less of my mama, not more. But my getting well matters almost as much to Mama as it does to me."

Susan did not want to lock her mother out at a time like this, and why should she have to? As I listened to her I began to privately simmer with indignation. I could say that the steam of my indignation rose from my commitment to systemic family therapy or to the notion that it is the client's privilege to bring whom she wants to her therapy. But honestly, the fire that made my pot boil was my own experience in mothering and dealing with "experts." I was thinking, "Where does this guy get off, deciding that Susan is overdependent and that her mother would be bad for her? How can he assume that only he knows best about who should be involved in her treatment? Susan and her mother solved many problems before he came along. Good for her that she has decided to lose the expert and keep working on this with her mother!"

Susan interrupted my thoughts: "I brought you something." She pulled a book from her purse. The title was something like *The Christian Answer to Anxiety*. I squirmed, not wanting to dishonor Susan, but also not wanting our therapy to be programmed by ideas I might find hard to swallow.

"So when I realized that I could not go to the specialist, I started reading this wonderful book that Mama got for me. I read and I prayed, and I decided to come to you. I don't know if you will agree with this man's methods, but he has some good, sound Christian ideas. If I'm going to get over this, I will need all the support I can get—Mama, you, and God."

I hesitated, fearing I could not satisfy Susan and remain true to myself. Then the perfect solution occurred to me. I could refer her to a reputable, local seminary-based family counseling program that I believed would parallel the ideas of her book. "I don't know that I could learn and employ his methods, but since you find this book to be so valuable, may I connect you with a counselor who might have more expertise with this approach?"

"No, I don't want to do that. In fact, I called the author of this book in Oregon and asked him what I should do. He told me to come back to see you, because I said I was comfortable with you. He even said that we didn't have to use his methods, that we could just take what we want to use and leave the rest. I'm pretty sure that we can work it out. I just know that I need to depend upon the Lord, and that I can't do it alone."

Susan was asking me to include her God, not to obey this author. She just wanted me to be interested. This was really not so different than Susan asking the panic disorder specialist to include her mother. It made sense. So what had made hesitate? It was the same kind of knee-jerk thinking, I am embarrassed to say, that gave the specialist pause. When I saw the book title, I thought I *knew* about the God to whom she related. I *knew* that this was going to be an authoritative, inflexible God who would require not only Susan but also myself to be unquestioning and submissive to his authority. Because of what I thought I knew, I almost lost this opportunity to work with Susan, her mother, and her God, who actually turned out to be concerned, calming, and one whose quiet, gentle voice she could hear the most clearly, calling her to self-acceptance and health.

This and many other cases repeatedly teach me that if "I think I know" the basic story of someone's experience with God, I am probably beginning to close off therapeutic possibilities. I then risk joining those forces of cultural oppression that would instruct and censor what might be spoken. Resistance to these forces is possible only to the extent that I can discover and depart from my own certainties.

I am interested in the never-ending process of discovering "stories of certainty" that lure me into "already knowingness," away from curiosity and creativity. I want to open these certainties to the refreshing breezes of wonder, in which multiple realities can coexist and relationships can evolve. Both clinical work and research work (Tingle et al., 1993) have helped me to move from certainty to curiosity. I have discovered some of the "stories of certainty" that intrude upon, oppress, and constrain the possibilities for conversations with God in therapy. Surely, readers will see certainties I continue to employ that I am unable to see. Or perhaps the reader may discover certainties of his or her own.

## FROM CERTAINTY TO WONDER

I offer some "certainties" that I have recognized in my work, then I offer ways to open them to curiosity.

### Certainty 1: I know what God is like for you, because I know your religious denomination.

When Southerners meet one another for the first time, denominational affiliations may well be part of our initial exchange of information. Knowing this classification cues us into the worship style and behavioral code of that group. It tells us how to be hospitable. For instance, because I know that the Southern Baptist[2] denomination traditionally opposes alcohol, if my guest said she was a Southern Baptist, I would offer her a cup of coffee. If she said she was an Episcopalian, I would offer her a glass of wine. Of course, it could be that the Episcopalian was a member of Alcoholics Anonymous and that the Southern Baptist would quite like a glass of wine, but a curious outsider would be more likely to ask about this than would a fellow Southerner. And in so doing that outsider might be a more hospitable host than I.

Likewise, we are cued into images of what God is like for different denominational groups. The fellow Southerner might imagine the God of the Southern Baptist to be a close but strict father, and might imagine the God of the Episcopalian to be a remote, more lenient parent. These assumptions are often as faulty as the one about who would enjoy that glass of wine, and these assumptions render our therapy conversations less hospitable.

Our research (Tingle et al., 1993) has borne out the fallacies of these kinds of assumptions. For example, there was no correlation between measures of religious fundamentalism and the extent to which the God portrayed by an individual showed qualities of acceptance or flexibility. Denominational group beliefs, and even individually stated beliefs, were often poor predictors of a person's experience of God. Many clinical experiences have confirmed this for me. The most memorable, perhaps because he was one of the first people to challenge my assumptions, was Thomas.

When I first met Thomas, I feared his religious doctrine might never allow him to feel forgiveness. As he told me his story, I found myself wishing he were an Episcopalian, so that he might have a lenient God—but he wasn't. He was a loyal member of a conservative religious denomination. Members of his group believe in sanctification and obedience to a strict moral code. They are known to be as clean and honest in appearance as in behavior. Thomas said that he felt unclean because of an affair with a married woman. He had ended the relationship, but his longings and fantasies persisted. His secrecy about it had separated him from his faith community and from his God. According to his stated belief, he could not approach God until he was clean because "God cannot look upon sin." Yet he could not change his ways without God's help.

"I am in quicksand," he said, "and I did this to myself. There were warning signs all around—DANGER, DO NOT ENTER—but I went into the swamp anyway, willfully. Now I am stuck in the quicksand. The more I try to get out by my own efforts, the deeper I get. It is a toxic place, too poisonous for any person to enter, and too filthy for the Lord to even look on." We talked about his dilemma from many perspectives, all along wondering what his Lord's perspective might be. Actually, he said, he knew the Lord would rescue him. He had before. It's just that he had seen such disappointment and weariness in the Lord's face. Thomas couldn't ask him to make the sacrifice of coming to this vile place to save him. For several weeks thereafter neither he nor I could see a way for him to be true to his beliefs and to escape from this bind, and the bind continued to isolate and depress him.

Then one day Thomas entered my office, visibly lighter. He described an experience "like a very real daydream." In truth, Thomas's vision was as surprising to me as it was to him. He said he saw the Lord walking toward him, past the danger signs, walking boldly into the swamp, into the muddy, smelly quicksand. The Lord bent down and lifted him up, carrying him in his arms to a cool, clear stream. He dipped him and cleansed him, then carried him out, with words of comfort, not of reproof.

"And what of the mud and the filth in that place?" I asked. "Did the Lord walk through it with disgust or did he walk above it, untouched by it?"

Thomas paused to reflect. "He was in the midst of it, not above it. But it didn't seem to be a problem. I couldn't see him react to it at all, because his eyes were on me."

"And did he look disappointed and weary?" I asked.

"No, he honestly just looked peaceful, genuinely happy to find me and to cleanse me and to give me rest."

The wonderful surprise to Thomas was not that his Lord would help in time of need but that his Lord would walk through the filth without disgust. With this new knowledge, he could reconnect with members of his faith community. He started by forming one new friendship there that was dominated neither by a need to confess nor a need to hide. Later he informed me about many trusting friendships made possible because of his felt knowledge of the grace of his Lord. What I learned from Thomas was wonderful for me also. It enabled me to connect more creatively with other persons from conservative denominations, to be ready for surprise.

## Certainty 2: I know what God is like for you, because I know what your language about God means.

As people gather in churches to worship, they speak together the words of a liturgy, the common words that bind them together. In unison the congregation utters, "Our Father who art in Heaven," to begin the Lord's Prayer. When individuals of this congregation are asked what God is like, several might say, "like a kind heavenly father," and the inquirer may conclude that the congregation members have very similar experiences of God.

Our research conversations suggest, however, that these phrases are more like a door, and although the doors to people's hearts may look the same, the insides are wonderfully different. In the first segment of the research project, participants reviewed a list of different descriptions of God (masculine, feminine, harsh, kind) and selected one that fit their experience. Almost all participants circled "God is like a kind father." In the second and third parts of the project, in the interviews about their actual experiences of God, they conveyed a wide range of images and spoke with new words. The research question that brought forth those varied images is forever in my front file as a therapy question. It reliably moves me away from certainty and toward curiosity: "In those moments when God is most real to you, when you know you are with God, what do you hear or see or feel that tells you what God is like?" Here are some of the responses:

"Like a warm cocoon, enclosing me as the world falls in around me."

"Like an exasperated mother whom I have disappointed and been ungrateful to too often."

"Like an Olympic coach who does not model my task for me, but delights in my potential and pushes me to it."

"Like a nourishing, flowing river that comes to me, the parched dry riverbed, and gives me life."

"Like a strict old grandfather, angry with my continual wrongdoing, who has finally turned his back on me."

"Like the silence in a deep, waterless cavern, where I finally arrive after swimming down through a troubled lake."

"Like a nursing mama who is happy to be close to me and always has plenty of milk. As I lay my head on her breast, I feel her breathing and hear her heartbeat, and I am calmed."

When asked, "What human relationship in your life most reminds you of the one you have described with God?," some research participants who had begun with a description of a kind, fatherly God did indeed recall their own kind fathers or grandfathers. Others who related to a kind, fatherly God associated him with their human relationships with women:

"My mother, who kept calm and kept things in perspective."

"Our housekeeper, who taught me about love that lasted through hard situations."

"My grandmama, who always had a lap available."

"My women friends who are closer than family, who confront me, encourage me, and support me no matter what."

"My other mama, my Irish Catholic neighbor lady, who always had
room at her table for one more, whose house was liberatingly messy
and filled with laughter, and who, when she gave of herself, became
more, not less, herself."

The research project suggested, and my clinical experience confirms,
that no language that therapists can employ—certainly including the word
*God*—is free from oppressive connotations. One participant, Priscilla, said,
"I don't use the word God when I can avoid it. That's the word I used for
the old 'Thou-shalt-not' God who stifled me for so many years. That word
almost makes me sit up straight at attention, be careful, not talk, and *certainly* not laugh. That word has nothing to do with the Spirit I know now,
the Spirit inside me and surrounding me, who invites me to open, to love,
to create, and to laugh."

"But," she smiled, "if you really need me to, I'll say *God* with you.
Just remember that it's shorthand, not the real thing." I was struck by her
words and in this slow and careful research conversation I stayed close to the
language she preferred. I'm sure, though, that in speaking of spirituality,
as well as other areas, I still sometimes impoverish therapy conversations
by unwittingly accepting, or inadvertently asking, that a client use "shorthand."

I could not ever have known what the word *God* was like for Priscilla,
nor can I know what any word means for another by knowing its dictionary
definition, or even its common cultural usage. Language, as the hermeneutic
philosophers have taught, is a way of being present with another person, a
way of touching the other (Heidegger, 1971; Gadamer, 1976). To Priscilla,
to say the word *God* was to touch her with a hard, cold thing, but to learn
and to say her words—*Spirit* and *Light*—was to touch her with a strong surrounding goodness; for her, "the real thing."

### Certainty 3: I know what God is like for you, because your image of God is a reflection of your early attachment figures.

My introduction to the psychological study of the development of the image
of God was the writings of an object relations theorist (Rizzuto, 1979). She
proposed that a child synthesizes parts of parental images to create their
experiential God image. But one need not read object relations theory to
learn this idea. In many churches, fathers are admonished with the warning
that they serve as their children's first models of God. Furthermore, one can
theorize that this image, especially if it is a shaming one, may be held and
interacted with so privately that it becomes reified and stabilized. These

theories could guide the therapist to a story of certainty, wherein the character of a person's God cannot transcend its resemblance to the character of the person's parents.

To counter this certainty I look not to the stability of the God image and the theories that explain it, but rather to the transformations, differences, and unique outcomes that could never be predicted by these theories. These latter elements deconstruct my certainty, and questions based on these elements free me to be curious.

Carol came to therapy for help with extreme anxiety symptoms. She was a brave and determined woman, working three jobs to support herself and her daughter. I often privately doubted that I could offer her anything in an hour that would be more helpful than the nap she sorely needed. "Must you work this hard? Could family or maybe bank loans help?" I asked.

"No," she replied, "there is no help, and, yes, I am physically exhausted, but I can handle it."

As we talked more it seemed that this philosophy had served her well through a difficult life. Her inner talk seemed to go something like: "This is tough, but I'm tough too, and I can handle it"; or, "If I *can* handle it, then I *should* handle it."

I asked whether, given a choice, this was a philosophy she would select to guide her life and work. Carol thought she would prefer in the future to ask herself, "Am I comfortable with this?" and "Is it worth my time and effort?" She anticipated this to be a difficult change because she received so much praise for her stamina. I began to inquire about her imaginal dialogues (Watkins, 1986). Who might encourage her to seek a more comfortable life, and who might bind her more to the "If I can, then I should handle it" lifestyle? As Carol reflected on these questions, I asked where God might be in this debate. I knew Carol to be a spiritual person who was a sensitive, comfort-giving woman to her daughter and friends. I expected her to say that God would want her to stop suffering and to have rest and comfort.

Her reply jolted me: "Well, this must be how God wants it, or he would change it. He would get some money to me, but obviously he doesn't want it to be any easier for now."

"So he wants it this way?" I asked.

"Yes, I think he could change it. I see him somehow getting money to my friends. But there are no family checks coming to me. There is no letup. I am suffering, and so is my daughter. It's like he's saying, 'I know you can work very hard, harder than most people, so I know you can do this.'"

I asked, "What is it like to hear these words from God? Do you tell him you're suffering?"

"It's lonely," she said. "I don't feel very close to him. I don't tell him anything. I'm not even sure he hears me."

"What do you sense from him, as he urges you to work hard? A tone of voice, a face, a posture? Could you show me?"

"I can't see his face, because his face is turned away. I can only see the side of it, like this," Carol demonstrated, standing erect, embodying a stone-faced God with arms crossed, head turned away.

"What does that face mean?" I wondered with her.

"I'm not sure—either anger or disappointment. He doesn't tell me what it means, but it feels awful to me."

We paused. I asked, "Has there been a human relationship in which you had this feeling of a face turned away, when you didn't know what it meant, but it felt awful to you?"

Her gaze drifted away. "Well, maybe with my grandfather. He was strict and very religious, but he was really good to me in lots of ways, the steadiest person in my life. I hated when he was angry with my cousins, though. He wouldn't say he was angry. He would just ignore them, not acknowledge them. Sometimes he would have gifts for the rest of us but not for the ones he disapproved of. That was awful."

I did not say a word. In a flash, Carol was aware of the parallels. "Wow," she said, "that's pretty similar. I mean, intellectually, I believe this is not all there is to God, but that's sure how he is for me right now, way out there, not very concerned about me, but he has gifts for those others."

At this point I could have asked Carol what she believed, what she knew intellectually that was different than her experience, but she had already said she *knew* this did not tell the whole story of God. Still, this was her experience. I was interested not so much in what she knew but in how she had come to know that "this is not all there is to God." As with any relationship, one could assume that Carol's experiences with God were broader and more varied than could be captured by any single story, including the one about her grandfather. I wanted to know not about similarities to the grandfather story, which seemed to be so limiting, but about times when Carol's experiences with God were unlike those with her grandfather.

So I asked, "Carol, has there ever been a time when you experienced God being with you in a different kind of way, a time when God surprised you?"

"Oh, yes, I can remember a time very clearly years ago. It was after I had stopped drinking, not long after I became a Christian. I was facing so much, sinking deep into depression, without the relief I once had from getting drunk. One night I decided I had to go drink. I couldn't take feeling this bad anymore. I got dressed to go. I knew that the Lord would be disapproving of me, maybe angry with me for doing this wrong thing, so I didn't want to think about him. But I sat down before I left and turned, and there was Jesus sitting beside me . . . weeping . . . not weeping in a way to make me feel guilty . . . just sad for me, deeply sad that I was about to do something to hurt myself and that I was hurting. He just didn't want me to hurt. It was like he took my hands and we wept together. I didn't need to go drink then. In fact, it was then that I first was able to ask for help for the depression and got some therapy, which did help."

I wondered aloud what was possible in the presence of the Jesus who wept with her that was not possible in the presence of the God who turned his face away. I also asked her, "If Jesus were here with you now, weeping, knowing your suffering, how would he talk with you about your life, your hurting now?"

"I'm not sure," she spoke quietly, "but it's enough just to have him near now. I haven't felt that presence in a long time."

Carol's quiet tone and her clarity that this presence was "enough" led us into some moments of silence. Whether my questions were answered, whether I learned about her experience of this presence was unimportant and would have been intrusive. What I did learn from this prompts my practice now. Whether a person's description of God is generous or stingy, kind or cruel, like or unlike early attachment figures, I always ask, "Is there any other way you have experienced God, any way that surprised you?" Almost always there is. If the person would like to be more with God in this way, this then can become a point of curiosity, a time to delight in, to historicize, and to expand this alternative and desired story (White & Epston, 1989).

It is still quite useful to hear the stories that people relate about similarities between experiences with God and experiences with early attachment figures. But if such a story is unwelcome, it can become less constraining when it is known to be only one of many stories of the person's relationship with God.

## Certainty 4: I know what God is like, and you need to know God as I do.

All of the stories I have written here end with a person describing an encounter with a loving and accepting God, a God of grace. I remember these stories because I love them.

I must then always ask myself whether I am imposing rather than co-creating these endings. I hope not, for a God of grace imposed is still imposed. I learned this many years ago from Mary.

Mary was in serious danger of death from self-starvation, entrapped in a vicious binge–purge cycle. She knew that she needed inpatient treatment but refused to consider it—not because she didn't want it, but because she felt she didn't deserve it, and that she didn't deserve to upset and worry and cost her parents more than she already had.

Mary mentioned that she had attended a church that was known for its acceptance, although she had always sat in the back row. I hoped that going to that church might show her a God who deemed her acceptable and worthy of living.

I asked, "Do you ever talk with God about your dilemma about going to treatment?"

"Of course not. It's no use."

"Why? What would happen if you did?"

"God," she said with a bitter tone of sarcasm, "isn't talking to me these days."

I asked her if she could show me what that was like. She showed me Mary, seated on the floor, head down, eyes looking down, and God, high up and far away, back turned completely to her, speaking these words grimly: "I have given you chances to change before, and you have failed. You have been selfish and stubborn. I have tried and tried to help you, but I have grown tired of you. You don't really want to get well, and you have used up your chances with me." God never flinched, never considered turning to look at her.

Mary stopped me short when I began to inquire whether she had any different experiences of God. She was very sure of how God was now. Previous experiences were rendered irrelevant. She had become unlovable and unbearable. She had worn God out, and he had given up on her.

The disgust and rejection Mary described from God horrified me. I felt my body stiffen and recoil. I could not let her go on. I interrupted her: "No, Mary, that's not God! I know it's not! Don't you see?"

Mary turned me off with a bored, cold stare and left the room. I don't know if she said with her eyes or her lips, "I didn't come here for preaching," but I knew I had betrayed her and had been untrue to what I had promised the therapy would be about.

In sessions after that I listened and tried to understand. We didn't stop talking about God, but our talk changed. With genuine curiosity I asked Mary what it was like sitting in the back row of her church, listening to others describe a God who would always forgive, yet finding for herself a God who had become fed up and turned his back on her. "It's like a thick piece of Plexiglas is between me and the rest of the church, not soundproof but feeling-proof glass. It gets thicker every week."

Then, one day she came into our appointment with light in her face. "I'm ready to go inpatient. I need to take care of myself. I want to live. Lots of other people want me to live, too. Even God wants me to live."

I was thrilled but flummoxed. "What happened? How can this be?"

"On the elevator coming up here, I ran into a little girl. Well, she's a big girl now . . . but she was little when I took care of her. I used to babysit her every day. I was so surprised to see her. It's been years."

"And what did she say?"

"Nothing, really. She just hugged me. She was so happy to see me! She loved me. She always loved me. Then, on the elevator, I suddenly realized that I was lovable. Somehow, I knew God loved me too and that I must get well."

Mary did get well. I'm not sure how to understand the role of the therapy as a part of it all, but she told me it helped her "get ready." What helped, she said, was that I did not get scared and did not try to take charge of her life. Mary didn't remember how close I came to trying that, but I do remember. If my anxious knowingness had charged me to persist in preaching—whether subtly or blatantly—my own God, I believe Mary might have left the therapy, if not physically, by the door, then psychologically, by false acquiescence.

It would not be true to my values to write only about Mary here, to omit my own context that gives birth to, delights in, and struggles with all this. For me, this work cannot be only therapy. It must be congruently connected with my own experience with God. When I hear descriptions that I feel could not possibly be God, I want to defend and correct, just as I would if I heard someone misunderstand and malign my sister. I would have to defend her—to say, "No, you're wrong. She's not like that. She's kind and good." So will I not do for God as much as I would do for my sister?

No. While my sister may need my defense, and I need to protect our relationship by defending her, the God I know neither needs my defense nor my limiting descriptions. When I assume a defensive, knowing stance about this with a person in therapy, I diminish the possibilities for that person's intimacy with his or her God, as well as our intimacy in the therapy.

## CONCLUSION

Undoubtedly, I will again become seduced into certainties. I will attempt more to provide than to co-create the meaning of a person's experience with God. The hope is that it is in the very acknowledgment of these breaches and their repair that intimate interaction can occur (Weingarten,

1992). Indeed, after I wrote this chapter I offered my telling of their stories back to "Thomas," "Priscilla," "Carol," and "Mary" for their repair and revision. Each of them gave me a new way of seeing the story, an expanded understanding of their evolving relationship with God, and of the part our therapy and research conversations played in that evolution. Each of these people has changed me, not only in how I see therapy but also in how I see God.

It is in the context of these intimate interactions that a person continues to co-create an evolving story with God that is uniquely his or her own. Such a story cannot be dominated by my story. My listening cannot limit it to a chronicle of psychological development, the elaboration of religious teaching, or the constraints of culture and language. Though these other stories may compete for space in the discourse and may influence the evolving narrative, primacy must be given to how the individual describes his or her experiences. It must be given to the words and the meanings the person teaches us, to the possibilities and surprises we encounter together.

My tradition says, "The Holy One's name is Surprise." If one is too certain of one's specifications of God, one will miss God. A rabbi told me that the Israelites could not wholly name God. They said *Yahweh*, which meant "I am who I am, and I will be who I will be." Movement and mystery. Still, just as I sometimes get peace confused with safety,[3] I get faith confused with certainty. I do believe, though, that to search for the one is to lose the other.

## APPENDIX

The purpose of the Conversations with God Research Project, in the Department of Psychiatry at the University of Mississippi School of Medicine, was to study characteristics of intrapersonal dialogues with a personal God to suggest how they could best be employed as a resource in individual and family therapies. Thirty-two volunteers, each of whom considered his or her relationship with God to be a vital relationship, participated as research subjects. First, participants supplied self-report data on theological orientation, degree of fundamentalism, personality characteristics, characteristics of family of origin, and characteristics of self–God relationship. Second, in a videotaped psychodramatic role play, participants enacted a situation in which the presence of God was intensely experienced. Third, participants were interviewed as to whether the God they portrayed in the interview (the expressions, metaphors, posture, and stance) reminded them of any person in their life.

We analyzed the videotapes utilizing Structural Analysis of Social Behavior, a coding system for interpersonal communications. The preliminary findings were as follows:

1. All expressed images of God contained both maternal and paternal characteristics, with descriptions of God by persons who identified themselves as fundamentalists being the more paternal.

2. Fundamentalists and nonfundamentalists did not differ on measures of authoritarianism, self-esteem, locus-of-control, social support, or family environment scales, except that nonfundamentalists showed greater family participation in active recreational activities.

3. Although nearly all participants consistently referred to God as "He," about half associated specific attributes of God to particular memories of a mother or grandmother.

4. Most participants showed an evolution of relationship between self and their personal God that occurred primarily in adult life through discontinuous, transformational changes prompted by major losses and crises. This shift in relationship typically was a movement away from an emotionally distant or controlling self–God relationship that strongly resembled the childhood relationship with one or both parents to an intensely affiliative, intimate self–God relationship relatively free of dimensions of control and lacking characteristics of the early life relationship with parental figures (Griffith et al., 1992; Tingle et al., 1993).

Though the research participants were all either Protestant or Catholic Christians, the multiethnic research team included persons of Hindu, Greek Orthodox, Protestant, and Catholic traditions. Team members were Alexis Polles, Jeanetta Rains, Carol Tingle, Dinesh Mittal, Nancy Krejmas, James L. Griffith, and myself.

## ACKNOWLEDGMENTS

This chapter is a revision of an article first written for the *Journal of Feminist Family Therapy* [7(1/2), 123–142 (1995)] and copublished in K. Weingarten, Ed., *Cultural Resistance: Challenging Beliefs about Men, Women, and Therapy* (pp. 123–142, Binghamton, NY: Haworth Press).

I am indebted to the individuals who allowed me to share their stories, first in therapy and again in writing this article. I am grateful to my colleagues; to Kaethe Weingarten for helping me to reflect on this work as resistance to cultural oppression and for first encouraging me to write about it; to James L. Griffith for collaborating in further development of these ideas (Griffith & Elliott Griffith, 2002); and to Froma Walsh for including my voice in the rich and diverse chorus of contributors she has gathered for this book. I am especially grateful to Van Elliott Griffith for clarification and careful editing.


## NOTES

1. The Conversations with a Personal God Research Project was conducted in the Department of Psychiatry at the University of Mississippi School of Medicine. Researchers studied characteristics of intrapersonal dialogues with a personal God to learn how these dialogues could best be employed as a resource in individual and family therapies.
2. I hope these stereotyping views do not offend. I decided to choose the Episcopalians and the Southern Baptists because I have been a member of each of these groups. I have and still do benefit from both of these faith communities.
3. Dietrich Bonhoeffer (executed at Flossenburg Concentration Camp in 1945) was a pastor who stood firmly in resistance to Hitler. Addressing the Christian churches in Germany, he implored them to realize that the quest for their personal safety was counter to the quest for peace. He warned that the actions that might ensure their safety would be the very actions that would destroy God's peace; for God's peace could only come with justice (Glazener, 1992).


## REFERENCES

Bakhtin, M. M. (1981). *The dialogic imagination* (M. Holquist, Ed.). Austin: University of Texas Press.

Elliott, M. (2007, August). *Encountering the sacred in the clinical encounter.* Presidential Address, Division of Family Psychology, 115th Annual Convention of the American Psychological Association, San Francisco, CA.

Elliott Griffith, M., & Griffith, J. L. (1997). Coming to peace: Dialogues on survival, suffering, and death. In B. Doherty, S. McDaniel, & J. Hepworth (Eds.), *The shared experience of illness.* New York: Basic Books.

Gadamer, H. G. (1976). *Philosophical hermeneutics.* Berkeley: University of California Press.

Glazener, M. (1992). *The cup of wrath: The story of Dietrich Bonhoeffer's resistance to Hitler.* Savannah, GA: Beil.

Griffith, J. L., & Elliott Griffith, M. (2002). *Encountering the sacred in psychotherapy: How to talk with people about their spiritual lives.* New York: Guilford Press.

Griffith, J. L., Elliott Griffith, M., Rains, J., Tingle, C., Krejmas, N., Mittal, D., et al. (1992, November). *Quality of relationship between self and a personal God: Its narrative history and relationship to individual and family variables.* Paper presented at the American Family Therapy Academy/George Washington University Research Conference at Captiva Island, FL.

Heidegger, M. (1971). *On the way to language.* New York: Harper & Row.

Rizzuto, A. M. (1979). *The birth of the living God.* Chicago: University of Chicago Press.

Tingle, C. V., Griffith, J. L., Elliott Griffith, M., Rains, J., Mittal, D., & Krejmas, N. (1993, May). *God–person relationships: Their character and relation to individual and family system variables.* Paper presented at the 146th Annual Meeting of the American Psychiatric Association, San Francisco, CA.

Watkins, M. (1986). *Invisible guests: The development of imaginal dialogues.* Hillsdale, NJ: Erlbaum.

Weingarten, K. (1992). A consideration of intimate and nonintimate interactions in therapy. *Family Process, 31,* 45–59.

White, M., & Epston, D. (1989). *Literate means to therapeutic ends.* Adelaide, South Australia: Dulwich Centre.

# Stretching to Meet What's Given
## Opportunities for a Spiritual Practice

### KAETHE WEINGARTEN

Listening began the original version of this chapter: worry that readers would not listen carefully to me and memories of how I had to learn to listen well myself. Listening dominated my thinking about a spiritual practice of therapy 10 years ago, when I wrote that chapter, just as hope dominates it now. I suspect an intersection of life cycle and life events can account for the shift.

In Part I of this chapter, I present a shortened version of the original chapter in the first edition of this volume. Part II is a current update. The two are linked by tone and my willingness to reveal the narrowest places to show how I have tried to create more space, for myself and for others. Indeed, stretching to meet what's given.

### PART I

*Listening*

My mother was diagnosed with a terminal cancer in 1974. We were told, but she was not, that she had only a year to live. The challenge for me was how to stay in intimate connection when the ground for it—"truth"—seemed pulled from underneath us by her doctor and my father who, in those years, was willing to adhere to whatever their experienced and wise physician told him was the right course. I learned during this time of the mutability of truth, of the wonders of listening empty of preconceptions, expert knowledges, and facts. I learned that listening this way opens me to reverence and awe, such that they form a conversational net, a matrix within which talk of pain and joy, grief and grind can proceed with some ease. Listening this way provides comfort.

Comfort, care, connection, commitment, and compassion. These are a few of the words in my spiritual lexicon. Listening and love. These are a few of the practices I embrace in my clinical work. I am willing to face anguish and joy with others. This, to me, is the heart of a spiritual practice.

I did listen my heart out when my mother was dying. It started the very evening I learned that she might die soon, soon enough so that she would never become an old lady and I would never sit on a porch with her, looking over at her protectively, asking her if she needed a cup of tea or a shawl to keep her warm. On the bus ride to the hospital that winter evening after my shattered father had told me—"It's everywhere. Go. I can't go. You go. Don't tell her. Say nothing. She expects to see you. Go."—I repeated the same question to myself over and over. How can I lie to my mother? Only days later did my thinking become more nuanced and the questions I posed more textured. What if my father can't bear to talk with my mother about her dying and she is alone with her fears? What if we disagree as a family about what should be done, about what is right? Only years later, in my theoretical work, did I pose the question: What if voice is dependent on audience (Weingarten, 1997)? What if a person can only speak what she believes others can bear to hear?

I didn't have to lie to my mother that night. She was groggy and in pain. She dozed, I sat dazed. I suppose I did start to listen in a new way that night. I listened to her breathing. I listened to my breathing. I noticed that when I breathed along with my mother's breath, my breath settled and, for a moment, I was less afraid. This was a clue.

My mother survived for 2½ years. My family lied to her for one of those years. During the year I was not supposed to tell her the "truth," I learned to listen. I banished what I thought I knew about her tumor and her lifespan in order to be fully present without hypocrisy to what she had to tell me. My few "facts"—that no one with her tumor had survived longer than a year, that they had *not* gotten it all—faded in importance compared to the rich tapestry my mother wanted to discuss. I entered her territory and navigated with her map. This way of listening, antithetical to most of my professional training that encouraged *me* to be the expert, created my mother as the expert on her life and her dying. My "knowledge," besides being wrong, was a distraction. I was full of feeling about the "when," the time frame, which I thought I knew. Had we focused on "when," we would have lost the opportunities in the now to be together much more.

And there were many opportunities. Certainly, imminent loss contextualized much of our time together. But loss was the background, and pleasure in each other's company was the foreground. The kind of listening I learned to do helped make this possible for me. This listening allowed me to still my own thoughts in order to hear my mother's. This kind of listening brought me in touch with a spacious calm I could tap for myself and offer to others. It helped me ride the swells of pain and loss, grief and rage, sorrow and joy, that, eventually, taught me patience. Any down would rise up. There was always a metaphorical shore. I came to believe this. These are beliefs that are now stitched into the fabric of my awareness, and they inform my spiritual practice.

I would not wish the death of a loved one on anyone, although death will come to everyone, but I also know that the hours spent loving and listening to my mother, opening myself to sorrow and finding connection in loss, have stood me in better stead as a clinician and a person in the world than any professional training I have ever had.

### Fear

Both of my children were born with birth defects. My older child Ben had a ventricular septal defect that closed when he was 2 years old, was heard again when he was 12, and closed again when he was 14 years of age. Although the first year of adjusting to my worries about him were difficult, I know from my experiences with our daughter Miranda that I didn't really know the taste of fear.

Miranda was born 8 minutes after noon on the eighth day of the month—auspicious numbers. During the hours before we learned that Miranda had a rare genetic disorder from which she might die, I talked to family and friends, describing our new baby as beautiful and adorable, as any new mother would, and remarking on three features that later would become the cornerstones of a medical diagnosis. I went on and on about these features, never once imagining that my rapturous descriptions of these three observed phenomena would be redescribed by a medical language that would transform these already-beloved features from sources of joy to sources of worry.

Four hours after her birth, the pediatrician who had been present at her delivery nervously walked into the hospital room and, with photocopies of three articles in his hand about her genetic disorder, informed us that our daughter had been transferred to the special care nursery. They were uncertain that she would be able to feed and, he cautioned us, she might not live.

My husband Hilary and I wept, and, as has become the pattern of our lives, we quickly made a plan. Still loopy from the postcesarean anesthesia, I worked the phones. Hilary went directly to the nursery, where he spent the next 12 hours rocking Miranda, singing to her, and working with her and a bottle until he could report to me and the staff that she was an avid, agile nurser. These hours were decisive in setting our course with Miranda, a course in which we scrutinized carefully every bit of professional knowledge, trusting only those who, like we, observed Miranda herself with exquisite care. We learned to value what narrative therapists call "local knowledge" (White & Epston, citing Foucault, 1989). I began to trust our experience of our daughter over the doctors' pessimistic assessments of her. I learned to distinguish partial observations from ones that seemed to match our more in-depth knowledge of her. We came to value experience-near wisdom (White, citing Geertz, 1998): our own, and those who worked closely with us and with Miranda.

The first 6 years of Miranda's life taught me a great deal about the vicissitudes of fear. I could chart the differences between mind-numbing panic, acute terror, and chronic, corrosive fear. Fear made me heavy; the object of that fear, Miranda herself, made me light. Being with her was like the meditation practice I learned later. It forced attention to the present, to the now, where teaching, laughing, cajoling, and shepherding were as necessary as tending and ministering. It taught me to release vigilance in her presence, and it taught me humility about what I could not do.

In high school, I read all I could of the poet John Keats, including commentaries and biographies. I circled around his letter on negative capability, intuiting that I would find it apt for years to come. In this letter he writes, "*Negative Capability*, that is when man [*sic*] is capable of being in uncertainties, Mysteries, doubts, without any irritable reaching after fact & reason" (Bate, 1963, p. 249). Being with Miranda exercised my negative capability; it stretched me to live with uncertainties. This is something I can now do and, at my best, I can do so without "irritable reaching." This quality, too, is part of my spiritual practice.

### White Chocolate

Listening to others without my own agenda, opening myself to intense emotion, learning how to be still in the presence of uncertainty without any irritable reaching, riding out the turns of fear, and showing up in the present have all been lessons learned from life that I use daily in my clinical practice. They are what I bring to my relationships with clients that create, I believe, a sense of spaciousness for others. In my office there is world enough and time. I, at least, have a sense of the sacred. I feel my breathing slow, my focus heighten, and an immense respect for the people who gift me with opportunities for transformative conversation. This is what I mean by a spiritual practice.

Slowing down, moving to the heart of the matter is what I do for myself, for my family, and for my clients. I needed to do this one June day in 1991. Miranda was 12.

*. . . I am taking Miranda, age 12, to the dentist where she will learn whether or not she needs braces. When we go home, she must grab something quickly for dinner because she has her school's Spring concert this evening. The dentist seats us in an alcove and begins to tell her his conclusions. I observe that on the front of her chart, as we have requested, are the words, in capitals, "DO NOT DISCUSS GENETIC DISORDER WITH CHILD." The dentist begins. "On a scale from 1 to 10, your mouth is an 11," he says. "You have the worst alignment of your teeth that it is possible to have and you will most certainly need braces." Miranda is stunned. "But I brush my teeth every day," she asserts, irrelevant to the situation, but an act of resistance nonetheless to this brutal, totalizing presentation of an opinion. "Why?" she asks. "Because of your disorder," he tells her. "Your lower jaw has grown disproportionately, and this is just one of the consequences." I am gesticulating wildly and then, not caring if I am rude, I stand up and tell the dentist we will discuss this at another time.*

*By the time we reach the sidewalk of the large, urban street we are on, Miranda is howling in rage and distress. She is running down the street, with no regard for the heavy rush hour traffic alongside us. I run after her, pulling her writhing body to mine, holding her tightly in an embrace. She is pouring out questions. "Why did he say that to me? What is happening to my body? Is something bad happening to it all over? Is there more I don't know?" And much more.*

*"Look," I say to her. "This sucks. What he did to you was wrong and it's a big problem. Your disorder is a big problem, too. But we can't do anything about either of them right now. You have 1 hour to get to your concert. I know that's important to you. Your job now is to figure out what you know about yourself that will help you pull yourself together so you can do the concert. What will work? What will help?"*

*With some hesitation, and with her eyes doing a quick movement, suggesting that an interior search is taking place, she says, "White chocolate. White chocolate will help."*

*We search. We find. In the store, well-brought up as she is, she takes one large bar of white chocolate. "No," I say, as I take the bar from her hand and put it back on the shelf. "You have a job here, too. You have to figure out how many bars of white chocolate this event has been. How many bars of white chocolate do you need now and for later to manage what's just happened?"*

Five times she reached for the large, paper-wrapped bars of white chocolate. Each time, she paused and contemplated, assessing, I imagine, the damage to her and the need for repair.

Today, I regard white chocolate as her sacrament. The image of her removing the bars is continually present for me, confirming my belief that in times of trouble, with love and support, people can access what sustains them and it can make a difference. Believing this in the face of unrelenting trouble—events and feelings that press on persons beyond what it would seem the spirit can bear—is a hard-won spin-off of my own efforts to keep faith with the possible. It allows me to feel certain that if I ask, "Is there something that provides solace that is available now?" then the direction of this inquiry, and the conviction I bring to the questioning, will construct the possibility and the actuality of solace for those in the heart of pain. This is a belief I have practiced in my own life. It is one of the ways my struggles have stretched me.

## Aloneness

I have asked myself the question I asked Miranda many times, perhaps most memorably one dark night in December 1988, several days after learning I would need chemotherapy and radiation to treat a newly diagnosed breast cancer. "What can you access now that is already available to you that will staunch this pain?" I answered, "Spirituality." I then asked myself this: "What do you understand about your spirituality? What will make it present for you now?"

My answer did not surprise me. Connection. I did not invoke a connection to a God who might comfort and accompany me. Instead, I turned to people I knew, and to some I did not know. I called people and wrote them; people called and wrote me back. I asked certain people to be my witnesses. Everyone I asked agreed to do so. A man who owned a bed-and-breakfast at which I had stayed recently, once informed, sent me a poem every week. Tom Andersen sent me a picture of a mountaintop that I keep in my glove compartment to this day. Friends gave me amulets and healing stones.

These connections were sustaining. They sustained hope and they provided comfort. The relational matrix within which I did the rituals of daily life and ceremonial life mostly held terror at bay.

Mostly. Nights, connection dissolved and I faced what cancer's bottom line is for me: You die alone. Alone. For a person who has devoted herself to the care of others and for whom intimacy has been a passion, the idea of death/disconnection is intolerable.

I panicked. I obsessed. I railed against it. I also practiced meditation, breathing, and mindfulness. I exercised daily. I took hot baths. I struggled and I gradually came to live with the idea of aloneness, both my own everyday aloneness and my own Ultimate Aloneness. I confronted aloneness in the context of my own mortality. I tried to fight it and found that I could not. I didn't accept it either. I learned that I would have to live with it and manage it somehow.

From this struggle, I learned what many of my clients come into therapy already knowing: There is a darkness that no love will ease. I am able to sit with them, in the void that this knowledge illuminates, and talk about what can coexist with—not ease—the void. For me, connection remains the answer. I value connection, although I know that I will not always have it. Stretching to face the inevitability of my death, not just once, but recurringly, forced a relationship to aloneness. Tending to this relationship is part of my spiritual practice.

## Intimacy and Collaboration

For all of Miranda's life, my skills as a psychologist, child therapist, and family therapist have been invaluable. I have used what I have learned not from an expert position but from a side-by-side position, trying to make my skills visible to her, so that they would transfer more quickly and easily. From the beginning, my immersion in a strength-based, nonpathologizing theoretical model stood us all in good stead. Believing that through the alchemy of love and listening, pain can transform itself into resilience, I never feared that her multiple hospitalizations, procedures, or chronic discomfort would diminish her.

In 1993, when Miranda was 14, her disorder shifted from an intermittent to a steady presence in her life. She entered a phase of constant pain. Plagued by loose connective tissue, including that of the blood vessels, she would have sudden dislocations of her joints, and fainting. At age 17, Miranda dislocated both of her shoulders so severely that they couldn't be repositioned. For treatment, she was encased in a metal and plastic brace from her pelvis to her neck, with her arms kept rigidly in place by steel supports from shoulder to fingertips. She required 24-hour face-to-face care. Offered a home tutor, she insisted that she would go to school. Despite excruciating pain, despite an inability to read because the muscle relaxants and pain killers she took affected her eye muscles as well, despite having to have a personal care attendant with her at all times, Miranda went to school every day for the 6½ weeks of this ordeal. She told us: "The only way to change people's attitudes to disabled people is to expose them to us."

Concurrently, at the time that this happened to Miranda, I was working with a middle-aged woman who had become suicidal again. This time, she was able to ask for help, and I told her that far from finding her phone calls intrusive, I saw them as evidence that she believed she was worthy of care and support, two experiences that had been lacking in her bleak and damaging childhood. These phone calls, in my view, were evidence that what she desired—comfort—was not only possible but also that she already had the ability to secure it for herself.

My client, I call her L, described herself as living under a "blanket of pain." I was able to reach her there. Having spoken to her about this chapter, I knew that she would say that a sense of possibility was present in our work together. She would also say that the space between us often felt intimate. In articles I have written about intimacy (Weingarten, 1991, 1992), I propose making a distinction between intimate interaction, in which meaning is co-created or shared, and nonintimate interaction, in which meaning is rejected, provided, or misunderstood. I suggest that intimate interaction between clients and therapists is therapeutic and that nonintimate interaction rarely is. However, I make clear that in the inevitable lapses of intimate interaction that occur between therapists and clients, there is an opportunity for profoundly meaningful collaboration.

A therapist who has a child with a serious medical condition that flares up erratically cannot always be available to clients. Intimate interaction at the level of conversation may be present, but it is always likely that an appointment will have to be canceled at the last moment. A conscientious person, disciplined and reliable to a fault, I struggled with this: how to care for clients when Miranda needed my attention urgently and immediately.

Interruptions were particularly difficult for L during this time. I wanted to respond openheartedly to her phone calls, but caring for Miranda eventually made me realize this would not be possible. Knowing that the cost to myself was too great, that the calls were not pro forma but hard-won efforts to reach out for comfort from a desperate woman who needed my concentrated presence which I could not give, I scheduled a session with L and her husband to tell them I could no longer take her calls, framed so positively in our work together, and that I could only meet with L for our regularly scheduled appointments.

The session was difficult. Having slept very little in the previous 2½ weeks, miserable that I could not provide what my client needed and deserved, I was nonetheless clear that I had reached my limit. I explained briefly what had happened to Miranda and her requirements now for round-the-clock care. I explained that I would still meet with L, but I could no longer return her phone calls.

In this session, I acted on my belief that the process of being included in meaning making—that is, the sharing of meaning that creates intimate interaction—is a process that can contain terrible pain and unhappiness. It was not "natural" for me to share my daughter's troubles, but it seemed clinically necessary to create the conditions for L to manage the loss of our phone contact. I trusted that by being included in my process, she would feel respected and valued at the level of our relationship, even though, at the level of my behavior, I was setting a limit on my contact with her.

That session was a turning point. It has also taught me about the sturdiness of the human soul and the will to feel strong and whole. Rather than feeling that I had abandoned her for Miranda, L felt that I cared deeply for them both. Identifying herself along with Miranda as a person I was intent on helping, L released herself to have empathy for herself, as well as my daughter. I have L's permission to reproduce excerpts from a letter she wrote Miranda hours after our session.

> Dear Brave Fighter:
>
> This is for you and for me. It's a pep talk from a moment of calm to remind the courageous one inside that pain, suffering, and despair pass. . . . We will survive it. And make meaning of it. It will be the texture and richness of that which fuels our passions. Our goals are made of this stuff, the stuff of surviving and surpassing.

I read the letter to Miranda and called L to let her know my daughter's reactions. Miranda was touched that compassion for her had triggered L's compassion for herself. It confirmed her worldview that one person's suffering can have value to others. It made her feel useful not helpless. I felt awe that a circle of caring had created such a positive effect all around.

As for L, there have been struggles since, but she has never lost her compassionate connection to herself. She is working on making self-care and self-empathy steadfast companions. A few months later, L wrote me a letter describing vividly her view of that time. The following is an excerpt:

> . . . For me to be in so much pain and hear you say you felt concerned about my needs in the face of your own need to be less available because of Miranda's situation made me feel at once understood (you got where I was at) and respected (you shared significant personal material) and concerned (because it brought me out of my pain and into my caring place). Knowing the seriousness of the situation and feeling great empathy for you and Miranda, I felt

a yearning to respond. The parallel of seeing myself and Miranda as both suffering from uninvited troubles created movement. In empathy for her, my self-empathy expanded. . . . That you as therapist centralized all this pain and in setting boundaries for managing it (availability to me, taking care of yourself, responding to your daughter) created some kind of opportunity for us all. When I wrote my letter to Miranda it was from a place of identification and deep caring of her (as another suffering person, as a child of someone I care deeply about) and of caring for myself too. It was a mutual pep talk. In talking to her, I could hear myself and really take it in.

## Conclusion

These continue to be core elements of my spiritual practice: listening without my own agenda; opening myself to sorrow; finding connection in loss; attending to the present; resting within uncertainties; accepting fear; tending my relationship to aloneness; believing that there is always something that can be sustaining; working for a preferred identity; and relating intimately and collaboratively.

Each element has a tale attached, fragments of which have made their way into this chapter. Each one is a lesson I have taken from life experiences that I would never have wished on myself, but from which I have become the person I am. Lessons like these accrue. They start off like drips of water during a spring thaw after a heavy snowfall, relentless and steady. And they create a substantial runoff, a flow.

So too my lessons have started from single moments of pain and worry and have gained mass and meaning. There have been no sudden blinding revelations when I knew what to do and knew what was "right." Rather, I suffered a long time and then gradually, because I was desperate to turn sorrow into sense, I gathered ideas that sustained.

I hope that my story—a story of suffering and sustaining practice—will be of some help to others. If it is, meaning will have sprung from sorrow.

## PART II

Reading this chapter 10 years after I first wrote it has been a powerful experience. I am now older than my mother when she was first diagnosed with cancer, and my children are older than I was at that time. I myself have had cancer three times and survived, so far, for 18 years. I have been sick for two-thirds of my children's lives; for many of my clients, I have always been a therapist who has had cancer. L, who is no longer my client, is thriving. We sat together recently at a film event I moderated.

When I contemplate what to add to this chapter, whose points I heart-ily endorse, I would say that two concepts that I referred to casually in Part I, witnessing and hope, have become the center of my professional and personal life. I have written about both at length elsewhere (Weingarten, 2003, 2004a, 2004b, 2005a, 2005b, 2005c, 2007), but I wish to include them in this chapter, which may be as close as I ever come to a spiritual autobiography. I will no doubt write about hope and witnessing differently here, because the entry point I have chosen for each idea in this chapter—listening, fear, white chocolate, aloneness, intimacy and collaboration—is so deeply, nakedly personal.

In fairness, the reader should know that I am suffering from a grave, incurable but not fatal lung infection at this moment. I have been on intra-venous antibiotics every few hours for the last 5 months, and this has taken a toll on me. I am exhausted. I have had to jettison most of my professional work—although I work about 10 hours a week, teaching, supervising, and seeing clients—so that I can administer the infusions and manage my own case. I spend time wrangling with systems to get the care I need, not writing about the meanings I can extrapolate from my experience. I do so here for the first time. As ever, I wish that there were other domains of my life about which I could write: Joy would be nice.

Still, I remain "upbeat," as one of my stable of doctors recently described me; I think I can explain why. I am *doing hope* with others, as I have come to understand and disseminate this interpretation of it. I do hope in so many ways, big and small, that my life is an annotation of the concept as I con-ceptualize it.

I think of hope as a verb, not a noun. It is something we do. Of course, hope may be a feeling, but I am concerned mainly with the practice of hope. In any case, I believe that feeling follows action. The practice of hope provides a profound spiritual satisfaction, almost contentment. It connects one to the webs of meaning and relationship that make life purposeful and meaningful. It gives one something to do.

But what we do depends on our position in relation to hope. Those who are hopeless and those who witness their despair have different tasks. Some people, some groups of people, some nations even, lack and need hope; others, with hope intact or untested, are witnesses. For however long these circumstances obtain, they position us differently and call for different actions.

*Hopeless, we must resist isolation. As witnesses to despair, we must refuse indif-ference.* Neither is easy.

Those who are hopeless must resist the temptation to withdraw from others. *The task is to resist isolation.*

## Witnessing

The task of witnesses is a related one. In the face of calamities and tragedies that happen over and over again, in our homes and on our planet, we must reject indifference. Indifference exerts a persuasive pull, roping us in by our feeling first inadequate, then overwhelmed. Recognizing these seductions is the first step of *refusing indifference.*

For most of my life, I have chosen to be a witness to despair. I started on this path as a child, before I fully understood the implications of my choice. It looked like I was an empathic child, but it was more than that.

James Hatley (2000, pp. 3, 5) writes of the witness in a way that I find rich and compelling.

> By witness is meant a mode of responding to the other's plight that . . . becomes an ethical involvement. One must not only utter a truth about the victim but also remain true to her or him. In this latter mode of response, one is summoned to attentiveness, which is to say, to a heartfelt concern for and acknowledgment of the gravity of violence directed toward particular others. In this attentiveness, the wounding of the other is registered in the first place not as an objective fact but as a subjective blow, a persecution, a trauma. . . . We find that our witness of the other who suffers is itself suffered. But this suffering is not one of empathy, which is to say a suffering that would find in its own discomfort a comparison to what the victim has suffered. . . . We suffer, so to speak, the impossibility of suffering the other's suffering.

I chose to enter the phenomenal world of the other and I intuited the distinction made by Hatley about the "impossibility of suffering the other's suffering." As a child, perceptive enough to grasp this, but too naive to appreciate its inevitability, the impossibility made me sad. Yet I stayed loyal to my awareness that I could never truly know what the other suffered, try as I might. Later, this insight inspired my developing a typology of witnessing positions, believing that witnessing, like hope, is done from different positions, not one.

The four witness positions of my typology arise from the intersection of two dimensions: awareness and empowerment (see Figure 18.1). Position 1 occurs when one is an aware and empowered witness to violence or violation. Taking action, and clarity about what actions to take, goes along with the experience of this witness position. A person is likely to feel competent and effective in position 1; it is definitely the position for which I strive. Position

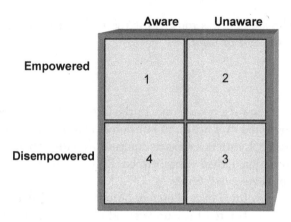

**FIGURE 18.1.** Witness positions. From Weingarten (2000). Reprinted with permission from Wiley–Blackwell.

2 may be the position that is most dangerous to others. People who witness violence and violation, who are clueless about its significance or implications but nonetheless respond as if they know what they are doing, will be misguided. Their actions will be ineffective at best and harmful at worst. The negative impact of witnessing from this position may be far-reaching, particularly if the person witnessing occupies a position of power or is perceived as having power. Position 3 warrants a certain amount of pathos, except that the effects on others, not just the self, are so disastrous. If one is unaware and disempowered, the potential for being nonprotective when one should be protective and passive when one should be active is so great as to make it a near certainty. A professional who is unaware of and, thus, passive in relation to the urgent need of a client has abandoned that client. This abandonment may be a form of malpractice, as harmful as the misguided efforts stemming from actions taken from position 2. Position 4, alas, is the one I most often hear described. In this position, a person is aware but uncertain what to do or lacks the resources to act exactly as he or she knows to do. With regard to illness, the domain in which I so often find myself a witness to others and to myself, awareness conjoined with helplessness is all too familiar and devoutly to be resisted. Mounting resistance to the feelings of helplessness that so often accompany illness has been a life's work for me.

In 2003, diagnosed with cancer for the third time, I had to summon the energy to resist again. Due to a surgical complication, my wound would not heal; I had to change dressings every 20 minutes. I was unable to continue working and even had to cancel a tour for my latest book, *Common Shock:*

*Witnessing Violence Every Day: How We Are Harmed, How We Can Heal.* I was unmoored from the daily challenges that make my life feel purposeful.

On December 1, International AIDS Day, I was in the audience for a Grand Rounds I was supposed to have helped prepare, but had not. Part of my work involves consulting to colleagues in South Africa who are deeply involved with the AIDS pandemic. I had hoped to contribute some insights from their work to this Grand Rounds, but I had not been able to pursue this plan. Listening to the talks, connecting to the immensity of the problem, and noticing my upsurge of gratitude toward my South African colleagues, I had an epiphany. True, my work was lying in the bowels of a hospital getting zapped by electron particles. But, strapped to the table, as stripped down as one can get, I still had something to offer others: those very same particles that were entering my body and, I hope, giving me a chance for a long and productive life. How different from the people my South African colleagues were helping, who weren't being given state-of-the-art treatment. I saw a path toward action.

After radiation that day, my eighth session, I sent off e-mails to four of my closest South African colleagues.

> As you know I am undertaking radiation treatment. While there are discomforts, I am mindful of how fortunate I am to be able to receive treatment. I am dedicating my next session to the four of you for all that you do for those who suffer with AIDS and for those families, caretakers, and communities that suffer as well. In deep gratitude for all that you do.

Sending off the e-mail, I felt back in my life for the first time in months. A few hours later, I devised a plan. Each day I would dedicate my radiation treatment to people or a cause whose work in relation to violence I wished to honor. I hoped that the knowledge that someone cared enough about the work they were doing to dedicate their treatment to them would encourage them in the daily challenges they faced.

For the remaining 25 days of my treatment I researched people and organizations to whom I would write letters, and worked on how those letters could truly witness their work. I labored over each letter, explaining why their work moved me to link them to my daily work of being radiated. I wrote to the Medical Foundation for the Care of Victims of Torture, the Mandela Foundation, and a reporter based in Iraq. I sent the letters off with no expectation that I would hear back, although I did hear—and was touched when I did—from over half of my dedicatees. Writing the letters helped me to focus on one aspect of global violence each day and to believe that I was making a positive contribution. Dedicating my treatments made the radiation sessions themselves tolerable. I was doing my work, on and off the table, by transforming my private pain into an opportunity to recognize others' efforts to transform violence. In focusing so intently on the people, organizations, and causes I had chosen to honor, I felt connected to them, defeating the feeling of isolation that grinds down people living with cancer.

Months after treatment ended, I turned my private experience of treatment dedication into the Treatment Dedication Project (*www.witnessingproject.org/treatded.html*). I wrote two guides, one for those undergoing treatment and the other for those who wish to facilitate the dedications. Many people who receive treatment for cancer would love to do something like this, but they do not have the energy or focus to take it on themselves. Although I believe I would have had a keen interest myself 18 years ago, my first time around, I doubt I would have had the time or personal resources to do it alone, while I was managing work and caring for two young children. With help, I might have been able to dedicate my treatments.

### Hope

I have written a lot about hope (Weingarten, 2000, 2004b, 2007). Expecting people who are sick and scared to feel hopeful may be expecting too much. I prefer to think of hope as the responsibility of the community. Hope is something we do together. The latest research makes it clear that hope is essential to health (for a review, see Groopman, 2004). This makes it even more crucial that hope be available to all, not just those few robust people who can summon hope under the most challenging circumstances.

I believe that hope *can* be made available to all, because we can do hope together. Hope is helping people feel connected when life's blows make people feel isolated. Hope is resisting indifference to the plight of those who are sick and diminished. Hope is doing what one can for others.

These days my position with regard to hope is no longer the position of one who must resist indifference. Now it is the position of one who dreads that others will show indifference. It is the position of one who works to believe that she is still worthy of attention, although she can contribute so much less than she did before. It is the position of one who must find purpose and meaning on a canvas suddenly not large. I am a person who must believe that small actions need not be trivial.

To do this, I strive for realistic hope, the same kind of hope I have conceptualized as crucial to the people with whom I have worked. Realistic hope is not hearts and flowers; it is not "the thing with feathers / that perches in the soul . . . and never asks a crumb of [us]" (Dickinson, 1997). On the contrary, it demands a great deal of us. It requires that that we think about hope in very specific ways that open us to the complexities and contradictions of our lives. It is the "tough love" version of hope.

Realistic hope accommodates doubt and despair. It is not rolled up with optimism. As Vaclev Havel says in *Disturbing the Peace,* hope is "definitely not the same thing as optimism. It is not the conviction that something will turn out well, but the certainty that something makes sense, regardless of how it turns out" (1991, p. 181). Havel points to what we must do: make sense of the cornucopia of feelings we all have that mess with us, particularly when we are discouraged and most in need of hope. Doubt and despair are inevitable when we are down. Looking at them full on and not losing hope is the challenge. In fact, it is precisely when we suppress doubt and despair or push them away that we are at risk of making tragic errors in our lives. Doubt and despair are worthy signals whose messages need to be considered and incorporated into our lives. Hope scrubbed of despair is really childlike innocence. It is rarely a form of hope on which a solid foundation of human relationship can be built.

As appealing as innocent hope may be, there are problems with it. It prefers the straight line, the black or white, the simple form. Realistic hope is comfortable with a mess. It accepts that chaos can assort itself into order, eventually. It embraces contradiction, which is one hallmark of a rich life.

Innocent hope is full of idealism. Realistic hope is pragmatic; it seeks goals and pathways to them. People tend to feel buoyed, hopeful, when the goal is clear, the pathway known, and hopeless when the way is blocked, the goal obscure. Despair is the conviction that nothing one wants is within reach, whether love or security or clean water or health. The task is to cultivate a practice of clarifying goals and identifying pathways toward them.

Doing this is not necessarily simple. First, there is often a lot of trial and error to define goals and pathways that will succeed. Goals, and pathways to them, may have to replace each other at a rate one would never have expected or wanted. Second, life deals us circumstances in which we have to select goals and pathways we never thought we could accept. Yet the practice of re-forming goals and cultivating pathways to them, stretches us, helping us sustain realistic hope.

My mother died decades ago. During her time of dying she was rarely hopeless, a gift that has continued to unfold in the lives of her children and grandchildren to this day. I, who had wanted to grow old with my mother, at first, wanted her to avail herself of any treatment that might extend her life. Ultimately, in the final hours of her life, I wished her dead. I saw that my hope for connection to my mother would forever be in my dreams and in my heart, and never with the unconscious body lying inert in the hospital bed. In one excruciating 24-hour period my hope tumbled through four phases: "Please don't let her die" became "Please don't let her suffer," which passed on to "Please let her die comfortably," which then morphed the most inconceivable thought into a conceivable wish, "Let her die now." Realistic hope depends on a path to an achievable goal, whether that goal breaks our heart or not.

So many of us have grown up on the popular tropes about hope: It is butterflies and rainbows, a lilting sound. Hope's story line is invariably portrayed as a progressive narrative, a straight line up. Life, this narrative shape implies, gets better and better over time. Hope is always on an upward flight. The story line for realistic hope, my kind of hope, is determined less by the outcome of events than by the responses of the communities of people who support each other through the events. In community, any narrative form—including uncertain ones—can be borne.

## Conclusion

I can now add four other spiritual practices to the ones I have written about in Part I: two of which I have already introduced—doing hope and witnessing—and two of which I describe below. To do hope, one must have others, even one other, or the memory of one other. Doing hope is a relational activity. It is a commitment to staying in relationship despite the pull of withdrawing into isolation. Despair tugs us away; hope pulls us toward. In the midst of anguish, it is a spiritual practice to go toward, especially when one desires to back away.

Doing hope during an illness of any kind is both imperative and challenging. Connecting to community when one's life has taken a direction wildly different from that of others, whether because one is depressed, traumatized, ill or disabled, is not easy, practically or emotionally. During this recent illness, some aspects of attending to community I could do myself. I sent out e-mail updates to various lists of people from different sectors of my personal and professional life. Other tasks were too much for me to do. My son set up a calendar, so that people could sign up to be with me for one of my four intravenous infusions a day. My husband requested poems from close friends. People dropped off food when we needed it. Establishing connections to manage the pragmatics of daily life is an important feature of doing hope but not all of what it can be.

Doing hope in community also entails being receptive to the kinds of spontaneous witnessing that comes from being observed at close range. Hearing observations from family and friends about the arduousness of my life, really our lives, Hilary's and mine, was always eye opening, sometimes distressing, and often profoundly acknowledging. As part of my spiritual practice, I tried to ensure that those who offered their witnessing of me felt aware and empowered in doing so, regardless of how close their witnessing "hit the mark." The fact that people offered witnessing was what mattered. I wanted those who were willing to resist indifference to feel that their efforts were appreciated.

I did not have to act. One of the skills I have developed over the years, a spiritual practice like the others, is a willingness to feel gratified by moments of intimate connection. It is an ability I have honed over the years of struggle, and it expresses a commitment I have made to be sustained by what is on offer. I can make a moment open up inside me and expand to fill my needs. This means that even small gestures of others make a difference. This practice creates a positive synergy: Gratitude follows giving, which sparks more giving.

Finally, I work at creating continuous loving contact. "Obstructed love makes us ill," sagely notes Humberto Maturana (in Linares, 2006, p. 111). While I may have diseases, I do not contend with feeling ill. For a sick person, I feel well; I attribute this to the health of my relationships. I work at creating unobstructed love in all facets of my life. This too is a spiritual practice.

Doing hope, witnessing and being witnessed, feeling gratified by receiving even brief moments of what I need, and smoothing away obstructions so that I can feel unimpeded love in all my relationships are the additional components of my spiritual practice. They permeate my life, whether in my home, the classroom, or my clinical office. I offer what I am, what I have become. For, although illness has been my bane, it has also been my goad. It has spurred me to develop these practices. I am grateful.

## REFERENCES

By convention one cites those books and articles that are clearly "referenced" in the text. I have done so here. However, there are other passages that have so informed, impressed, and inspired me that I have them in my very cells. These sources are immanent in the text but not visible on its surface. For these, I am profoundly grateful and, as well, for the reliable resource that reading has been for me.

Bate, W. J. (1963). *John Keats*. Cambridge, MA: Harvard University Press.

Dickinson, E. (1997). *The complete poems of Emily Dickinson*. Boston: Back Bay Press.

Groopman, J. (2004). *The anatomy of hope*. New York: Random House.

Hatley, J. (2000). *Suffering witness: The quandary of responsibility after the irreparable*. Albany: State University of New York Press.

Havel, V. (1991). *Disturbing the peace.* New York: Vintage.

Hoyt, M. F., & Combs, G. (1996). On ethics and spiritualities of the surface: A conversation with Michael White. In M. F. Hoyt (Ed.), *Constructive Therapies 2.* New York: Guilford Press.

Linares, J. L. (2006). Complex love as relational nurturing: An integrating ultra-modern concept. *Family Process, 45,* 101–115.

Weingarten, K. (1991). The discourses of intimacy: Adding a social constructionist and feminist view. *Family Process, 31,* 285–305.

Weingarten, K. (1992). A consideration of intimate and non-intimate interactions in therapy. *Family Process, 32,* 45–59.

Weingarten, K. (1997). *The mother's voice: Strengthening intimacy in families* (2nd ed.). New York: Guilford Press.

Weingarten, K. (1998a). The small and the ordinary: The daily practice of a post-modern narrative therapy. *Family Process, 37,* 3–15.

Weingarten, K. (1998b). Review of *The shared experience of illness: Stories of patients, families, and their therapists. Families, Systems, and Health, 16,* 179–182.

Weingarten, K. (2000). Witnessing, wonder, and hope. *Family Process, 39,* 389–402.

Weingarten, K. (2003). *Common shock—witnessing violence every day: How we are harmed, how we can heal.* New York: Dutton.

Weingarten, K. (2004a). Commentary on Candib (2004): What Is at the center, and what is at the edges, of care? *Families, Systems, and Health, 22,* 152–157.

Weingarten, K. (2004b). The ripple effect. *Hope, 44,* 34–37.

Weingarten, K. (2005a). A guide to dedicating cancer treatments. Available at *www.witnessingproject.org.*

Weingarten, K. (2005b). The companion guide for volunteers facilitating the treatment dedication project. Available at *www.witnessingproject.org.*

Weingarten, K. (2005c). Cancer, meaning making, and hope: The treatment dedication project: Comment. *Families, Systems, and Health, 23,* 155–160.

Weingarten, K. (2007). Hope in a time of global despair. In C. Flaskas, I. McCarthy, & J. Sheehan (Eds.), *Hope and despair in family therapy: Reflections on adversity, reconciliation and forgiveness.* London: Routledge.

Weingarten, K., & Worthen, M. E. W. (1997). A narrative analysis of the illness experience of a mother and daughter. *Families, Systems, and Health, 15,* 41–54.

White, M. (1995). *Re-authoring lives: Interviews and essays.* Adelaide: Dulwich Centre.

White, M. (1998). *Narratives of therapists' lives.* Adelaide: Dulwich Centre.

White, M., & Epston, D. (1989). *Literate means to therapeutic ends.* Adelaide: Dulwich Centre.

# Heart and Soul
## Experiential Exercises for Therapists and Clients

### JANINE ROBERTS

The healing spirit will elude those who have an agenda to impose. Men and women who want to proclaim their private truths at the vulnerable and ill are not physicians (*or therapists*).
—PAUL R. FLEISCHMAN (1994, p. 20; emphasis added)

I worked with a client, Yvette, who told me that when she and her husband fought, the figurines of saints on top of the TV cabinet moved. They turned their faces to the wall; they fell over. She interpreted this as a sign that something was wrong in the house. I was raised Catholic, but not Italian Catholic like Yvette. I was in a quandary. Should I treat her beliefs as delusional or as a resource in therapy?
—CHRISTINE (therapist, age 32)

One of my clients, Ron, aged 47, was recently diagnosed with colon cancer and is facing surgery and possibly chemotherapy and/or radiation treatments. His view of why he got it is that it is a random event—"things happen." His wife, Alisa, has a very different take on it. She's wondering, "What is the universe trying to tell me? What lessons do we need to learn? How is this my Karma?"
    I'm doing couples therapy with them. They are already in a lot of conflict. I don't know how to manage the fact that they have such different views.
—JAMES (therapist, age 41)

## BELIEFS: YOURS, MINE, AND OURS

The spiritual and religious beliefs of clients are seldom addressed directly in family therapy training (Abbott, Berry, & Meredith, 1990; Prest & Keller,

359

1993; Taibbi, 1990, Weaver, Koenig, & Larson, 1997). Yet, as the preceding two vignettes show, they are often very present in the issues that people bring to therapy. Spiritual beliefs[1] can be both a tremendous resource in treatment and a constraint. Rachel and George, dealing with the loss of their only son when he was 16 in a car accident, believed that he was so perfect that God wanted him by his side. Their therapist listened carefully to their convictions and helped them to articulate these beliefs clearly, as well as find ways to share them with others. For instance, they made up photo cards of their son with a quotation about what a gift he was to God, to send to friends thanking them for their support after his death. Respect for the beliefs of Rachel and George gave them comfort and helped them with their deep grief and sorrow.

A survey of 1,225 Latina women in California, funded by the National Cancer Institute, was conducted to find out why Latina women underutilized preventive services for cervical cancer: Nearly 25% of the women believed that cervical cancer is God's punishment for an immoral lifestyle. Among first-generation Hispanic immigrants, the figure rose to 43% (Cooper, 1997). In this case, beliefs act as a constraint against people having regular Pap smears or seeking out other preventive services. One of the researchers, a physician, noted that people who wish to inform Latinas about the need for Pap smears "may actually drive patients away, if they are not aware of the shame-laden perception" (p. 17).

If family therapists are not aware of the worldviews of clients about life's purpose, guilt, fate, afterlife, or other beliefs that have a spiritual component, they may be missing key elements that impact on issues people are trying to sort through in therapy.

The spiritual beliefs of therapists are addressed even less in training or in clinical work (Anderson & Worthen, 1997). Reasons for this include worries about imposing ideas on clients and the secular–religious boundaries in Western societies. For example, as indicated in a recent survey of 138 randomly selected members of the American Association of Marriage and Family Therapy (AAMFT), the more respondents were asked about the importance of directly bringing up religion in sessions and other specific interventions, the less people responded in the affirmative (Carlson, Kirkpatrick, Hecker, & Killmer, 2002). There is also pressure in the mental health field to be seen as "scientific."

But clinicians' spiritual beliefs can also be a constraint or a resource in treatment; if they go unexamined, the therapist does not have help identifying blind spots, or have access to how being transparent about his or her own values may be useful in therapy (Roberts, 2005). For instance, a therapist who is an agnostic may not ask about religious beliefs or church, mosque, temple, or synagogue connections, which may be a key community link for a family. Or a religious therapist may not ask about pagan beliefs.

A person who is familiar with various views and religious groups may be able to work with clients quite differently than someone without that information. Kevin, raised a Unitarian, was having a difficult time understanding why a client, Anne, raised Irish Catholic but no longer practicing, was agonizing over whether to have an abortion. In seeking supervision on the case, Kevin talked with a Catholic colleague. She explained to him how having an abortion was still considered a sin by the Catholic church, that some factions viewed it as akin to killing someone, and that it was an affront to God as well, because it meant that a woman was taking God's work into her own hands. Kevin was able to go back and ask very different kinds of questions of Anne about guilt, sin, autonomy, sexuality, pregnancy, and beliefs in her relationship to Catholicism and to God. As the conversation opened up, Anne felt more understood and found it easier to make a decision.

Being more cognizant of both clients' and therapists' spiritual and/or religious beliefs can make them more available (when appropriate) as part of the therapy process. Interestingly, in the previously mentioned survey of AAMFT members, "a surprising 95% of the respondents believed in the relationship between spiritual and mental health" (Carlson et al., 2002, p. 166). In the rest of this chapter, I share six exercises I have developed that can be used in training and supervision, as well as clinical practice, to learn more about when, where, and how to work with or not work with spiritual beliefs.

A safe area in which to explore this aspect of life is with other trainees and colleagues. They can bring to bear on the discussion their listening, reflective, and analytical skills to examine what it means to cross boundaries into this topic. Also, generally, in therapeutic work, it is important that therapists have some informed experience with the kinds of things they ask clients to examine. This means not only knowing a variety of techniques but also personally working with them in some fashion, so that therapists have empathy for the intricacy of lived experiences, as well as ideas on how to work with contradictory responses that may come up. This is important to balance curricula that are starting to be published about spiritual issues in family therapy (Patterson, Hayworth, Turner, & Raskin, 2000) that heavily emphasize clinical study and application.

Six exercises are presented in a sequence in which they build upon and complement each other. They are offered as starting points for designing and adapting one's own exercises to fit with one's context. Each exercise is described, with directions and time needed for them. Ideas are also introduced about ways to adapt some of the exercises for use with clients. This is a key part of the process, because it keeps linking the experiential work done by people to therapy. Thus, the focus is kept on becoming better clinicians.

The first exercise, "Out in the Open," invites participants to complete unfinished sentences, such as "Spiritual beliefs in my life. . . ." It is intended as a warm-up. In dyads, participants can help each other sort out and articulate their thoughts about the place of spiritual convictions in their lives, as well as make distinctions between what they see as religious experiences and spiritual ones.

The next exercise, "On the Line," brings in ideas of others in the family therapy field and is structured to facilitate a series of minidialogues with a number of people. This can quickly open up the discussion to a wider range of issues.

The third exercise, "Rituals," looks at the sacred aspects of family rituals. All families have rituals. Examining spiritual beliefs and practices through looking at daily rituals, such as mealtimes and bedtimes, or family traditions, such as birthdays and anniversaries, can be a gentle entrance into and a different perspective on the topic.

The fourth exercise, "Through the Ages," uses a genogram as an anchor point for some guided imagery and poses questions, such as "What is your first memory of what you would call a spiritual or religious encounter?" This exercise can help participants examine familial patterns over time.

The fifth and sixth exercises move closer to therapeutic practice. "Questions, Questions: Who's Got the Questions?" includes several inquiries about how appropriately to introduce ideas about spirituality into therapy. The final exercise, "Role Plays," offers suggestions about ways to structure role plays to simulate sessions.

For all of the exercises, the facilitator should say the phrases, questions, or ideas slowly, repeating them so people can mull over them. Help people to concentrate by creating a focused and contemplative atmosphere with your voice.

## OUT IN THE OPEN: UNFINISHED SENTENCES

This exercise can be a good warm-up, because it helps people start to name, explore, and explicate the context for their beliefs. It is also very open-ended, which can aid people in discovering what may be important themes for them. Done in dyads, it is a safe format in which disclosure is with only one other person and choices can be made easily by the partners about how much to disclose.

About 40 minutes are needed to do the exercise. For a group in which people do not know each other at all, it may be important to work through any issues of trust and boundary setting before beginning. For example, you might talk about what people need to feel safe in disclosing information (e.g., partners will not share things with the larger group without checking it out with the other person first, or nothing will be shared outside of the workshop). There might also be some discussion about what kinds of verbal and nonverbal responses are important, so that people feel they have been heard by others and/or what helps participants to build trust. A key role for the facilitator in this discussion is modeling respect for the range of ideas that might emerge, as well as helping people to give concrete examples.

To begin the actual exercise, the facilitator says the first unfinished sentence (see Box 19.1) and asks each member of the dyad to finish it with the first thing that comes to mind. Ask people not to edit or think about their response too much. Then, give the dyads 3–4 minutes to talk with each other about why they completed the sentence in that way.

People may want to write down their initial responses to be able to go back to them after they listen to their partners. This can free them to be

---

### BOX 19.1. Out in the Open: Unfinished Sentences

1. Spiritual beliefs in my life (as a child, adolescent, young adult—choose different time frames) . . .

2. Learning about spirituality . . .

3. Therapy and spirituality . . .

4. Religious beliefs in my life . . .

5. My mother's (stepmother's, aunt's, or other person who took on this role) religious life . . .
   My father's (stepfather's, uncle's, or other mother, if raised in a lesbian family) religious life . . .
   My grandparents' religious life . . .

6. The spiritual beliefs of my clients . . .

7. The role of my spiritual and/or religious beliefs in therapy . . .

better listeners. The important thing is to keep and support the energy that can get generated between two people interacting. If they are looking down and writing too much, this can detract from dynamic interaction. Having the unfinished sentences up on an overhead can support those who have a visual learning style. Giving participants a handout of the sentences afterward can make them less concerned about writing things down exactly.

Sophie completed the first sentence as follows: "Spiritual beliefs in my life as a child were unsettled, and as an adolescent, even more unsettled." Her partner Brad completed the same sentence with "Spiritual beliefs in my life as a teenager were sunk in guilt." They then went on to discuss with each other what they had said. Sophie commented, "My family was Jewish, but I didn't feel as if they practiced Judaism, because it meant particular things to them and it helped them know how to lead their lives. Rather, it was because they were supposed to do it because 'that's what good Jews did.' I heard that phrase a lot. On the one hand, I had the words that these were important spiritual practices; on the other hand, I watched the behaviors, which were quite different. It was very unsettling."

"That clicks with what I experienced," said Brad. "I was raised Episcopalian, but it was like we went to church out of guilt—because that's what it meant to be a good person. If you didn't go, you were bad. But it was not as if my parents believed in the church because it comforted them. It was more because it made them virtuous."

Have participants go through all the sentences, as in the preceding example. If you wish, you can add an eighth sentence to complete this exercise: "Doing this exercise was. . . . " This can help to provide closure to doing the sentences, as well as help the partners in the dyad to see their own experience against the backdrop of someone else's. The juxtaposition of different people's reflections can help participants to notice new things about their experience, flesh it out more, and make more detailed distinctions. For example, Sophie got clearer about why her experience was so unsettling by hearing Brad talk about how his family did not seem to take pleasure in churchgoing. "We had too many 'shoulds,' too," said Sophie. "We had to dress up, sit for hours in the synagogue. We weren't allowed to drive or use any mechanical things. It was a tense time in the family."

When the dyads have completed the exercise, ask the partners to give each other any affirmations and appreciations for things they have shared. This can be another way to provide closure for the exercise.

To encourage some group interchange, you can ask people to come back together and see whether there are several dyads who are comfortable sharing both what it was like to do the exercise and what issues came up for them that seemed particularly knotty, juicy, or useful to explore more. It can also be productive to ask people how they might adapt this exercise to use with clients as a way to keep making links between their own experience and clinical practice. For instance, Hwei Ling was fascinated by how her spiritual and religious ideas had shifted over her life. She said, "I think it would be useful to offer clients four or five unfinished sentences about their beliefs and experiences at different time periods. It would give them a structure to reflect back on and a sense of how they came to their current views. I think I would add another phrase, too: 'My spiritual beliefs in the future. . . . ' This could help people clarify aspects they might want to be moving toward."

Abdul commented, "I think I would, for some clients, use phrases that separate out religious practices and spiritual beliefs. I think these can be quite distinct, and contradictions and tension points between them might be important for family members to understand."

## ON THE LINE: VIEWS AND VOICES

This second exercise is intended to open up the dialogue more broadly and move beyond personal experiences and ideas. What theorists and clinicians have said about the role(s) of spirituality and religion in family therapy is introduced, and people are invited to react to these statements by placing themselves on an imaginary line depending on whether they agree or disagree with the statement. People then take a few minutes to discuss with others on the line why they put themselves there.

This is a good exercise to do after the unfinished sentences; it is more contemplative and lays a foundation for understanding the context of individual beliefs. "On the Line" provides a format for people to move out with their beliefs into a wider arena of ideas in a relatively short period of time that makes for a vibrant interchange (see Box 19.2).

Clear space in the room and ask people to pretend there is a line across it from one corner to another. Tell the participants that you will read a statement, and that they are then to put themselves on the line based on whether they agree or disagree with it. The closer they stand to one corner (identified as the "agree" corner), the more they agree with the statement, and vice versa. After people have placed themselves, give them 3–4 minutes to talk with others in dyads or triads about why they placed themselves where they did. Encourage people at opposite ends of the line to talk to each other. These are often some of the liveliest discussions, and they help people to gain different perspectives. Some 30–40 minutes are needed to do this exercise in its entirety.

---

### BOX 19.2. On the Line: Voices and Views

1. All persons, even those who consider themselves agnostic or atheistic, are spiritual, whether or not they choose to express their spirituality through religious language or practice. (p. 4)

2. *Spirituality* is defined as subjective engagement with a fourth, transcendent dimension of human experience. (p. 3)

3. Three basic assumptions of spiritually based therapy are the following:
   (A) God (or a Divine Being) exists.
   (B) Human beings have an innate yearning for connection with this Divine Being.
   (C) This Divine Being takes an active interest in human beings and acts upon their relationships to promote beneficial change. (p. 3)

4. Hart (1994, p. 48) suggests that the therapist's deepest vocation may be to serve as an embodiment of divine love, in effect, as an "incarnation of God." (p. 11)

*Note.* All quotes are from Anderson and Worthen (1997).

---

The statements that I have chosen to have people react to are from a lead article on spirituality in the *Journal of Marital and Family Therapy* by Anderson and Worthen (1997), two pastoral counselors. Let people know the source of the statements. Read the first statement several times and encourage people to move onto the "line." You can also have the statements on an overhead or PowerPoint slide, showing each one as you say it out loud.

One group generated a lively discussion about the differences between spirituality and religion. "The third statement was the most provocative one for me," said Eunice. "I felt like it was way too narrow of a definition. Those assumptions to me were religious tenets for Christian-based therapy, not spiritual tenets."

"I reacted to them, too," said Manuel. "They did not reflect different cultural or spiritual beliefs from around the world."

"Many of the ideas in the quotes felt imposed, like prayer in the schools. Like in #2, I don't think you have to be in some fourth plane to have a spiritual experience. It might be as simple as a walk in the woods," added Andrea. "To me spirituality is more open than a lot of the ideas expressed."

Other statements can be chosen for this exercise and used with the same format. People in a class or training group can be asked to bring in possible quotes. What is important is that they not be personal statements from anyone in the group, because this would affect the group dynamics and participants' freedom to openly agree and disagree.

This exercise generates a lot of ideas quickly. As Andrea said, "Being able to talk to so many people in such a brief period of time opened up a lot of new perspectives for me." Guillermo commented, "Each statement gave me a holding point to examine, move around, and go off from. Having to explain to others where I put myself helped me to clarify what my responses and ideas were."

To adapt this exercise for use with clients some changes need to be made. First, rather than using quotes from professional literature, statements need to be more generic and open-ended, and drawn from typical family experience (e.g., "Many things in life are predetermined by fate, and there is not much you can do about them"; "An important part of healing for me is my spiritual beliefs"; "Within a family there should be room for different religious and spiritual ideas"). Second, this should only be done with clients when the intent is to open up dialogue, not to stir up contentious debate. Thus, there needs to be basic tolerance and trust within the family.

Finally, because the family you are working with will likely be smaller than a training or supervision group, and part of the potency of this exercise depends on having a number of people articulate different views, you may need to ask clients to imagine where others who are close to them, or are in their extended kin network, or their community, might place themselves. Discussion can then ensue about how those other perspectives make them feel about their own beliefs.

## RITUALS: A GENTLE INTRODUCTION

A low-key entrance into the theme of spirituality can be via a look at family rituals. All families have rituals: They provide a window into central values and beliefs, and often express what families consider as sacred (see Imber-Black, Chapter 12, this volume). Rituals can be resources for meaning making in common situations that we all face, such as illness (Roberts, 2003a, 2003b).

Many exercises have already been developed to help people understand the role of ritual in their lives (Imber-Black & Roberts, 1998; Roberts, 1999). These can be easily adapted to focus more primarily on rituals with a spiritual component. The exercise presented here helps people scan and identify across the four different types of family rituals—day-to-day rituals, family traditions, holiday celebrations (or holy day observance), and life-cycle rituals—in which spiritual aspects are central.

About a half-hour is needed for this exercise. Ask people to get comfortable and do whatever will help them to focus on their memory and interior experience (rather than the noises and stimuli around them). This might mean removing things from their laps, breathing more slowly, putting feet flat on the floor—or perhaps closing their eyes or just focusing on one place in the room. Once people have begun to relax, here are some suggestions for how you might guide them through their memories.

### RITUAL REMEMBERING

I am going to ask you to scan across different types of rituals, both in your life as a child and currently, and to think about what spiritual and/or religious aspects of them have been or are important to you. I would first like to ask you to think about daily rituals like mealtimes, bedtimes, how you say hello and good-bye. You may have a meditation in the morning when you wake up, or practice yoga in some way—or have a moment of silence at meals, prayers at nighttime. How have these been important to you in your life? Who are others who join you or do not join you in these practices? What impact does that have on your relationships? Are there aspects of these rituals that feel obligatory or hollow? What changes might make them more meaningful?

The second kind of ritual I would like to ask you to think about is family traditions. This includes events like birthdays, anniversaries, vacations, and reunions. Where do spiritual expressions come into play in them? Perhaps a family prayer at a reunion, or a remembrance of family members who have died. Or some way in which the sacredness of life is acknowledged at birthdays, or birthing stories are told. Or perhaps it is vacationing in a place of particular spiritual or religious significance to you. Or an anniversary marked of an important transition in the family.

Which family traditions have more spiritual components to them—birthdays, anniversaries, reunions, vacations? Why do you think that is?

Holiday celebrations are the third type of family rituals. As I name a range of celebrations that occur as we pass through the year, I would like to ask you to think of any spiritual/religious practices that go along with them. There might be special foods, music, mantras that are said, prayers, gathering with other people. Think about these elements as I name any holidays that were and/or are important to you: New Year's Day, Three King's Day, Chinese New Year, Ramadan, Passover, Memorial Day, Fourth of July, Rosh Hashanah (Jewish New Year), Yom Kippur, Halloween, Divali (Hindu New Year), Thanksgiving, Hanukkah, Christmas, Kwanza.[2]

What memories of different holiday celebrations have stayed most vividly in your mind? How are these connected or not to spiritual and/or religious practices? What is the significance of these memories to you?

The last kind of family rituals I am going to ask you to explore are life-cycle rituals—ones that take us on our journey from birth to death. These include events like engagements, showers, commitment ceremonies, weddings, baby-naming ceremonies, adoption day parties, rituals for pregnancy loss, leaving home, divorce, graduations, retirements, funerals, and other new rituals for today's life-cycle passages. As you think about them, what spiritual aspects of them come to mind? How do these elements help transitions and changes over the life cycle?

I would like to ask you to think back over the four different types of rituals: daily rituals, family traditions, holiday celebrations, and life-cycle rituals. In which area do you or did you have the richest examples of spiritual and/or religious practices that were meaningful to you? Which areas were not as rich? Where might you like to amplify any practices? What might you like to change about other practices? When you are ready, please come back to this time and space.

Thinking about family rituals is a very accessible manner to explore spiritual and religious ideas, beliefs, and practices. This exercise can be a good way for people to step into that area, because work with rituals may be something that they are already using as a resource in therapy. This exercise can also help people be more aware of spiritual aspects of rituals that they have not focused on or named as such.

## THROUGH THE AGES: RELIGION, SPIRITUALITY, AND THE GENOGRAM

This exercise helps participants look at larger patterns in their extended family over time. It uses people's genogram as the anchor point for leading them into some guided imagery, and to consider some questions about spiritual beliefs and practice in their lives (see Box 19.3).

You will need approximately an hour: 10–15 minutes for the introduction and the drawing of the genogram; 15–20 minutes to add to the genogram as the facilitator asks participants the questions in Box 19.3; 15 minutes for dyad partners to give each other a tour; and 10–15 minutes to process the exercise overall and brainstorm ways to use it with clients. Participants first sketch a basic genogram of three or four generations (McGoldrick, Gerson, & Petry, 2008), noting ethnic background of family members

## BOX 19.3. Genogram Questions and Guided Remembering

1. What is your first memory of what you would call a spiritual or religious encounter?
   - Where does that memory sit within you?
   - What kinds of feelings does it bring up?
   - In what ways does that memory inform you now?
   - How can you show this in some way on the genogram with color, a symbol, a phrase?

2. What was passed down through the generations to you about religious and/or spiritual beliefs?
   - By what people did?
   - By what they said?
   - By what they gave to you?
   - By religious or spiritual events you were asked to participate in or were excluded from?
   - What gender messages were embedded in these actions?

   How can you indicate some of the key things passed down to you on your genogram?

3. What rituals of life-cycle changes were marked by some kind of ceremony and/or religious event (e.g., baby naming, bar or bat mitzvah, Confirmation, Brahmin thread ceremony, weddings, or funerals)?

4. What were major shifts in religious/spiritual identification for various family members?
   - How can you indicate these on the genogram?
   - What was the impact on one or two key relationships with these shifts?
   - How can you show this?

5. How do various people in your extended family use or not use religious/ spiritual beliefs and practices to get them through difficult times?
   - Which of these strategies have you incorporated the most yourself into your life, or pushed against the most?
   - How can you show any of this with a word or phrase, a symbol, different colors?

and religious or spiritual beliefs. Each person needs a large piece of paper and colored crayons, markers, or pencils. With completed genograms in front of them, ask participants to think about the genogram questions given in Box 19.3.

When people are done responding to the questions and suggestions of things to ponder, ask them to take a partner on a tour of their genogram. Keeping in mind the things they have been asked to consider, each member of the dyad should walk the other through their history. It can be helpful to have the prompts visible on an overhead. This can facilitate asking more process questions, such as "Which of the questions or comments by the facilitator were the most provocative for you? Or the most disturbing? Or opened up the most things for you to consider?"

It can be instructive to ask people to hold up their genograms to share with the rest of the group or tape them up on the walls. Clinicians can learn more ways to help clients indicate patterns on genograms from the sharing of imaginative participant ideas. For example, Mara, whose family was predominantly Irish Catholic, but with varying degrees of commitment to the church, colored in crosses to indicate strong believers, crosses that were just outlines to represent tentative believers, and crosses with an x through them to represent those that had left the church. This enabled her to see some very interesting generational patterns, with dramatic shifts over four generations to many fewer connections to the church. Randall put in letters for the range of different groups represented in his genogram: B for Baptist, M for Muslim, L for Lutheran, and NA for New Age. KoKwang, who had come to the United States from South Korea, indicated how he felt about being Buddhist in such a predominantly Christian society by drawing a small temple besieged by crosses.

Besides stimulating ideas on how to help clients creatively show their family's spiritual history, this exercise aids people in seeing larger patterns beyond their own direct experience. Lise, whose family was predominantly a mixture of Jewish and New England Yankee Protestant, saw links she had not made before with the legacy of her English forebears fleeing England in the 1600s, seeking religious freedom, and her Jewish grandparents fleeing religious persecution in Europe in the 1930s. As she said, "I've always thought of them as two very distinct heritages, but there is this thread that connects them—they both wanted freedom for their beliefs."

Joseph, an African American man, told the story of his uncle, who returned to Alabama after serving in World War II, having had a dream that he should return home and serve the community. He came back to his small town, and did just that. Joseph went on to become a psychologist and also dedicated his life to helping others: "Like my uncle. I made this association for the first time today when I looked at what my relatives modeled for me about spirituality."

Therapists are more likely to inquire about and add information about spiritual and religious beliefs of clients on genograms if they see the importance of that realm in their own lives. Being exposed to other people's experience can also pique their interest and inform them about other ways to think about spirituality. Having prior experience in ways to integrate information into a genogram or show it can also increase therapists' comfort level and the likelihood that they will incorporate this theme into any gathering of family history. Frame's article (2000) provides other suggestions on doing a spiritual genogram with clients, and using it as an organizing tool to talk about religion and spirituality in therapy.

## QUESTIONS, QUESTIONS:
## WHO'S GOT THE QUESTIONS?

The fifth exercise is a series of questions about therapists' spiritual values, as well as how they come into play or not in therapy (see Box 19.4). In training people to work with these issues, I think it is important to keep finding ways to link what they are exploring and discovering with therapeutic process. These questions should be done in small groups of two, three, or four people.[3] The size of the group depends partly on available time and on whether you want people to get to know others more intimately in a small group. If you have done some of the previous exercises primarily with dyads, it can be instructive to have a larger group sharing responses for exposure to a variety of experiences and ideas.

A warm-up for this exercise can be a brief guided remembrance in which participants are asked to recall a time or times when they felt some kind of spiritual solace or connection. Who or what was around them? What feelings did they have? What do they carry with them now from this memory? What would be one way to express it to others with words, with a gesture, or movement? As a way to begin, you can ask the participants to share briefly the feelings that were evoked for them with others in their group either nonverbally or verbally.

These questions are meant to be a general guide. People are encouraged to explore other questions that they find interesting, drop ones that do not draw their attention, and stay with those they find more intriguing. Groups can be asked to work with the questions by letting one person at a time

BOX 19.4. Spirituality and Religious Beliefs
in Families and Family Therapy

1. Who taught you the most about spiritual/religious beliefs as a child?
   - Did you learn different things from men? From women?
   - From people inside your family? People outside your family?
   - How were your beliefs then looked upon by the larger society?
   - In what ways were social class issues reflected in membership in different religious/spiritual groups?

2. What did you learn about yourself as a boy/girl through your experiences of spirituality and/or religion?

   What has been the influence of religion and/or spirituality on major adult decisions in your life or in the lives of other key family members (e.g., abortion, choice of people to date, partner with, and/or marry, circumcision, or divorce)?

3. What ways have any of the various identities you have (as a divorced person, married person, gay person, heterosexual, woman or man, person with some physical challenge, parent, etc.) been supported by religious scripture/doctrine/tradition? Or not supported?

   What has been difficult for you personally about spiritual and/or religious beliefs? What has been healing? When is a time in which you think you appropriately introduced ideas (or can imagine appropriately introducing ideas) about spiritual and/or religious beliefs into the therapy process?

   What helped to make it appropriate?

5. Values, beliefs, and biases are all embedded in different spiritual and/or religious practices.

   What is a way (or ways) you check to make sure you are neither imposing nor ignoring key belief systems as either a resource or a constraint in therapy?

   Can you state this as a guideline for others?

respond to questions under the first theme and then go onto the questions under the following themes (2–5). Or one person could go through all of the questions of personal interest, while the partner(s) are the listeners. A useful way to keep building a good community of listeners is to ask partners to share what resonated for them when they heard others talk. Again, the group can be brought together as a whole to share experiences of the exercise and ideas generated.

As with the previous exercises, participants are asked to come up with links to practice as a way to keep a focus on providing good treatment. One group came up with the following guidelines for ways to introduce ideas appropriately about spirituality into therapy:

1.  Do it in a frame of open inquiry about clients' beliefs, not sharing your own (which could be seen as proselytizing).
2.  Ask clients if this feels like an area they want to explore more. Take your cues from their energy and interest level.
3.  Be attuned to circumstances of people's lives that might bring up and/or pull for attention to spiritual and/or religious beliefs.
4.  Be sensitive to the biases of the larger culture about religious and/or spiritual beliefs. For instance, the unfounded accusations that people at first made in the Oklahoma City bombing incident, that it was done by Muslim terrorists, reflected prejudices against that religion.

## ROLE PLAYS: WAY ON INTO IT

The closest approximation to actual work is to do role play. Scenarios can be written up to act out, or people can be asked to improvise them. Often the most active role plays are ones that people just make up, because issues they present are often at the core of things that are the most meaningful to them. Here is one scenario written out:

### DENIAL HAS ITS PLACE: A ROLE PLAY

*Father*—early 40s, tax accountant. Works both outside home and has home office. He is spending more and more time in his home office.

*Mother*—late 30s. Works outside of home as monitor for the state for family day care centers. Used to run a day care center in the family home. Has been taking some leave time to be at home.

*Oldest son*—14, diagnosed with leukemia a year and a half ago. Avid baseball player before the illness and solid student.

*Second son*—13, not doing particularly well in school. Lot of conflict with older brother both before and after illness.

*Youngest child*—a girl, age 5. Seems to be disoriented, not at all sure about what is going on in the family.

The therapist wants to support the hopes of the family for a remission for the oldest son. At the same time, every couple of weeks, when she sees the family, the son is visibly weaker to the point that family sessions need to be moved to the home. No one talks about the possibility that he might die. The therapist is concerned about the impact this is having on all of them, especially given the father's withdrawal, the younger son's history of conflict with his brother, and how disconnected the daughter seems.

The next therapy session ends up being in the oldest son's bedroom, because he is too weak to get up out of bed. While the mother is gathering the rest of the family, the oldest son makes it clear to the therapist that he thinks he is going to die.

The therapist wants to help them talk about this together and learn more about their beliefs about death, loss, life after loss, and life after death. She is afraid to upset the parents' denial about how ill their son is, as the denial certainly seems to be giving them the fortitude to get through a very difficult period.

Crucial to working with role play is building in structures to support people as they are doing it, as well as analysis and discussion of what people are learning from it. For instance, the role play can be done with a live supervision or reflecting team format (Anderson, 1987; Roberts, 1997) so that the therapist and family can get immediate feedback and the benefit of ideas from the team. Also, observers can be asked to watch for specific things, such as issues and questions that arose in the previous exercises.

Another possible format is to have reflections on the role play given by teams afterward. Rich information can also be obtained by interviewing the people who played the different roles in the role play. This is a good way to help de-role people as well, an often neglected aspect of role plays. Family members can be asked to comment on their responses to things the therapist tried; the therapist and family members can share times when they felt engaged and connected. Suggestions can be given for other ways to address interactions. It is important to be as attentive to how you set up this part of the experience as the actual role play itself. Good working structures for analysis and discussion enables participants to get the most out of the actual scenario.

## MOVING BEYOND

These exercises are intended as "starter yeast" for your own ideas. Try parts of them yourself. Adapt and change ideas around to fit situations in which you are working. Experiment with others; ask participants for feedback; rework the exercises based on their input. Bring in other family therapy techniques. For example, you might have people make a floor plan (Coppersmith, 1980) of a place of worship that has been important to them, or sculpt (Papp, 1976) their relationship to spiritual and/or religious beliefs over time. Spiritual ecomaps (Hodge, 2000) can focus people spatially on current connections to faith communities, members of them, and/or beliefs. Read widely in the literature. For example, in the *Journal of Refugee Studies*, De Voe (2002) writes thoughtfully about Muslim beliefs, the *hijab* (veil), and Somali families in the United States, and Dwyer (1999), in *Gender, Place, and Culture: A Journal of Feminist Geography*, looks at British Muslim families.

## ACKNOWLEDGMENTS

Thanks to Don Banks, EdD, Deborah Berkman, PhD, Stephen Blane, EdD, Julie Cox, MS, Rich McKeown, LICSW, Jessica Morris, PhD, Laurie Ostendorf, PsyD, and Donna Volpe, PsyD, for feedback and ideas on these exercises.

## NOTES

1. The term *spiritual* refers broadly to personal beliefs and practices that may be experienced within a formal, organized religion or in nonreligious spiritual nourishment (e.g. through contemplative practices, nature, the arts, or social activism; see Walsh, Chapter 1, this volume). It is useful to highlight these distinctions.
2. It is important to have a range of holidays that reflects the constituency of your group.
3. You may also give this exercise to ongoing groups in training or practice.

## REFERENCES

Abbott, D., Berry, M., & Meredith, W. H. (1990). Religious belief and practice: A potential asset in helping families. *Family Relations, 39*, 443–448.
Anderson, D., & Worthen, D. (1997). Exploring a fourth dimension: Spirituality

as a resource for the couple therapist. *Journal of Marital and Family Therapy, 23*, 3–12.

Anderson, T. (1987). The reflecting team: Dialogue and meta-dialogue in clinical work. *Family Process, 26*, 415–428.

Carlson, T., Kirkpatrick, D., Hecker, L., & Killmer, M. (2002). Religion, spirituality, and marriage and family therapy. A study of family therapists' beliefs about the appropriateness of addressing religious and spiritual issues in therapy. *The American Journal of Family Therapy, 30*, 157–171.

Cooper, G. (1997, May/June). Network briefs: Cancer is punishment. *Family Therapy Networker*, p. 17.

Coppersmith, E. (1980). The family floor plan: A tool for training, assessment and intervention in family therapy. *Journal of Marital and Family Therapy, 6*, 141–145.

De Voe, P. A. (2002). Symbolic action: Religion's role in the changing environment of young Somali women. *Journal of Refugee Studies, 15*(2), 234–246.

Dwyer, C. (1999). Veiled meanings: Young British Muslim women and the negotiation of differences. *Gender, Place, and Culture: A Journal of Feminist Geography, 6*(1), 5–27.

Fleischman, P. R. (1994). *Spiritual aspects of psychiatric practice*. Cleveland, OH: Bonne Chance Press.

Frame, M. W. (2000). The spiritual genogram in family therapy. *Journal of Marital and Family Therapy, 26*(2), 211–216.

Hodge, D. R. (2000). Spiritual ecomaps: A new diagrammatic tool for assessing marital and family spirituality. *Journal of Marital and Family Therapy, 26*(2), 217–228.

Imber-Black, E., & Roberts, J. (1998). *Rituals for our times: Celebrating, healing, and changing our lives and our relationships*. Northvale, NJ: Jason Aronson.

McGoldrick, M., Gerson, R., & Petry, S. (2008). *Genograms: Assessment and intervention*. New York: Norton.

Papp, P. (1976). Family choreography. In P. J. Guerin (Ed.), *Family therapy: Theory and practice* (pp. 465–479). New York: Gardner Press.

Patterson, J., Hayworth, M., Turner, C., & Raskin, M. (2000). Spiritual issues in family therapy: A graduate-level course. *Journal of Marital and Family Therapy, 26*(2), 199–210.

Prest, L. A., & Keller, J. F. (1993). Spirituality and family therapy: Spiritual beliefs, myths, and metaphors. *Journal of Marital and Family Therapy, 19*, 137–148.

Roberts, J. (1997). Reflecting processes and "supervision": Looking at ourselves as we work with others. In C. Storm & T. Todd (Eds.), *The complete systemic supervisor* (pp. 334–348). Boston: Allyn & Bacon.

Roberts, J. (1999). Beyond words: The power of rituals. In D. Weiner (Ed.), *Action methods in psychotherapy: A practical guide* (pp. 55–78). Washington, DC: American Psychological Association.

Roberts, J. (2003a). In sickness and health: Ice bells ringing. *Families, Systems, and Health: Journal of Collaborative Family Health Care, 21*(4), 441–448.

Roberts, J. (2003b). Rituals and serious illness: Marking the path. In E. Imber-Black, J. Roberts, & R. Whiting (Eds.), *Rituals in families and family therapy* (pp. 237–252). New York: Norton.

Roberts, J. (2005). Transparency and self-disclosure in family therapy: Dangers and possibilities. *Family Process, 44*(1), 45–63.

Taibbi, R. (1990, July/August). The uninitiated. *Family Therapy Networker,* pp. 31–35.

Weaver, A. J., Koenig, H. G., & Larson, D. B. (1997). Marriage and family therapists and the clergy: A need for clinical collaboration, training, and research. *Journal of Marital and Family Therapy, 23,* 13–25.

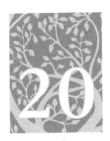

# The Therapeutic Benefits
# of a Justice-Seeking Spirituality
### Empowerment, Healing, and Hope

ALICE DE V. PERRY
JOHN S. ROLLAND

She first came to therapy to talk about her marriage unraveling. Within a few weeks Mary Ann found herself facing the possibility of her whole life unraveling. This 39-year-old mother of three (two daughters ages 11 and 13, and a 10-year-old son) was diagnosed with breast cancer so aggressive that she needed 3 months of "life-saving" chemo before she had a bilateral mastectomy. The diagnosis devastated and terrorized Mary Ann, but she vowed, "If I have to do it, I will do this with grace." And over the next many months she did. "I had a very unconventional approach to the illness and treatment," she explained. She dressed up for the chemo treatments and brought roses, starting with one, then two, and so on, to mark each session in succession. She shared Krispy Kreme donuts with the other women at the clinic and told dirty jokes.

Prominent in Mary Ann's story is her spirituality. An active Catholic laywoman, she drew strength from a close relationship with God. She understood that in all choices she was to trust in God's love and to keep focused on the service to others that was, for Mary Ann, the essence of her spirituality and faith. She thought of her daughters, she thought of other women, and she thought about how, through her choices, she might help to make things better for others. She refused to let cancer get the better of her. She took initiative. Anticipating the loss of her hair, she asked her priest to shave her head and then let her children paint her bald scalp with colorful, decorative designs. She agreed to have herself photographed, documenting every stage of her treatment (the chemo treatments, the mastectomy, and the several surgeries for breast reconstruction), providing for other women the in-the-flesh photographs that she would have found so helpful for herself. Initially she rejected the photography project. "I didn't want to show others. I didn't want to see myself like this." But she relented when in prayer she heard God say, "I need you to do this. You've been listening to me all your life. You're going to stop listening to me now?" In addition she recently started a nonprofit foundation, Get in Touch, to educate preteen girls and habituate them to the practice of breast self-examinations and to connect women going through breast cancer treatment.

Mary Ann experienced, and expressed in our (Perry) therapy sessions, the predictable range of responses: terror, sadness, grief, anger, and distress. She also expressed a fierce determination to live and to be well, especially for her children. She understood wellness and healing to be spiritual and emotional, as well as physical. This larger understanding and experience of wellness "lifted me up and carried me and still carries me along," she explained. It carried her through getting "kicked in the teeth many times": a stroke during a chemo treatment; the consequent discovery of, and surgery for, a congenital hole in her heart; and the news that the cancer was indeed in both breasts. For Mary Ann, wellness "is nurtured by reaching out," "finding life right in the midst of the struggle," and working passionately and persistently to make things better for others. She is committed to such social justice activism. It is deeply rooted in her spirituality and has been for her a lifeline. It has helped (and continues to help) to generate hope for others, as well as hope, and a sense of purpose and healing, for herself. "I have never been more alive than I am now."

This chapter examines spirituality as it inspires and finds expression in social activism like Mary Ann's. Such activism constitutes an intervention in the dominant social order, with the goal of seeking to repair the hurts and harm of social injustices and to "make things better for others." The societal benefits of such activism are obvious, but of interest to us as well are the distinct therapeutic benefits, specifically, a sense of purpose and empowerment, and the concomitant generation of hope and well-being for those engaging in the activism. We know and recognize these benefits because we have experienced them in our respective lives.

For the past four decades, social justice activism has been for the two of us definitional, a focus of our work and the locus of our own sense of purpose and meaning, as well as the generator of hope and vitality. We have each been involved principally in the work of peacemaking and disarmament, and variously in the work of welfare reform, health care reform, violence prevention, the abolition of torture, family and community recovery in the aftermath of genocide, the promotion of active nonviolence, gender equity, reproductive rights, and economic and ecological sustainability. Underlying—indeed, motivating—our activism have been, on the one hand, anger in response to troubling and painful disorders in the social fabric and, on the other, determination to reach out and to make things better.

## SOMETHING AMISS:
## SEEKING TRANSFORMATION, PURSUING JUSTICE

Anger, writes the feminist theologian Beverly W. Harrison, "signals something amiss in relationship" (1989, p. 220). The heartache of "something amiss," its pain keenly felt, is typically what brings individuals and families into therapy, seeking transformation. Similarly, "something amiss" propels the work of social justice, mobilizing individuals like ourselves to engage the community (local, national, and/or global) with the goal of its transformation. Activism has many expressions, but its singular goal is the establishing of justice, that is, the restoration of right—respectful, equitable, loving, caring, reconciled, and mutual—relations. Thoroughly woven into activism is hope. To step out and challenge the way things are not only requires a vision alternative to the present order but also generates hope in the belief that such imagined and preferred alternatives can and will be made real, that what is amiss can and will be set right. Hope, as the Biblical scholar Walter Brueggemann describes it, offers a "promissory call to a new future" (2001, p. 64). It "is the refusal to accept the reading of reality which is the majority opinion" (p. 65).

Given the potential societal and therapeutic benefits of activism, it is critical, we believe, for practitioners of family therapy to be conscious of, inquire about, and support the social justice activism, or possibilities for activism, of those with whom we work. We need to recognize that such activism is integral to spirituality and an essential expression of it. Such activism is spirituality in full bloom. Every major religious tradition, for example, emphasizes the translation of religious or spiritual beliefs into acts of mercy and justice. Judaism calls for *tikkun olam*, the repair of the world. The central practice of Christianity is Jesus's love ethic extended to the stranger and even one's enemy, with the goal of creating what Martin Luther King, Jr. called "the beloved community," a realm of loving, in effect, without borders. At the heart of Buddhism is compassion. Charity (*zakat*) or service to others is one of the five pillars of Islam.

At the same time, activism can constitute a primary form of spiritual expression. For many, spirituality is less informed by a specific religion or religious practice. Rather, it is more guided by an internal moral compass often informed by witnessing social injustice.

I (Rolland) was taught by my mother that the accentuation of "differences" among humans was a fundamental lethal step toward seeing an "otherness" among humans, which then created the context for a hierarchy of human worth and the expression of power through sociopolitical oppression, violence, and ultimately genocide. The reification of otherness was fuel for the rupture of right relations leading to injustice and evil.

My parents, German Jews, migrated to the United States in 1936, barely escaping the growing atrocities toward Jews, but leaving their parents and other relatives behind, some of whom, including my father's parents, were exterminated in concentration camps. This family history profoundly influenced the development of my spirituality (for me, a moral compass) and its expression through my commitment to social justice and activism. I also learned to appreciate a distinction: to condemn heinous acts by individuals or social/political systems without condemning an entire culture for eternity. I came to see part of my life's work as helping others to recognize the value of this difference, so we don't perpetuate a culture of retribution where as Gandhi recognized, "An eye for an eye makes the whole world blind." This has included my work with family therapy colleagues in Kosovo, developing the Kosovar Family Professional Education Collaborative, which has provided family-centered professional mental health training and services to assist families in recovery from the "ethnic cleansing" campaign against the Muslim ethnic Albanians. I heard stories from Kosovar families that could be interchangeable with any people who had suffered genocide because of their culture and faith. It was like hearing my own family's stories.

## SPIRITUALITY: RECOGNITION OF OUR PROFOUND INTERCONNECTEDNESS

The imperative to "do justice" (Micah 6:8b) and the desire to make things better for others stems from and points to a defining characteristic of spirituality: the recognition of a profound interconnectedness, an intricate interrelatedness, at the heart of human existence and of all creation. "We are caught," as Martin Luther King, Jr. said, "in an inescapable network of mutuality, tied in a single garment of destiny" (Washington, 1986, p. 290). We "cannot be selves," asserts H. Richard Niebuhr, "save as we are members of each other" (1978, p. 52). In Africa, the reality of our interrelatedness is captured in one word, *ubuntu*, the concept that "I am because we are." As the South African theologian, Denise Ackerman writes, "We live in a web of relationships" (cited in Botman & Petersen, 1996, p. 49). Bellah, Madsen, Sullivan, Swidler, and Tipton in *Habits of the Heart*, remind us that we "need to remember that we did not create ourselves, that we owe what we are to the communities that formed us, and to what Paul Tillich called 'the structure of grace in history'" (1985, p. 295). In short, we are dependent on one another and because of this mutuality and interdependence we, as the Russian monk in Dostoevsky's *The Brothers Karamazov* taught, "are each responsible to all for all" (1880/1950, p. 356). The perils of global warming and the events of September 11, 2001, with the consequent and costly wars in Afghanistan and Iraq, are crises that have "writ large" and are heightening awareness of the reality of our interdependence and our responsibility "to all for all."

The lens of spirituality brings into sharp focus this profound interdependence—this is our human condition—and the existence of an energy field, a sacred power, and creative life force or spirit that infuses, suffuses, connects and courses through all that is. This power or force is variously named in different religious traditions: God, Spirit, Chi, Divinity, Mystery, Jesus, Allah, Love. In every instance the language points to a spirit-filled reality that is beyond yet within and between ourselves, creating, connecting, and inspiring (literally in-spiriting) the created order and each creature within it.

Although some people experience and express spirituality as if it were only a private and personal enterprise, "me and my God," often otherworldly, abstracted, and uprooted from the socioeconomic and political context of day-to-day living, spirituality as we understand it is down to earth. It is the experience of spirit immersed, embodied, incarnated, and encountered in the nitty-gritty of life. As Robert McAfee Brown observes, "All the domains of human existence—ecology, economics, health, prayer, politics, sexuality, and education—are the province of spirituality" (1988, p. 117). Spirituality thus understood locates "divine revelation. . . . in the concrete struggles of groups and communities to lay hold of the gift of life and to unloose what denies life" (Harrison, 1989, p. 214).

Such an understanding of spirituality calls into question practices of separation, division, exclusion, and hierarchy, as well as the various barriers and divides (and conflicts over the same) that "Balkanize" our world. Such practices lead to and in turn are aggravated by the various "isms"— nationalism, classism, sexism, heterosexism, racism, and ageism, to name a few. When people are spiritually aware and alive, they discover (recover) themselves as connected to and engaged in the web of life (or "network of mutuality") rather than insulated and isolated. "The life of spirituality," writes theologian Robert McAfee Brown, "will be located in the midst of the world's turmoil, rather than in safe havens of disengagement" (1988, pp. 118–119). Spirituality by its very nature not only inclines but requires one to engage the world with a sense of responsibility for the well-being of creation, and with a commitment to repair what is amiss and to act in defense of the creation. Spirituality and justice seeking are thus inextricably tied; like a Möbius strip, they are not distinct realms, but flow seamlessly one into the other.

How is this inextricable, intimate relationship between spirituality and social justice activism, or what we refer to as *justice-seeking spirituality*, relevant to the practice of family therapy? As Mary Ann's story exemplifies, activism—"reaching out" to make things better for others—has distinctly therapeutic benefits. In her case, drawing on the resources of her spirituality and faith, she found herself compelled to go public with her personal pain and suffering, to use her experience to connect to, empathize with, and advocate for others struggling with cancer. She committed herself to addressing the larger systemic issues of breast cancer treatment and women's health care. As she engaged with other women, she became increasingly aware and troubled by disparities in our society in terms of access to quality and affordable health care. Even as her life was being threatened, Mary Ann chose to engage in a spiritually inspired activism and to lay "hold of the gifts of life," specifically, a community of love and support, renewed and relentless hope, and an impassioned and empowered sense of purpose. Such a justice-seeking spirituality can offer for families and individuals (and communities) a pathway to meaning, hope, empowerment, community, and healing. It is a critical therapeutic resource to which we as family therapists need to pay attention.

## OPENING THERAPEUTIC CONVERSATION TO JUSTICE-SEEKING SPIRITUALITY

In practical terms then, how are we to attend to justice-seeking spirituality as a therapeutic resource and incorporate it as an awareness into our work?

## Exploring and Encouraging a Family's Activism

First, as mentioned earlier, we need to be conscious of and inquire about the spiritual convictions, commitments, and practices of the individuals and families with whom we work. It is important to explore and bring forth the activism that is often already part of a family's spiritual practice and meaning making, and make space for that within the therapeutic conversation. Such activism may be an aspect of involvement in a faith community or may be inspired by one's personal faith or spiritual belief system. This can take varied forms, locally or globally, as consonant with people's values and priorities (e.g., volunteering to meet human service needs; organizing afterschool and mentoring programs for inner-city children; advocating for medical research; pressing for health care reform; working for human rights; joining in public witnesses against war; assisting in disaster relief; advocating for same-sex marriage equality; and promoting environmental policies to counter global warming).

There is much for us as therapists to be curious about. What spiritual convictions and values are family members expressing through their activism? How are or might these shape and sustain the families with whom we work? How does their activism speak of what they believe and hold precious? Does it contribute to the family's sense of purpose, well-being, and hope? Does it connect them with others and strengthen community? Does it create or contribute to a sense of empowerment? The resources of a justice-seeking spirituality all too often can be eclipsed by the presenting problems and discounted or overlooked altogether by the individual or family, and even by the therapist. Interest and curiosity on the part of therapists can open up space for families to recognize, draw on, and extend the benefits of these resources.

> A case at point is Mary Beth, a married woman in her early 40s, mother of two adolescent boys, director of a credit union in a community hospital, and a recently enrolled student in a state university. Embarrassed by her lack of a college degree, she had tended to get easily separated from her sense of competency. Feelings of failure often overtook her. She had struggled with, and was being treated for, depression and anxiety. In the context of therapy, she voiced self-hatred and often harshly criticized herself for not being "good enough." When her 12-year-old son, who had been acting out at school, was diagnosed with depression, she found herself feeling responsible for his depression.
>
> By chance, early on in the therapy, I (Perry) noticed a letter that Mary Beth had written to the editor of a local religious paper. She was protesting the decision by a diocesan authority to evict a soup kitchen from a local church. The letter was strong and impassioned, reminding

the religious authorities of the Scriptural mandate to serve the poor. Here, I thought, was a voice of conviction and compassion, stunningly clear and empowered, beyond anything I might have expected based on the self-deprecating voice I had heard in the therapy sessions.

I became curious about the boldness and clarity of Mary Beth's convictions, the depth of her compassion, and the spiritual values that motivated her. Might these not be resources for her to draw on, and for the work of therapy to draw out? When I expressed interest and curiosity, Mary Beth began to thicken the story of putting her convictions into action and reaching out to make things better for others. She and her son Timothy had begun volunteering, she told me, once a week for an organization called Our Daily Bread. Together they delivered an evening hot meal and breakfast makings for individuals of modest means, recently discharged from local hospitals and recovering from or struggling with health problems such as AIDS. I asked Mary Beth to reflect on her commitment to this activism, its meaning for her, and its effects on her.

She invited me to accompany her and her son one day, and I did. I was immediately struck by how self-assured, engaged, and animated Mary Beth was as she delivered the meals. It was as if she had broken free of the burdens that so often oppressed her spirits. When talking with the recipients of the meals, and later with me, she was enthusiastic and gracious, expressive of a caring and compassionate self. She was very clear that she and her son delivered not only nutritional but also emotional sustenance. The shared work clearly also provided relational sustenance for their mother–son bond.

Mary Beth does this kind of community service, she explained to me, because she is concerned about people who fall through the cracks in our society. She feels called by her personal faith to offer support. The work has had particular benefit and meaning for her, keeping alive the memory of a very dedicated physician cousin who died at a young age with AIDS. Volunteering for others with health problems has been a way to heal her grief. Her cousin would be, she believes, "very proud" that she is "helping in this way." "People still need to be touched; people still need to be hugged," she said. Mary Beth does both.

It was important to recognize, honor, and make room, in the context of therapy, for the convictions and faith that inspired Mary Beth's commitment to activism. That recognition helped Mary Beth to recover belief in her own value as a person, to embrace herself as someone who cares and makes a difference, even in the midst of her own struggles and hardships, and to experience for herself the healing benefits of her passion and compassion.

## Understanding Oppressive Cultural Practices: Connecting in Community

Second, to incorporate a justice-seeking spirituality into our practices, it is imperative to be cognizant of and vigilant about the larger cultural context and how unjust societal structures and practices oppress and harm, creating pain and suffering, effectively dispiriting and disempowering persons. So often families experience their struggles as individual and idiosyncratic, as if they are unique to them. They can feel ashamed of, to blame for, guilty about, and isolated by problems, such as the traumatic effects of sexual abuse, which more often than not have roots in what Christie Neuger identifies as "the variety of power systems that organize the culture into systems of dominance and subordination" (2001, p. 7). Typically power systems—patriarchy, racism, classism, heterosexism, militarism, even professionalism—seek to render themselves "invisible," as if normal (how things are) and normative (how things should be). The real effects of these systems of dominance and subordination are anything but invisible for families who suffer personally, sometimes privately, often concluding that they are flawed and deficient. However, as Howard J. Clinebell has argued, "Behind every personal problem is a cluster of societal problems" (1983, p. 189). Therapists have a responsibility to help the individuals and families with whom we work recognize and analyze the "cluster of societal problems" that lie behind, contribute to, and cause that which hurts and disrupts their lives. Our responsibilities are several: to help individuals and families to understand the operations of the wider culture's oppressive practices; to support families in exploring possibilities for taking action to resist that which is oppressive and to reclaim their own agency and dignity; and to encourage them to connect, empathically and actually, with others in communities of solidarity and advocacy.

> Such empathetic connecting helped one family break free of shame and feelings of powerlessness. In therapy, they had disclosed to me (Perry) that a close adult male family friend, a lay member of their faith community, had used his position as a church youth leader to initiate numerous inappropriate communications with their teenage daughter and to engage in predatory sexual behaviors. The daughter had grown alarmed and told her parents, who then turned to me. They were furious but also shell-shocked; how could a friend, an admired member of their congregation, do this? The daughter was traumatized, frightened, and embarrassed. The whole family was in anguish, distraught with feelings of betrayal, anger, and hurt. When I explained that, as a thera-

pist and a clergy person, I was a mandated reporter, the mother looked stricken. The parent's first priority was their daughter's safety, and they wanted the offending behaviors stopped immediately, but they did not want this matter reported. They felt ashamed, and they did not want others to know. I reflected with them on predatory sexual behaviors, expressed the concern that this situation might not be isolated, and explained the imperative to investigate, to protect their daughter and also to protect others. "I can't bear to have others go through the hell we are going through," responded the mother. "I don't want anybody else to have to feel this pain." The parents began to empathize with imagined other victims and from that connection drew strength, feeling joined with and responsible to others and thereby less isolated. They recognized this as a justice issue, then felt empowered to act. I proposed that they could report to the Department of Children and Families, I could report, or we could report together. Their choice was to report together, with their daughter present. The benefits to her of this intervention were immediately obvious; she could "breathe again," knowing that her parents had acted to ensure her safety. She felt relieved to learn subsequently that her church community, in response to this situation of exploitation, had committed itself to creating a genuinely "safe church."

To consider another clinical example, advocacy became the pathway for Meghan to move toward empowerment and healing. An officer in the military, she had been raped by a male superior officer. She brought charges, but the response was the proverbial slap "on the wrist"; he was allowed to resign. When, a year later, another male superior officer was arrested for soliciting sex from minors, she was retraumatized and felt raped all over again. She was so enraged at this second perpetrator, and also at the military leadership for its complicity, that she wanted to hurt somebody. Her anger was understandable and justified, but when she realized its corrosiveness for her, she turned to the resources of her faith to calm herself down, specifically reflecting on the practices of nonviolent love. From that perspective, her rage combined with courage and paved a way for her to begin to feel compassion for this second perpetrator. She saw him as a complex human being filled with good and evil, as a child of God just like herself, with his own wounds. She channeled her anger at her perpetrators, including the military leadership, into naming the sexual violence of the military and speaking publicly about its "war" on women. She organized, and joined cause with, others to advocate for justice for military women, and through that activism she recovered her sense of power, purpose, and dignity.

By encouraging families to engage in justice-seeking activism, therapists can also help families to expand their family narratives to larger system and community narratives, thereby helping to strengthen a collective sense of responsibility and empowerment. As family therapists, we are ideally situated to help to promote precisely those connections with community that help to rebalance scripts skewed too narrowly toward individual responsibility (and blame). The following case illustrates this approach.

Residents in one economically depressed working-class neighborhood sought help from the community-based satellite clinic of a regional mental health center for problems with an adolescent gang that was disrupting and vandalizing the local library after school hours. Initially, the solution was defined in terms of intervention at the individual level, blaming the troublemaking adolescents and their dysfunctional families, who were viewed as unable to provide adequate structure and control. Introducing the perspective of a wider angle lens, one clinician noted that the city had several years earlier entertained a request to develop a youth community center for this area of the city and had endorsed the idea, but it had never provided the necessary funding. This lack of follow-through had reinforced the community's view of itself as marginal and powerless. The individual acts of violence had developed in this larger context.

As an alternative to traditional therapeutic intervention, a team of three clinicians, including myself (Rolland), approached these adolescents to engage them in pursuing the city's original commitment to develop a youth center. We invited the "troublemakers" to provide leadership to resurrect this idea and press the city to honor its commitment. This intervention succeeded. Gradually, the initial core group of adolescents recognized the need for a larger critical mass; they began to mobilize their own families, other adolescents and their families, local churches, and other neighborhood organizations in a community-organizing effort. The connection with community went still further. Aware that annually, the first-year students at the Yale School of Architecture would design and help to build a worthy project in New Haven as a community service, I suggested linking the community need with this University commitment. Besides the enormous cost savings, I saw this as an opportunity for collaboration between parts of the larger community that were normally far apart geographically, socioeconomically, and culturally. The Yale students and the Architecture School embraced the project. Public hearings and media attention brought final approval and funding. Adolescents (including the original gang members), their siblings and parents, other members of the community, and Yale students worked alongside each other in building the youth center. In addition, adolescents were included in the advisory committee to help develop and oversee the future of the youth center.

We viewed the problem behavior systemically as an expression of dysfunction at the level of this neighborhood's lack of adequate services and their marginalized, inequitable status within the city. As mental health professionals, we redefined the problem so as to facilitate the process of empowerment for the adolescents, their families, and the community at large, and to enable actions toward achieving greater social justice and community well-being.

Another way to foster connection and community is through the use of time-limited or ongoing monthly, multiple family discussion/support groups (Gonzales & Steinglass, 2002). They can serve as a cost-effective, powerful therapeutic approach for families facing similar life challenges, such as health and mental health problems (Rolland, 1994). Resilience-oriented, collaborative psychoeducational groups more readily engage families than does traditional therapy. A major benefit is their ability to counter isolation by establishing networks that extend well beyond the group meetings. This is particularly important in helping to empower families with major mental health conditions, which are prone to patterns of secrecy, and fears of stigma and discrimination (McFarlane, 2002).

Social class and race-based health care disparities complicate family challenges in their lack of access to affordable quality care, lack of health care insurance, or unequal coverage for mental health services. These groups can empower families in their struggles with other systems. For example, a time-limited group (six sessions) was offered to families coping with occupationally related respiratory diseases resulting from chemical sensitivity. For many, inadequate workplace health safety precautions to toxic chemical exposure were significant in causing their conditions. Many of the cases involved discrimination and litigation with previous employers, who were economically driven to disavow responsibility. The group meetings, which included discussion of faith-based convictions regarding social justice, were empowering for participants. At the last meeting of this psychoeducational series, the group members decided to form an information, advocacy, and self-help network for themselves and other, similarly affected families throughout the state.

As family therapists we have an obligation to recognize the debilitating effects of socioeconomic–cultural disorders on personal vitality and spiritual well-being. We need to help those we work with understand the interplay of the systemic and the individual, the real ways in which the personal is political and the political is personal. This kind of social justice critique and commitment to activism are important if therapy is to be socially responsible and contribute to genuine transformation and restoration to health and wholeness for persons, and indeed for the social order. Otherwise, we risk, in the words of the Biblical prophet Jeremiah, "heal[ing] the wound of. . . . people lightly" (Jeremiah 8:11). We risk simply accommodating people to the way things are. As Christie Neuger points out, "Helping people to adapt to an unhealthy culture is not ethical" (2001, p. 40).

In *Care of Persons, Care of Worlds*, Larry Graham observes, "The destiny of persons and the character of the world are intertwined" (1992, p. 13). In the same vein, Chellis Glendinning suggests, "In a kind of interplay of mutual causation, the themes we play out in our private lives mirror those we are exposed to in our society, and vice versa. Could there be a relationship between nuclear war and wife battering? Between alcoholism and toxic contamination? Between global warming and workaholism?" (1994, p. xii).

Nevertheless the practice of some therapies has sometimes been decontextualized and disconnected, without adequate attention to this "interplay of mutual causation," to the intertwining of "the destiny of persons and the character of the world." In recent years many family therapists and larger systems-oriented clinicians have broadened our range of vision to include the powerful influences of culture, social class, race, gender constraints, and social systems, such as the workplace and health care (Aldarondo, 2007; Almeida, Parker, & Dolan-Del Vecchio, 2007; Boyd-Franklin, 2006; Doherty & Carroll, 2002; Falicov, 1995; Flores & Carey, 2000; Imber-Black, 1988; McGoldrick & Hardy, 2008; Mirkin, 1990; Rojano, 2004; Rolland, 1997; Walsh, 2006; Waldegrave, 2003; Weingarten, 2004). Also, collaborative models, such as the use of narrative approaches (Freedman & Combs, 1996; Madsen, 2007; White & Epston, 1990), are congruent with and expressive of a justice-seeking spirituality. The major focus of these models is to move the therapist away from the expert-in-charge stance toward a more egalitarian partnership with clients. The hope in this process is to empower families and transform therapy into a mutual search for new options and understanding. Even so, in mainstream clinical practice, some interventions still focus too much on individual client families, failing to attend sufficiently to the family's place and interaction within the larger community and the real effects (for good and for ill) on the family of the larger community, often the very same communities that therapists share with them.

## Standing on Common Ground: Resisting Societal Counterspiritualities

This final observation points to a third consideration for incorporating justice-seeking spirituality into our therapeutic conversations: recognition of and honesty about the common ground we stand on and share with those with whom we are working. There is no hermetic seal between us as therapists and those who come to us. We are not immune from the varieties of power systems that organize the culture into systems of dominance and subordination. We all are living in this context; these systems permeate our world. Although the degrees of exposure to the brunt of what the Biblical scholar Walter Wink (1992) calls the "domination system" vary and, indeed, some benefit from it, none are exempt; we are all affected (and infected) in real ways. Its operations are pernicious: intimidation, creating a fear-based (terrorized) culture of malleable and easily manipulated people; isolation, undercutting a sense of community and communion, creating pervasive mistrust of the "other" and separating people through a mentality and strategy of "divide and conquer"; constriction of imagination and of an alternative consciousness that challenges what is; and the promulgation of despair. It has been argued that the spirituality of domination is despair (see also Aponte, Chapter 6, this volume).

Despair serves domination systems because along with its defining characteristic of hopelessness comes powerlessness, the loss of confidence in one's own power, agency, value, and capacity to act, to change the way things are, to set right what is "amiss," to restore justice, and to make any kind of a difference at all. Disempowered people often become docile or resigned, acclimated or numb to the way things are, thereby tolerating the intolerable (e.g., the U.S. government's practice of torture) and no longer believing in the possibilities for transformation. In short, they learn to accommodate injustice, and in some cases even accept it as if it were the norm. They abandon hope.

As therapists we need to recognize the ways we, too, succumb to the adverse effects of systemic domination and what one might call its "counterspiritualities," specifically, despair, but also violence, hierarchy, consumerism, and even individualism—all cultural practices that damage community, undercut mutuality and collaboration, gradually erode human rights and dignity, and foster "I–it" relationships, rather than the I–Thou relationships that are the heart and soul of justice-seeking spirituality. These systemic counterspiritualities not only threaten but also are themselves threatened by the real benefits of justice-seeking spirituality: connectedness, mutuality, compassion, and caring, inclusive, in some religious traditions, of the consciousness of divine spirit infusing and sacralizing all that is.

It is important for us as therapists to admit our own susceptibility and vulnerability (and sometimes blindness) to the constrictions and constraints of counterspiritualities. It is imperative that we be vigilant and honest. As professionals, it is vital that we be mindful, to avoid an elitist culture of professionalism that promotes "otherness" and disconnects us from our client families and their communities. By being vigilant about such counterspiritualities, we promote right relations that facilitate an egalitarian collaborative relationship with families and community. And it is important for us to become activists in our own right and in our professional capacity, advocates for not only those who come to us but also ourselves. If we are to resist the adverse, but often seductive, effects of counterspiritualities that threaten to undo the well-being of all, we need to do precisely what we encourage the families seeking our help to do: find our voice and embrace our power, take action to restore justice, connect with others, ground ourselves in communities of support, embody in all we do the ways of love and compassion, and work for the healing of all.

As mental health and health care professionals, we can foster our own connections with wider justice-seeking communities by forming coalitions with consumer advocacy organizations that serve the needs of populations related to our areas of expertise. Many such organizations have professional experts on their advisory boards. In my (Rolland) involvement in serving families with serious illness and disability, I have forged collaborative relationships with consumer organizations such as the National Family Caregivers Association, the Well Spouse Foundation, the National Alliance for the Mentally Ill (NAMI), and illness-specific organizations, such as Y-ME (the national breast cancer organization), empowering both families and professionals. Many such organizations have extensive experience with policy formulation and gaining access and influence in policy and funding processes for research, treatment, and prevention. Building coalitions of professionals and consumers can have far-reaching benefits.

As therapists, we can band together to advocate for social justice concerning issues of discrimination toward couples and families, especially the poor and marginalized groups in our society. The Council on Contemporary Families (CCF), an information and advocacy organization, was formed by leading family scholars, educators, and therapists to promote the strength and welfare of all families through research-informed, constructive discussion of contemporary families and how their needs might best be met. It counters moralistic, politicized rhetoric and erroneous claims, under the rubric of "family values," characterized by simplistic diagnoses, and one-size-fits-all prescriptions. This harms many people by stigmatizing and pathologizing couples and families that differ from the traditional, idealized norm (Walsh, 2003). The CCF provides accurate information, grounded in systematic research, to the media and public sector on which to base public policy and programs responsive to the diversity, strengths, and challenges of today's families.

Our current health care crisis is a prime example illustrating a need for professional alliances, consumer initiatives, and professional–consumer coalitions. The fact that 47 million United States citizens lack any health care coverage; the fact that minority families and the poor suffer gross disparities in access to health care and a disproportionate rate of major health problems and mortality; the fact that family caregivers to the chronically ill sap family financial and emotional resources, creating the largest cause of personal bankruptcy; and the lack of parity for mental and physical health care are just a few expressions of the gross inequities affecting families in our current corporate, profit-oriented, health care system. Therapists can themselves join, and encourage affected client families to join, like-minded consumer–professional groups, local and state initiatives (e.g., Healthcare for All Illinois), or professional organizations, such as Physicians for a National Health Program, which advocates universal health care through a single-payer system, akin to an expanded Medicare program for all. Such activism goes beyond the traditional therapeutic mandate of helping families one by one, toward collaborative efforts to transform larger systems to benefit all.

## CONCLUSION

The justice-seeking spirituality we have described and advocated in this chapter promises expansive therapeutic benefit. It offers an antidote to our culture's counterspiritualities. At the same time it offers encouragement and an approach for fostering the connections and community, the right relations, that are intrinsic to and vital for the liberating experiences of hope, empowerment, and healing. A justice-seeking spirituality helps people move from separation to belonging, from disconnection to community, from powerlessness to empowerment, from complicity to compassion, from unjust relations to right relations, from despair to hope. A justice-seeking spirituality promises to be healing and vitalizing for not only our client families but also ourselves as family therapists and as human beings.

## REFERENCES

Aldarondo, E. (2007). *Advancing social justice through clinical practice.* London: Routledge.

Almeida, R., Dolan-Del Vecchio, K., & Parker, L. (2007). *Transformative family therapy: Just families in a just society*. Saddle Brook, NJ: Pearson.

Bellah, R. W., Madsen, R., Sullivan, W. M., Swindler, A., & Tipton, S. M. (1985). *Habits of the heart*. Berkeley: University of California Press.

Botman, H., & Petersen, R. (Eds.). (1996). *To remember and to heal*. Cape Town: Human & Rousseau.

Boyd-Franklin, N. (2006). *Black families in therapy: Understanding the African American experience*. New York: Guilford Press.

Brown, R. (1988). *Spirituality and liberation*. Philadelphia: Westminster Press.

Brueggemann, W. (2001). *Prophetic imagination*. Philadelphia: Fortress Press.

Clinebell, H. J. (1983). Toward envisioning the future of pastoral counseling and AAPC. *Journal of Pastoral Care, 37*(3), 180–194.

Doherty, W. J., & Carroll, J. S. (2002). The citizen therapist and family centered community practice. *Family Process, 41,* 561–568.

Dostoevsky, F. (1950). *The brothers Karamazov* (C. Garnett, Trans.). New York: Modern Library. (Original work in Russian published 1880)

Falicov, C. J. (1995). Training to think culturally: A multidimensional framework. *Family Process, 34,* 373–388.

Flores, M., & Carey, G. (2000). *Family therapy with Hispanics: Towards appreciating diversity*. Boston: Allyn & Bacon.

Freedman, J., & Combs, G. (1996). *Narrative therapy: The social construction of preferred realities*. New York: Norton.

Glendinning, C. (1994). *My name is Chellis and I'm in recovery from Western civilization*. Boston/London: Shambhala.

Gonzalez, S., & Steinglass, P. (2002). Application of multifamily groups in chronic medical disorders. In W. F. McFarlane (Ed.), *Multifamily groups in the treatment of severe psychiatric disorders* (pp. 315–341). New York: Guilford Press.

Graham, L. (1992). *Care of persons, care of worlds*. Nashville: Abingdon Press.

Harrison, B. W. (1989). The power of anger in the work of love. In J. Plaskow & C. Christ (Eds.), *Weaving the visions: New patterns in feminist spirituality*. San Francisco: Harper & Row.

Imber-Black, E. (1988). *Families and larger systems: A family therapist's guide through the labyrinth*. New York: Guilford Press.

Madsen, W. (2007). *Collaborative therapy with multi-stressed families: From old problems to new futures*. New York: Guilford Press.

McFarlane, W. F. (Ed.). (2002). *Multifamily groups in the treatment of severe psychiatric disorders*. New York: Guilford Press.

McGoldrick, M., & Hardy, K. V. (Eds.). (2008). *Re-visioning family therapy: Race, culture, and gender in clinical practice* (2nd ed.). New York: Guilford Press.

Mirkin, M. (1990). *The social and political contexts of family therapy*. Boston: Allyn & Bacon.

Neuger, C. C. (2001). *Counseling women: A narrative, pastoral approach*. Minneapolis: Fortress.

Niebuhr, H. R. (1978). *The meaning of revelation*. New York: Macmillan.

Rojano, R. (2004). The practice of community family therapy. *Family Process, 43*(1), 59–77.

Rolland, J. (1994). *Families, illness, and disability: An integrative treatment model.* New York: Basic Books.

Rolland, J. (1997). The meaning of illness and disability: Sociopolitical and ethical concerns. *Family Process, 36*(4), 437–441.

Waldegrave, C. T. (2003). *Just Therapy: A journey: Collection of papers from the Just Therapy Team.* New Zealand: Dulwich Centre.

Walsh, F. (2003) *Normal family processes: Growing diversity and complexity* (3rd ed.). New York: Guilford Press.

Walsh, F. (2006). *Strengthening family resilience.* New York: Guilford Press.

Washington, J. (Ed.). (1986). *A testament of hope: The essential writings of Martin Luther King, Jr.* San Francisco: Harper & Row.

Weingarten, K. (2004). *Common shock: Witnessing violence every day: How we are harmed, how we can heal.* New York: New American Library.

White, M., & Epston, D. (1990). *Narrative means to therapeutic ends.* New York: Norton.

Wink, W. (1992). *Engaging the powers: Discernment and resistance in a world of domination.* Minneapolis, MN: Fortress Press.

# Index